T0337470

AVOIDING COMMON ERRORS IN PEDIATRIC EMERGENCY MEDICINE

ASSOCIATE EDITORS

Maybelle Kou, MD, MEd

Landon A. Jones, MD

Andrea Fang, MD

Keith Borg, MD, PhD

Michael H. Greenwald, MD

Christopher S. Amato, MD, FAAP, FACEP

Madeline M. Joseph, MD, FACEP, FAAP

James C. O'Neill, MD, FACEP

Matthew Neal, MD, MBA

Jean Klig, MD

Chad Scarboro, MD, FACEP

Jessica Wall, MD, MPH, MSCE, FAAP

Jenny Mendelson, MD

Lucas Friedman, MD, MEd

Whitney Minnock, MD

Debra S. Rusk, MD

Anna McFarlin, MD

Jennifer E. Guyther, MD

Marla C. Levine, MD

Dina Wallin, MD

Sheryl E. Yanger, MD

Julia N. Magana, MD

Anupam B. Kharbanda, MD, MSc

Mark S. Mannenbach, MD

Emily Rose, MD, FAAP, FAAEM, FACEP

Paul Ishimine, MD

AVOIDING COMMON ERRORS IN PEDIATRIC EMERGENCY MEDICINE

DALE P. WOOLRIDGE, MD, PHD

Professor of Emergency Medicine, Pediatrics, Chemistry and Biochemistry
Department of Emergency Medicine and Pediatrics
University of Arizona, College of Medicine
Tucson, Arizona

SECTION EDITORS

SEAN M. FOX, MD

Professor of Emergency Medicine
Professor of Pediatrics
Program Director, Emergency Medicine Residency Program
Department of Emergency Medicine
Carolinas Medical Center
Charlotte, North Carolina

JAMES (JIM) L. HOMME, MD

Assistant Professor of Pediatrics and Emergency Medicine
Division of Pediatric Emergency Medicine
Department of Emergency Medicine
Mayo Clinic College of Medicine and Science
Rochester, Minnesota

AARON N. LEETCH, MD

Assistant Professor of Emergency Medicine and Pediatrics
Program Director, Combined Emergency Medicine and Pediatrics Residency
Departments of Emergency Medicine and Pediatrics
University of Arizona, College of Medicine
Tucson, Arizona

TIMOTHY K. RUTTAN, MD

Assistant Professor of Pediatrics
University of Texas at Austin Dell Medical School
Department of Pediatrics
Dell Children's Medical Center of Central Texas
Pediatric Emergency Medicine
Austin, Texas

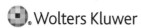

Philadelphia · Baltimore · New York · London
Buenos Aires · Hong Kong · Sydney · Tokyo

Executive Editor: Sharon Zinner
Senior Development Editor: Ashley Fischer
Editorial Coordinator: Blair Jackson
Production Project Manager: Bridgett Dougherty
Design Coordinator: Stephen Druding
Manufacturing Coordinator: Beth Welsh
Prepress Vendor: SPi Global

Copyright © 2021 Wolters Kluwer

All rights reserved. This book is protected by copyright. No part of this book may be reproduced or transmitted in any form or by any means, including as photocopies or scanned-in or other electronic copies, or utilized by any information storage and retrieval system without written permission from the copyright owner, except for brief quotations embodied in critical articles and reviews. Materials appearing in this book prepared by individuals as part of their official duties as U.S. government employees are not covered by the above-mentioned copyright. To request permission, please contact Wolters Kluwer at Two Commerce Square, 2001 Market Street, Philadelphia, PA 19103, via email at permissions@lww.com, or via our website at shop.lww.com (products and services).

9 8 7 6 5 4 3 2 1

Printed in China

Cataloging-in-Publication Data available on request from the Publisher

ISBN: 978-1-9751-3833-2

This work is provided "as is," and the publisher disclaims any and all warranties, express or implied, including any warranties as to accuracy, comprehensiveness, or currency of the content of this work.

This work is no substitute for individual patient assessment based upon healthcare professionals' examination of each patient and consideration of, among other things, age, weight, gender, current or prior medical conditions, medication history, laboratory data and other factors unique to the patient. The publisher does not provide medical advice or guidance and this work is merely a reference tool. Healthcare professionals, and not the publisher, are solely responsible for the use of this work including all medical judgments and for any resulting diagnosis and treatments.

Given continuous, rapid advances in medical science and health information, independent professional verification of medical diagnoses, indications, appropriate pharmaceutical selections and dosages, and treatment options should be made and healthcare professionals should consult a variety of sources. When prescribing medication, healthcare professionals are advised to consult the product information sheet (the manufacturer's package insert) accompanying each drug to verify, among other things, conditions of use, warnings and side effects and identify any changes in dosage schedule or contraindications, particularly if the medication to be administered is new, infrequently used or has a narrow therapeutic range. To the maximum extent permitted under applicable law, no responsibility is assumed by the publisher for any injury and/or damage to persons or property, as a matter of products liability, negligence law or otherwise, or from any reference to or use by any person of this work.

shop.lww.com

To Kirsten my wife, my best friend, and the MVP of the Homme household.
Without you, nothing productive would ever happen.

To my children Jack, Katie, Natalie, Sarah, and Megan—
you inspire me to be more than I am.

To George Lucas, J. R. R. Tolkien, and Walt Disney—
for a lifetime of imagination and wonder.

Most importantly—Jesus Christ—for saving what was lost (Luke 19:10).
—James (Jim) Homme, MD

This book is dedicated to Sarah for her support and partnership
as well as to my children, Isaac and Claire, for reminding me of what matters
most and for always being ready with love and hugs. A special thanks to the
patients, students, residents, fellows, and faculty with whom I have had the
honor to work, teach, and learn alongside as we all strive to serve others in the
emergency department and make the world a little better each day.
—Timothy K. Ruttan, MD

Maneesha Agarwal, MD, FAAP, FACEP
Assistant Professor
Departments of Emergency Medicine and
    Pediatrics
Children's Healthcare of Atlanta
Emory University School of Medicine
Atlanta, Georgia

Mahsa Akhavan, MD
Associate Director, Pediatric Emergency
    Medicine Fellowship
Attending Physician, Pediatric Emergency
    Medicine
Morristown Medical Center, Goryeb Children's
    Hospital
Morristown, New Jersey

Sabreen Akhter, DO, DTM
Associate Professor
Division of Emergency Medicine, Department
    of Pediatrics
University of Washington School of Medicine/
    Seattle Children's Hospital
Seattle, Washington

Christopher S. Amato, MD, FAAP, FACEP
Associate Professor
Department of Emergency Medicine &
    PediatricsSidney Kimmel Medical College
Director
Pediatric Emergency Medicine Fellowship
Goryeb Children's Hospital/Morristown
    Medical Center
Pediatric Medical Director
Atlantic Ambulance Company
Morristown, New Jersey

Minal Amin, MD, FAAEM
Interim Program Director
Altieri Pediatric Emergency Medicine
    Fellowship
Department of Emergency Medicine
Inova Fairfax Hospital/Inova Children's
    Hospital
Falls Church, Virginia

Nicky Amin, MD
Pediatric Emergency Medicine Fellow
Department of Emergency Medicine
Goryeb Children's Hospital
Morristown, New Jersey

Andrea P. Anderson, MD
Pediatric Emergency Medicine Fellow
Division of Emergency Medicine
Department of Pediatrics
University of Washington School of Medicine/
    Seattle Children's Hospital
Seattle, Washington

Jana L. Anderson, MD
Assistant Professor of Emergency Medicine and
    Pediatrics
Department of Emergency Medicine
Mayo Clinic
Rochester, Minnesota

Joseph Arms, MD
Pediatric Emergency Medicine
Associate Fellowship Director in Emergency
    Medicine
Emergency Department Staff Physician
Children's Hospitals of Minnesota
St. Paul, Minnesota

Anthony Arredondo, DO, FAAP
Pediatric Emergency Medicine Fellow
Department of Pediatrics
The University of Texas at Austin Dell Medical
    School
Dell Children's Medical Center
Austin, Texas

Mary Asal, MD, MPH, FAAP
Fellow
Section on Pediatric Emergency Medicine
Department of Pediatrics
University of Oklahoma College of Medicine
The Children's Hospital at OU Medical
    Center
Oklahoma City, Oklahoma

Carmen Avendano, MD
Emergency Medicine Physician
Adjunct Assistant Professor of Pediatrics
University of Minnesota Masonic Children's
  Hospital
Pediatric Emergency Division Faculty
St Francis Regional Medical Center
Shakopee, Minnesota

Shad Baab, MD
Assistant Professor of Emergency Medicine
Section of Pediatric Emergency Medicine
Brenner's Children's Hospital
Wake Forest University School of Medicine
Winston-Salem, North Carolina

Seth Ball, MD
Emergency Medicine and Pediatric Resident
  Physician
Departments of Emergency Medicine and
  Pediatrics
University of Maryland School of Medicine
Baltimore, Maryland

Nicole Barbera, DO
Pediatric Emergency Medicine Fellow
Department of Pediatrics
Altieri Pediatric Emergency Medicine Fellowship
Inova Children's Hospital
Falls Church, Virginia

Sarah Becker, DO, FAAP
Assistant Professor
Division of Pediatric Emergency Medicine
Department of Pediatrics
University of Utah School of Medicine
Salt Lake City, Utah

Kelsey Ford Bench, MD
Resident Physician
Department of Emergency Medicine
LAC + USC Medical Center
Los Angeles, California

Kelly R. Bergmann, MD
Emergency Research Director, Staff Physician
Department of Pediatric Emergency Medicine
Children's Minnesota
Minneapolis, Minnesota

Alyssa Bernardi, DO
Pediatric Critical Care Fellow
Department of Pediatrics, Critical Care Medicine
Baylor College of Medicine
Houston, Texas

Nehal Bhandari, MD, FAAP
Assistant Professor of Pediatrics
Division of Pediatric Emergency Medicine
Emory University School of Medicine/
  Children's Healthcare of Atlanta
Atlanta, Georgia

Mary Bing, MD, MPH
Director of Preclinical Programs
Associate Clinical Professor
Department of Emergency Medicine
University of California, Davis
Sacramento, California

Sarah Bingham, MD
Pediatric Emergency Medicine Fellow
Department of Pediatric Emergency Medicine
Wake Forest Baptist Medical Center
Winston Salem, North Carolina

Amanda L. Bogie, MD, FAAP, FACEP
Professor of Pediatrics
Section Chief Pediatric Emergency Medicine
  and Fellowship Director
Department of Pediatrics, Pediatric Emergency
  Medicine
University of Oklahoma Health Sciences
  Center
Oklahoma City, Oklahoma

Keith Borg, MD, PhD
Professor, Department of Pediatrics
Medical University of South Carolina
Charleston, South Carolina

Rebecca C. Bowers, MD, FACEP
Associate Professor of Emergency Medicine
University of Kentucky
Lexington, Kentucky

Amy Briggs, MD
Fellow, Wilderness Medicine
Department of Emergency Medicine
University of California, Irvine
Orange, California

Cortlyn Brown, MD
Emergency Medicine Resident Physician
Department of Emergency Medicine
University of California, San Francisco
San Francisco General Hospital
San Francisco, California

Ryan D. Brown, MD, FAAP
Clinical Associate Professor
Department of Pediatrics, Section on Pediatric
    Emergency Medicine
University of Oklahoma College of Medicine
The Children's Hospital at OU Medical
    Center
Oklahoma City, Oklahoma

Kathleen Kinney Bryant, MD, FACEP
Children's ED Medical Director, Vidant
    Medical Center
Associate Program Director, ECU/VMC
    Emergency Medicine Residency
Assistant Professor, Department of Emergency
    Medicine
ECU Brody School of Medicine
Greenville, North Carolina

Zachary T. Burroughs, MD, FAAP
Clinical Assistant Professor
Pediatric Emergency Medicine Clerkship
    Director
Division of Pediatric Emergency Medicine
Department of Emergency Medicine
University of South Carolina School of
    Medicine Greenville
Prisma Health
Greenville, South Carolina

Carrie Busch, MD, MSCR
Assistant Professor
Divisions of Pediatric Emergency Medicine &
    Child Abuse Pediatrics
Department of Pediatrics
Medical University of South Carolina
Charleston, South Carolina

James Buscher, MD
Pediatric Emergency Medicine Fellow
Emergency Department
University of Florida College of Medicine–
    Jacksonville
Jacksonville, Florida

Rachel Cafferty, MD
Pediatric Emergency Medicine Fellow
Section of Emergency Medicine
Department of Pediatrics
University of Colorado Denver–Children's
    Hospital Colorado
Aurora, Colorado

Derya Caglar, MD
Associate Professor of Pediatrics
Fellowship Director, Pediatric Emergency
    Medicine
Division of Emergency Medicine
Department of Pediatrics
University of Washington School of Medicine/
    Seattle Children's Hospital
Seattle, Washington

Meghan Cain, MD
Senior Associate Consultant
Department of Emergency Medicine
Mayo Clinic
Rochester, Minnesota

Matthew Carlisle, MD, MAS
Program Director, Assistant Professor of
    Clinical Medicine
Department of Emergency Medicine
LSU Health Sciences Center
New Orleans, Louisiana

Carlee Carranza, DO
Resident Physician
Department of Emergency Medicine
Los Angeles County + University of Southern
    California Medical Center
Los Angeles, California

Craig T. Carter, DO
Associate Professor–Emergency Medicine and
    Pediatrics
Medical Director, EM Advanced Practice Providers
Program Director, EM Advanced Practice
    Provider Residency
University of Kentucky
Lexington, Kentucky

James Chamberlain, MD
Director, Data Analytics and Informatics
Associate Director of Research
Division of Emergency Medicine
Children's National Hospital
Washington, District of Columbia

Carol C. Chen, MD, MPH, FAAP
Assistant Clinical Professor of Emergency
    Medicine and Pediatrics
Department of Emergency Medicine
University of California at San Francisco
    School of Medicine
San Francisco, California

Cullen Clark, MD
Resident Physician
Emergency Medicine/Pediatrics Residency
Louisiana State University Health Sciences
  Center–New Orleans
New Orleans, Louisiana

Forrest T. Closson, MD
Department of Pediatrics
Division of Pediatric Emergency Medicine
University of Maryland School of Medicine
University of Maryland Children's Hospital
Baltimore, Maryland

Jessica L. Chow, MD, MPH
Emergency Medicine Chief Resident
Department of Emergency Medicine
University of California, San Francisco and
  Zuckerberg San Francisco General
  Hospital
San Francisco, California

Forrest T. Closson, MD
Director, Pediatric Emergency Educational
  Program
Division of Pediatric Emergency Medicine
Department of Pediatrics
University of Maryland School of
  Medicine
Baltimore, Maryland

Ari Cohen, MD, FAAP
Chief of Pediatric Emergency Medicine
Department of Emergency Medicine
Massachusetts General Hospital
Boston, Massachusetts

Stephanie G. Cohen, MD
Assistant Professor of Pediatrics & Emergency
  Medicine
Director of Pediatric Emergency Ultrasound
Department of Pediatrics
Emory University School of Medicine
Children's Healthcare of Atlanta
Atlanta, Georgia

Daniel K. Colby, MD
Assistant Professor
Division of Medical Toxicology
Substance Use Intervention Team
Department of Emergency Medicine
UC Davis School of Medicine
Sacramento, California

Gena Cooper, MD, FAAP
Assistant Professor
Assistant Medical Director for Pediatric
  Emergency Medicine
Division of Pediatric Emergency Medicine
Department of Emergency Medicine
University of Kentucky College of
  Medicine
Lexington, Kentucky

Rachel E. M. Cramton, MD
Associate Professor of Pediatrics
Associate Program Director, Pediatric
  Residency University of Arizona
GME Director of Wellness
Pediatric Hospitalist/Palliative Care
  Provider
Banner University Medical Center–Tucson,
  Diamond Children's
Tucson, Arizona

Quinn Cummings, MD
Assistant Professor
Department of Emergency Medicine
Medical University of South Carolina
Charleston, South Carolina

Kristol Das, MD, FAAP
Pediatric Emergency Medicine Fellow
Department of Emergency Medicine
Nationwide Children's Hospital
Columbus, Ohio

Anna Darby, MD, MPH
PGY-4 Resident Physician, Chief Resident–
  Recruitment
Department of Emergency Medicine
Los Angeles County + University of Southern
  California Medical Center
Los Angeles, California

Danielle Dardis, MD
Assistant Professor
Department of Emergency Medicine
University of Kentucky
Lexington, Kentucky

Angelica W. DesPain, MD
Pediatric Emergency Medicine Fellow
Division of Emergency Medicine
Children's National Hospital
The George Washington
University School of Medicine
Washington, District of Columbia

Gabriel Paul Devlin, MD/CM
Resident Physician
Department of Pediatrics
University of California, San Francisco
San Francisco, California

Amanda Dupont, MD
Pediatric Resident
Department of Pediatrics
William Beaumont Hospital–Royal Oak
Royal Oak, Michigan

Corey W. Dye, MD
Emergency Medicine Resident
Emergency Medicine Department
University of Florida College of Medicine–
  Jacksonville
Jacksonville, Florida

Clifford C. Ellingson, MD, FAAP
Emergency Medicine and Pediatrics
Alaska Emergency Medicine Associates
Providence Medical Center
Anchorage, Alaska

Candace Engelhardt, MD, FAAP
Clinical Assistant Professor
Department of Child Health, Complex Care
  and Adolescent Medicine
University of Arizona, College of Medicine
  Phoenix, Phoenix Children's Hospital
Phoenix, Arizona

Jasmin England, MD, FAAP
Attending Physician
Department of Emergency Medicine
Children's Hospital of Orange County
Orange, California

Ryan Ericksen, MD
Clinical Assistant Professor
Department of Pediatrics, Pediatric Emergency
  Medicine
University of Oklahoma Health Science Center
Oklahoma City, Oklahoma

Andrea Fang, MD
Program Director, Pediatric Emergency
  Medicine Fellowship
Department of Emergency Medicine
Stanford University School of Medicine
Stanford, California

Ashley L. Flannery, DO, FACEP, FAAEM
Department of Emergency Medicine
AHS–Morristown Medical Center
Morristown, New Jersey

Sean M. Fox, MD
Professor of Emergency Medicine & Professor
  of Pediatrics
Program Director, Emergency Medicine
  Residency
Adult & Pediatric Emergency Departments
Carolinas Medical Center
Charlotte, North Carolina

Lucas Friedman, MD, MEd
Director of Ultrasound Education
Department of Emergency Medicine
Riverside Community Hospital
University of California Riverside School of
  Medicine
Riverside, California

Julia Fuzak Freeman, MD, FAAP
Assistant Professor
Section of Emergency Medicine
Department of Pediatrics
University of Colorado Denver–Children's
  Hospital Colorado
Aurora, Colorado

Alison Gardner, MD, MS
Assistant Professor of Pediatrics and
  Emergency Medicine
Department of Emergency Medicine
Wake Forest Baptist Medical Center
Winston-Salem, North Carolina

Peggy Gatsinos, MD, FAAP
Instructor of Pediatrics
Department of Pediatrics
Northwestern University Feinberg School of
  Medicine
Ann and Robert H. Lurie Children's Hospital
  of Chicago
Chicago, Illinois

**Marianne Gausche-Hill, MD, FACEP, FAAP,
FAEMS**
Medical Director
Los Angeles County EMS Agency
Professor of Emergency Medicine and
  Pediatrics
David Geffen School of Medicine at UCLA
Clinical Faculty
Departments of Emergency Medicine and
  Pediatrics
Harbor–UCLA Medical Center
Torrance, California

Nicole Gerber, MD
Assistant Professor of Clinical Emergency
  Medicine and Pediatrics
Department of Emergency Medicine
New York-Presbyterian Hospital Weill Cornell
  Medical Center
New York, New York

Jason Gillon, MD, FAAP
Pediatric Emergency Medicine Fellow
Department of Pediatrics
Dell Medical School at The University of Texas
  at Austin
Austin, Texas

Kina Le Goodman, MD, FAAP
Fellow, Pediatric Emergency Medicine
Department of Pediatrics
Emory University School of Medicine
Atlanta, Georgia

Denisse Fernandez Goytizolo, M.D.
Pediatric Emergency Medicine Fellow, PGY-6
Department of Emergency Medicine
University of Florida College of Medicine–
  Jacksonville
Jacksonville, Florida

Jessica Kraynik Graham, MD
University of Colorado School of Medicine
Children's Hospital Colorado
Aurora, Colorado

Joyce Granger, MD, FAAP
Clinical Assistant Professor
Department of Emergency Medicine
University of South Carolina School of
  Medicine–Greenville
Greenville, South Carolina

Emily Greenwald, MD
Fellow Pediatric Emergency Medicine
Clinical Instructor, Pediatrics
Section of Emergency Medicine
University of Colorado School of Medicine
Children's Hospital Colorado
Aurora, Colorado

Michael H. Greenwald, MD
Associate Professor, Pediatrics and Emergency
  Medicine
Emory University/Children's Healthcare of
  Atlanta
Atlanta, Georgia

Kendra Grether-Jones, MD
Associate Professor
Department of Emergency Medicine
UC Davis Medical Center
Sacramento, California

Ayush Gupta, MD
Clinical Assistant Professor
Department of Pediatrics
Louisiana State University School of Medicine
New Orleans, Louisiana

Vinayak Gupta, MD
Department of Emergency Medicine
University of Kentucky
Lexington, Kentucky

Dhritiman Gurkha, MD
Pediatric Emergency Medicine
Fellow Beaumont Health
Royal Oak, Michigan

Jennifer E. Guyther, MD
Assistant Professor of Pediatrics
Bon Secours Hospital-Baltimore
University of Maryland Medical Center
University of Maryland Upper Chesapeake
  Medical Center
Baltimore, Maryland

Monica Hajirawala, MD
LSU Pediatrics Chief Resident
LSU Pediatrics Clinical Instructor
Department of Pediatrics
Louisiana State University School of Medicine
  at Children's Hospital of New Orleans
New Orleans, Louisiana

Gregory Hall, MD, MHA, FACEP
Assistant Professor of Emergency Medicine
Department of Emergency Medicine
Medical University of South Carolina
Charleston, South Carolina

Molly Hallweaver, MD
Global Health Fellow
Department of Emergency Medicine
University of California, Davis
Davis, California

Mahmoud Hamdan, MD, CDE, ABCL
Pediatric Endocrinologist and Clinical
  Lipidologist
Carle Foundation Hospital
New Orleans Louisiana

Anna Handorf, MD
Pediatric Resident
Department of Pediatrics
Massachusetts General Hospital
Boston, Massachusetts

Rosy Hao, MD
Pediatric Emergency Fellow
Department of Emergency Medicine
SUNY Downstate/Kings County Hospital
Brooklyn, New York

Michael Hardy, MD, FAAP
Pediatric Emergency Medicine Fellow
Division of Emergency Medicine and Trauma
    Services
Children's National Hospital
The George Washington University School of
    Medicine and Health Sciences
Washington, District of Columbia

William E. Hauda II, MD, FACEP, FAAP
Medical Director
Inova Ewing Forensic Assessment and
    Consultation Team Department
Inova Health System
Falls Church, Virginia

Geoffrey P. Hays, MD
Assistant Professor of Clinical Emergency
    Medicine and Pediatrics
Departments of Emergency Medicine and
    Pediatrics
Indiana University School of Medicine
Indianapolis, Indiana

Michael Hazboun, MD
Rady Children's Hospital—San Diego
San Diego, California

Heather A. Heaton, MD, FACEP
Assistant Professor of Emergency Medicine
Mayo Clinic College of Medicine
Department of Emergency Medicine
Mayo Clinic
Rochester, Minnesota

Rachel J. Heidt, MD
Title (at time of writing chapter): PGY-3;
    (at time of publication) General
    Pediatrician
Department of Pediatrics
UC Davis Medical Center
Sacramento, California

Jonathan Higgins, MD, FAAP
Fellow, Pediatric Emergency Medicine
University of Washington School of Medicine
    and Seattle Children's Hospital
Seattle, Washington

Eva Tovar Hirashima, MD, MPH
Assistant Ultrasound Director, Assistant
    Professor
Department of Emergency Medicine
University of California Riverside
Riverside, California

James (Jim) Homme, MD, FACEP
Assistant Professor of Pediatrics and
    Emergency Medicine
Program Director
Emergency Medicine Residency
Mayo School of Graduate Medical Education
Department of Emergency Medicine
Division of Pediatric Emergency Medicine
Mayo Clinic College of Medicine and
    Science
Rochester, Minnesota

Jason (Jay) Homme, MD, FAAP
Assistant Fellowship Program Director–
    Pediatric Hospital Medicine
Department of Pediatric and Adolescent
    Medicine
Mayo Clinic School of Graduate Medical
    Education
Rochester, Minnesota

Rebecca Hutchings, MD
Director of Medical Education
Division of Emergency Medicine
Children's Hospital New Orleans
New Orleans, Louisiana

Vivian Hwang, MD, FACEP, FAAP
Inova Pediatric Emergency Department
    Resident Rotation Director
Department of Emergency Medicine
Inova Fairfax Hospital
Falls Church, Virginia
Assistant Clinical Professor
The George Washington University School of
    Medicine and Health Sciences
Washington, District of Columbia
Virginia Commonwealth University School of
    Medicine
Richmond, Virginia

Paul Ishimine, MD
Clinical Professor
Departments of Emergency Medicine and
Pediatrics
University of California, San Diego School of
Medicine
San Diego, California

Benjamin F. Jackson, MD, FAAP, FACEP
Associate Professor of Pediatrics
Pediatric Emergency Medicine
Medical University of South Carolina
Charleston, South Carolina

Courtney Jacobs, MD
Pediatric Emergency Medicine Fellow
Department of Emergency Medicine
Eastern Virginia School of Medicine
Norfolk, Virginia

Priya Jain, MD, FAAP
Assistant Professor, Pediatric Emergency
Medicine
Department of Pediatrics
Feinberg School of Medicine, Northwestern
University
Chicago, Illinois

Angela Jarman, MD, MPH
Director, Sex & Gender in Emergency
Medicine
Assistant Professor, Emergency Medicine
University of California, Davis
Davis, California

Lily Anne Jewett, MD
Resident Physician
Department of Emergency Medicine
University of California Davis Health
Sacramento, California

Daniel L. Johnson, MD, MSEd
Emergency Medicine Physician
LAC+USC Emergency Medicine Program
Los Angeles, California

Landon A. Jones, MD
Associate Professor–Emergency Medicine and
Pediatrics
Medical Director, Makenna David Pediatric
Emergency Center
University of Kentucky
Lexington, Kentucky

Madeline M. Joseph, MD, FACEP, FAAP
Professor of Emergency Medicine and Pediatrics
Assistant Chair, Pediatric Emergency Medicine
Quality Improvement
Department of Emergency Medicine
Associate Dean for Inclusion and Equity
University of Florida College of Medicine
Jacksonville, Florida

Cree Kachelski, MD, FAAP
Pediatric Emergency Medicine Fellow and
Child Abuse Pediatrics Fellow
Department of Pediatric Emergency Medicine
and Child Adversity and Resilience
Children's Mercy Hospital
Kansas City, Minnesota

Kristin Kahale, MD
Emergency Medicine Resident
Oakland University William Beaumont School
of Medicine
Beaumont Hospital, Royal Oak
Royal Oak, Michigan

Rahul Kaila, MD
Assistant Professor of Pediatrics and
Emergency Medicine
Department of Pediatrics and Emergency Medicine
University of Minnesota Masonic Children's
Hospital
Minneapolis, Minnesota

Ian Kane, MD
Associate Program Director, Pediatric
Emergency Medicine Fellowship
Department of Pediatrics
Medical University of South Carolina
Charleston, South Carolina

Ryan Kearney, MD, MPH
Northampton Area Pediatrics, LLP
Boston Children's Hospital Community of Care
Member

Kathryn Kean, MD
Pediatric Emergency Medicine Fellow
Department of Emergency Medicine
Goryeb Children's Hospital, Morristown
Medical Center
Morristown, New Jersey

Samantha Kerns, MD
Resident, Emergency Medicine
Department of Emergency Medicine
University of California, Davis
Sacramento, California

Naghma S. Khan, MD, FAAP, FACEP
Associate Professor of Pediatric and Emergency
  Medicine
Department of Pediatrics and Emergency Medicine
Emory University School of Medicine
Atlanta, Georgia

Anupam B. Kharbanda, MD, MSc
Chief, Critical Care Services
Children's Minnesota Emergency Medicine
Associate Professor of Pediatrics
University of Minnesota
Minneapolis, Minnesota

Tommy Y. Kim, MD
Health Science Clinical Professor
Department of Emergency Medicine
HCA Healthcare, Riverside Community
  Hospital/UC Riverside School of Medicine
Riverside, California

Tyler Kingdon, MD
Resident Physician
Department of Pediatrics
LSU Health Sciences Center, School of Medicine
New Orleans, Louisiana

Sarah Kleist, MD
Pediatric Emergency Medicine Medical Director
Department of Pediatrics and Emergency Medicine
Grand Strand Regional Medical Center
Myrtle Beach, South Carolina

Jean Klig, MD
Assistant Professor of Emergency Medicine and
  Pediatrics
Department of Emergency Medicine
Massachusetts General Hospital
Harvard Medical School
Boston, Massachusetts

Adam Kochman, MD, FAAP, FACEP
Associate Director of Pediatric Emergency
  Medicine
Department of Emergency Medicine
Deputy Advisor for Pediatric Emergency
  Preparedness and Response
Inova Fairfax Hospital for Children
Falls Church, Virginia

Marie Kotenko, MD, MPH
Emergency Medicine Resident
Oakland University William Beaumont School
  of Medicine
Beaumont Hospital, Royal Oak
Royal Oak, Michigan

Maybelle Kou, MD, MEd
Associate Clinical Professor
Department of Emergency Medicine
The George Washington University School of
  Medicine
Washington, District of Columbia
Assistant Professor
Departments of Emergency Medicine and
  Pediatrics
Virginia Commonwealth University School of
  Medicine Fairfax Campus
Falls Church, Virginia

Ioannis Koutroulis, MD, PhD, MBA
Pediatric Emergency Medicine Attending
Assistant Professor of Pediatrics, Emergency
  Medicine, and Genomics and Precision
  Medicine
Division of Emergency Medicine
Children's National Hospital
The George Washington University School of
  Medicine
Washington, District of Columbia

Atsuko Koyama, MD, MPH
Clinical Assistant Professor
Department of Child Health
University of Arizona, College of Medicine
Phoenix, Arizona

Kevin Landefeld, MD
Chief Resident
Department of Emergency Medicine
LSU Health Sciences New Orleans
New Orleans, Louisiana

Sean Larsen, MD
Pediatric Chief Resident
University of Arizona College of Medicine
Tucson, Arizona

Simone L. Lawson, MD, FAAP
Assistant Professor of Pediatrics and
  Emergency Medicine
Division of Emergency Medicine and Trauma
  Services
Children's National Hospital
The George Washington University School of
  Medicine and Health Sciences
Washington, District of Columbia

Flavien Leclere, MD, MA
Resident Physician
Department of Emergency Medicine
LAC+USC Medical Center
Los Angeles, California

Hannah Y. Lee, MD
Pediatric Urgent Care Physician
Department of Pediatric Urgent Care
Children's Healthcare of Atlanta
Atlanta, Georgia

Jonathan Lee, MD, FAAP
Pediatric Emergency Medicine Fellow
Department of Pediatrics
Inova Fairfax Hospital
Falls Church, Virginia

Moon O. Lee, MD, MPH, FACEP
Quality Director
Pediatric Emergency Department
Department of Emergency Medicine
Stanford University School of Medicine
Stanford, California

Aaron N. Leetch, MD
Associate Professor of Emergency Medicine
    and Pediatrics
Program Director, Combined Emergency
    Medicine and Pediatrics Residency
Departments of Emergency Medicine and
    Pediatrics
University of Arizona College of Medicine
Tucson, Arizona

Beatrice Leverett, MD
Combined Pediatric & Emergency Medicine
    Residency Programs
University of Maryland Medical Center
Baltimore, Maryland

Marla C. Levine, MD
Assistant Professor, Department of Pediatrics
The University of Texas at Austin Dell Medical
    School
Pediatric Emergency Medicine Physician
Dell Children's Medical Center
Austin, Texas

Jenna Lillemoe, MD
Chief Resident of Pediatrics
Department of Pediatrics
Massachusetts General Hospital for Children
Boston, Massachusetts

Stephen Lim, MD, FAAEM
Director of Resident Research
Assistant Professor
Section of Emergency Medicine
Louisiana State University Health Sciences Center
New Orleans, Louisiana

Carly Loner, MD
Attending
Department of Emergency Medicine
University of Rochester Strong Memorial Hospital
Rochester, New York

Mimi Lu, MD
Adjunct Assistant Professor
Director, PEM Education
Department of Emergency Medicine
University of Maryland
Baltimore, Maryland

Stephen Mac, MD, FAAP
Director of Clinical Effectiveness
Department of Emergency Medicine
Children's Hospital of New Orleans
Louisiana State University
New Orleans, Louisiana

Emily C. MacNeill, MD
Associate Professor/Associate Residency
    Director Emergency Medicine
Director of Inclusion and Health Equity for
    Medical Education
Carolinas Medical Center

Marci Macaraeg, MD
Department of Pediatrics
University of Arizona
Tucson, Arizona

Julia N. Magana, MD
Assistant Professor of Emergency Medicine
Pediatric Emergency Medicine
UC Davis Children's Hospital
Sacramento, California

Akhila Reddy Mandadi, MD
Fellow in Pediatric Emergency Medicine
University of Florida College of Medicine –
    Jacksonville
Jacksonville, Florida

Mark S. Mannenbach, MD
Consultant, Division of Pediatric and
    Adolescent Emergency Medicine
Chair of Education and Faculty Development
Department of Emergency Medicine
Mayo Clinic
Rochester, Minnesota

Erica Marburger, MD
Emergency Medicine Resident, PGY-3
Department of Emergency Medicine
Beaumont Health System
Royal Oak, Michigan

Julia E. Martin, MD, FACEP
Professor of Emergency Medicine
Department of Emergency Medicine
University of Kentucky
Lexington, Kentucky

William Martin, MD
Chief Resident, 2019-2020
Emergency Medicine and Pediatrics Residency
    Program, PGY-5
Indiana University School of Medicine
Indianapolis, Indiana

Chad D. McCalla, MD
Assistant Professor of Emergency Medicine
Section of Pediatric Emergency Medicine
Wake Forest University School of Medicine
Winston-Salem, North Carolina

Anna McFarlin, MD
Assistant Professor of Clinical Pediatrics
Department of Pediatrics
LSU Health New Orleans
New Orleans, Louisiana

Kayla McManus, DO
Department of Pediatrics
University of Florida School of Medicine
Jacksonville, Florida

Ryley McPeters, MD
Department of Internal Medicine and
    Pediatrics
Louisiana State University Health Sciences
    Center, Children's Hospital of New
    Orleans
New Orleans, Louisiana

Kathleen Meadows, MD, FAAP
Emergency Department
Children's Hospital New Orleans
New Orleans, Louisiana

Jenny Mendelson, MD
Assistant Professor, Division of Critical Care
Departments of Pediatrics
University of Arizona, College of Medicine
Tucson, Arizona

Neethu M. Menon, MD
Assistant Professor
Department of Pediatrics
The University of Texas Health Science Center
    at Houston & McGovern Medical School
Houston, Texas

Collin Michels, MD
Resident, Stanford Emergency Medicine
Stanford University School of Medicine
Stanford, California

Elise Milani, MD
PGY-4
Section of Emergency Medicine
Louisiana State University Health Sciences Center
New Orleans, Louisiana

Whitney Minnock, MD
Director of Simulation Pediatric Emergency
Emergency Medicine
Oakland University William Beaumont School
    of Medicine
Rochester, Michigan

Carl Mirus IV, MD
Resident
Department of Emergency Medicine
University of Rochester Strong Memorial Hospital
Rochester, New York

Michael S. Mitchell, MD
Medical Director, Pediatric Emergency
Department at Brenner Children's Hospital
Assistant Professor of Emergency Medicine
Section of Pediatric Emergency Medicine
Wake Forest University School of Medicine
Medical Center Boulevard
Winston-Salem, North Carolina

Perry White Mitchell, MD
PGY-IV Resident
Department of Internal Medicine/Emergency
    Medicine
LSU Health Sciences Center
New Orleans, Louisiana

Matthew Moake, MD, PhD
Assistant Professor
Division of Pediatric Emergency Medicine
Medical University of South Carolina
Charleston, South Carolina

Sephora N. Morrison, MBBS, MSCI, MBA,
CPE
Associate Division Chief, Director of Clinical
    Operations EMTC
Director, Patient Experience & Clinical Service
    Innovation
Children's National Medical Center
Washington, District of Columbia

Amber M. Morse, MD, FAAP
Assistant Professor and Associate Fellowship
 Director
Department of Pediatric Emergency Medicine
University of Arkansas for Medical Sciences
Little Rock, Arkansas

David Muncy, DO
Department of Emergency Medicine
University of Kentucky
Lexington, Kentucky

Erin Munns, MD
Pediatric Emergency Medicine Fellow
Department of Pediatric Emergency Medicine
University of Texas at Austin Dell Medical School
Austin, Texas

Carrie M. Myers, MD
Resident Physician
Department of Emergency Medicine
Hennepin County Medical Center
Minneapolis, Minnesota

Kimberly Myers, MD
Assistant Instructor of Emergency Medicine
Department of Emergency Medic
Wake Forest Baptist Medical
Center Winston-Salem, North Carolina

Vishal Naik, MD
Chief Pediatric Resident
Department of Pediatrics
University of Minnesota Masonic Children's
 Hospital
Minneapolis, Minnesota

Nidhya Navanandan, MD
Assistant Professor of Pediatrics
Section of Emergency Medicine
University of Colorado School of Medicine
Children's Hospital Colorado
Aurora, Colorado

Matthew Neal, MD, MBA
Clinical Assistant Professor
Department of Emergency Medicine
Prisma Health
University of South Carolina School of
 Medicine, Greenville
Greenville, South Carolina

Mylinh Thi Nguyen, M.D.
Assistant Clinical Professor, Pediatrics
University of California San Diego
San Diego, California

Jonathan Nielson, MD
Department of Pediatric Emergency
 Medicine
Pediatric Emergency Medicine Fellow
Children's Minnesota
Minneapolis, Minnesota

Mahnoosh Nik-Ahd, MD, MPH
Pediatric Emergency Medicine Fellow
Department of Emergency Medicine
UCSF Benioff Children's Hospital Oakland
Oakland, California

Kimberly L. Norris, MD
Assistant Professor of Pediatric Emergency
 Medicine
Department of Pediatrics
Emory University School of Medicine
Atlanta, Georgia

Rachel O'Brian, MD
Pediatric Emergency Medicine Fellow
Department of Pediatrics
Inova Fairfax Hospital for Children
Falls Church, Virginia

Michelle Odette, MD
Resident Physician
Department of Pediatrics
University of California, Davis
Sacramento, California

James C. O'Neill, MD, FACEP
Associate Professor of Emergency
 Medicine
Department of Emergency Medicine
Wake Forest Baptist Health
Winston-Salem, North Carolina

Nicholas Orozco, MD MS
Resident Physician
Department of Emergency Medicine
Los Angeles County + University of Southern
 California Medical Center
Los Angeles, California

Jonathan Orsborn, MD, FAAP
Pediatric Emergency Ultrasound
 Co-director
Department of Pediatric Emergency
 Medicine
University of Colorado School of Medicine
Children's Hospital Colorado
Aurora, Colorado

Leslie Palmerlee, MD, MPH
Assistant Professor of Emergency Medicine
Associate Director
Division of Emergency Ultrasound
Department of Emergency Medicine
LSU Health Sciences/University Medical
    Center New Orleans
New Orleans, Louisiana

Devan Pandya, MD
Resident Physician
Department of Emergency Medicine
HCA Healthcare, Riverside Community
    Hospital/UC Riverside School of
    Medicine
Riverside, California

Kelly Patel, MD
Emergency Medicine Resident
Department of Emergency Medicine
Beaumont Health – Royal Oak
Royal Oak, Michigan

Saharsh Patel, MD
Clinical Instructor
Department of Pediatrics
Stanford University School of Medicine
Palo Alto, California

Amy Pattishall, MD
Associate Professor
Division of Pediatric Emergency Medicine
Department of Pediatrics
Emory University School of Medicine
Children's Healthcare of Atlanta
Atlanta, Georgia

Robert Peterson, MD
Assistant Professor
Department of Pediatrics
University of Washington School of
    Medicine
Seattle, Washington

Frederick Place, MD, FACEP, FAAP
Director of the Pediatric Emergency
    Department
Department of Emergency Medicine
Inova Fairfax Medical Campus
Fairfax, Virginia

Jennifer Plitt, MD
Assistant Professor
Department of Emergency Medicine
University of Arizona, Banner UMC

Nicholas Pokrajac, MD
Assistant Professor
Pediatric Emergency Medicine
Department of Emergency Medicine
Stanford University School of Medicine
Palo Alto, California

Adriana Porto, MD
Pediatric Emergency Medicine Fellow
Department of Emergency Medicine
William Beaumont Hospital
Royal Oak, Michigan

Jennifer K. Potter, MD
Resident Physician
Department of Emergency Medicine
Carolinas Medical Center, Atrium Health
Charlotte, North Carolina

Amanda Price, MD
Assistant Professor
Division of Pediatric Emergency Medicine
Director, Pediatric Simulation
Department of Pediatrics
Medical University South Carolina
Charleston, South Carolina

Nadira Ramkellawan, MD
Department of Emergency Medicine
Inova Loudoun Hospital
Leesburg, Virginia

Katie Rebillot, DO
Keck School of Medicine of the University of
    Southern California
Assistant Professor of Clinical Emergency
    Medicine
Department of Emergency Medicine
Los Angeles County + USC Medical
    Center
Los Angeles, California

Ryan J. Reichert, MD
Fellow of Pediatric Emergency Medicine
Department of Emergency Medicine
Wake Forest School of Medicine
Winston Salem, North Carolina

Lindsey Retterath, MD
Resident Physician
Departments of Emergency Medicine and
    Pediatrics
Banner–University Medical Center
Tucson, Arizona

Nicholena Richardson, MD
Department of Emergency Medicine
Carolinas Medical Center
Charlotte, North Carolina

Eddie G. Rodriguez, MD
Attending Physician
Department of Emergency Medicine
Ponce Health Sciences University/St. Luke's
 Episcopal Medical Center
Ponce, Puerto Rico

Blair Rolnick, MD, FAAP
Chief Pediatric Emergency Medicine
 Fellow
St. Christopher's Hospital for Children
Philadelphia, Pennsylvania

Emily Rose, MD, FAAP, FAAEM, FACEP
Director for Pre-Health Undergraduate Studies
Director of the Minor in Health Care Studies
Keck School of Medicine of the University of
 Southern California
Associate Professor of Clinical Emergency
 Medicine (Educational Scholar)
Department of Emergency Medicine
Los Angeles County + USC Medical Center
Los Angeles, California

Efrat Rosenthal, MD
Assistant Professor
Department of Emergency Medicine
University of California, San Francisco
San Francisco, California

Debra S. Rusk, MD
Assistant Dean for Career Mentoring,
 Educational Affairs
Assistant Professor of Clinical Emergency
 Medicine
Assistant Professor of Clinical Pediatrics
Indiana University School of Medicine
Indianapolis, Indiana

Timothy K. Ruttan, MD
Assistant Professor of Pediatrics
Pediatric Emergency Medicine Education and
 Clerkship Director
University of Texas at Austin Dell Medical
 School
Department of Pediatrics
Dell Children's Medical Center of Central Texas
Pediatric Emergency Medicine
Austin, Texas

Sami K. Saikaly, MD
Dermatology Resident
Department of Dermatology
University of Florida
Gainesville, Florida

Sandal Saleem, MD, FAAP
Pediatric Emergency Medicine Fellow
Department of Pediatric Emergency Medicine
Beaumont Health – Royal Oak
Royal Oak, Michigan

Nicholas Sausen, MD
Assistant Professor of Pediatrics
Division of Pediatric Emergency Medicine
Department of Pediatrics
University of Minnesota Masonic Children's
 Hospital
Minneapolis, Minnesota

Chad Scarboro, MD, FACEP
Associate Professor of Emergency Medicine
 and Pediatrics
Division of Pediatric Emergency Medicine
Department of Emergency Medicine
Atrium Health's Carolinas Medical Center/
 Levine Children's Hospital
Charlotte, North Carolina

Anna Schlechter, MD, FAAP
Fellow, Pediatric Emergency Medicine
Department of Pediatrics
The University of Texas at Austin Dell Medical
 School
Dell Children's Medical Center of Central Texas
Austin, Texas

Dr. Suzanne M. Schmidt, MD
Assistant Professor of Pediatrics
Department of Pediatric Emergency Medicine
Ann & Robert H. Lurie Children's Hospital of
 Chicago/Northwestern University Feinberg
 School of Medicine
Chicago, Illinois

Jennifer J. Schoch, MD
Assistant Professor of Dermatology
University of Florida College of Medicine–
 Gainesville
Gainesville, Florida

Daniel Scholz, MD, MPH
Department of Emergency Medicine
Mayo Clinic
Rochester, Minnesota

Paul Schunk, MD, FAAEM
Assistant Program Director
Madigan Army Medical Center
Fort Lewis, Washington

Julia Schweizer, MD, FAAP
Director of Outreach
Department of Emergency Medicine
Children's Hospital of New Orleans
New Orleans, Louisiana

Erica Scott, MD
Resident
Department of Emergency Medicine
ECU Brody School of Medicine
Greenville, North Carolina

Kara K. Seaton, MD, FAAP
Fellowship Director, Pediatric Emergency
    Medicine
Department of Emergency Medicine
Children's Minnesota
Minneapolis, Minnesota

Suzanne E. Seo, MD
Pediatric Emergency Medicine Fellow
Department of Pediatric Emergency
    Medicine
University of Washington School of Medicine/
    Seattle Children's Hospital
Seattle, Washington

Haig Setrakian, MD
Assistant Professor of Emergency Medicine and
    Pediatrics
Indiana University
Indianapolis, Indiana

Lekha Shah, MD, FAAP, FACEP
Fellowship Director, Pediatric Emergency
    Ultrasound
Departments of Emergency Medicine and
    Pediatrics
Emory University/Children's Healthcare of
    Atlanta
Atlanta, Georgia

Seema Shah, MD
Medical Director
Division of Emergency Medicine
Rady Children's Hospital San Diego
Clinical Professor of Pediatrics
University of California San Diego
San Diego, California

Supriya Sharma, MD, FAAP
Fellow, Pediatric Emergency Medicine
Fellow, Child Abuse Pediatrics
Harbor–UCLA Medical Center
Torrance, California

Matthew Shapiro, MD
Pediatric Hospital Medicine Fellow
Department of Pediatrics
Ann & Robert H. Lurie Children's Hospital of
    Chicago
Northwestern University Feinberg School of
    Medicine
Chicago, Illinois

Corinne Shubin, MD
Clinical Assistant Professor
Pediatric Emergency Medicine
University of Washington School of Medicine
Seattle Children's Hospital
Seattle, Washington

Joshua Siembieda, MD
Pediatric Emergency Medicine Physician
Department of Pediatric Emergency Medicine
CHOC Children's Hospital
Orange, California

David Skibbie, MD, MA, FACEP, FAAEM
Inova Fairfax Hospital
Falls Church, Virginia
Department of Emergency Medicine
Assistant Professor of Emergency Medicine
Virginia Commonwealth University
Richmond, Virginia

Morgan J. Sims, MD, FAAP
Assistant Professor of Pediatrics
Pediatric Emergency Medicine
University of North Carolina
Chapel Hill, North Carolina

Leah Sitler, MD
Resident Physician
Department of Pediatrics
University of California Davis Children's
    Hospital
Sacramento, California

Daniel Slubowski, MD
Pediatric Emergency Medicine Fellow
Department of Emergency Medicine
University of Texas at Austin Dell Medical School
Dell Children's Medical Center
Austin, Texas

Adrienne N. Smallwood, MD
Resident Physician, PGY-3
Department of Pediatrics
Ann & Robert H. Lurie Children's Hospital of
  Chicago/Northwestern University Feinberg
  School of Medicine
Chicago, Illinois

Anna G. Smith, MD, FAAP
Fellow, Pediatric Emergency Medicine
Department of Emergency Medicine
Ann & Robert H. Lurie Children's Hospital
Chicago, Illinois

Jeremiah Smith, MD, FAAP
GME Director for Pediatric Education for EM
  Residency
Department of Emergency Medicine
Prisma Health–Upstate, University of South
  Carolina–Greenville
Greenville, South Carolina

Kathleen M. Smith, MD, MPH
Attending Physician
Rady Children's Hospital–San Diego
Department of Emergency Medicine
UCSD School of Medicine
San Diego, California

Natasha Smith, MD
Resident Physician
Department of Emergency Medicine and Pediatrics
University of Maryland Medical Center
Baltimore, Maryland

David Soma, MD, CAQSM
Assistant Professor of Pediatrics
Departments of Pediatrics and Orthopedic
  Surgery
Mayo Clinic College of Medicine
Rochester, Minnesota

Rajesh Sood, MD, FAAP
Pediatric Emergency Medicine Fellow
Department of Pediatrics
Inova Children's Hospital
Falls Church, Virginia

Fernando Soto, MD, FACEP
Attending Physician
UPR Hospital–Dr. Federico Trilla
University Pediatric Hospital–Dr. Antonio Ortiz
Assistant Professor Emergency Medicine/
  Pediatric Emergency Medicine
Department of Emergency Medicine
University of Puerto Rico–School of Medicine

Samuel J Spizman, MD, FAAP
Assistant Professor
Children's Healthcare of Atlanta
Department of Pediatrics
Division of Pediatric Emergency Medicine
Emory University
Atlanta, Georgia

Kathleen Stephanos, MD, FAAEM
Assistant Clerkship Director
Departments of Emergency Medicine and
  Pediatrics
University of Rochester Strong Memorial Hospital
Rochester, New York

Josephine Stout, MD
Chief Resident
Department of Pediatrics
University of Arizona, College of Medicine
Tucson, Arizona

Ashley M. Strobel, MD, FACEP, FAAP
Director of Pediatric Emergency Education
Assistant Professor of Emergency Medicine
Department of Emergency Medicine
Hennepin County Medical Center
Division of Pediatric Emergency Medicine
University of Minnesota Masonic Children's
  Hospital
Minneapolis, Minnesota

Jonathan Strutt, MD, FAAP
Assistant Professor
Pediatric Emergency Medicine
University of Minnesota Masonic Children's
  Hospital
Minneapolis, Minnesota

Katina M. Summerford, MD
Pediatric Emergency Medicine Fellow
Department of Emergency Medicine
Phoenix Children's Hospital
Phoenix, Arizona

Scott W. Sutton, MD
Assistant Professor of Emergency
  Medicine
Section of Pediatric Emergency Medicine
Wake Forest Baptist Health Medical Center Blvd
Winston Salem, North Carolina

Yongtian Tina Tan, MD, MBA
Pediatrics Resident
Department of Pediatrics
University of California at San Francisco
San Francisco, California

Ankita Taneja, MD, MPH
Pediatric Emergency Medicine Fellow
University of Florida, Jacksonville
Jacksonville, Florida

Joseph Abraham Tanga, MD
Resident Emergency Medicine Physician
Department of Emergency Medicine
PRISMA Health at the University of South
    Carolina School of Medicine–Greenville
    Campus
Greenville, South Carolina

Getachew Teshome, MD, MPH
Associate Professor and Division Head
Pediatric Emergency Medicine
Department of Pediatrics
University of Maryland School of
    Medicine
Baltimore, Maryland

Lindly A. Theroux, DO
Pediatric Emergency Medicine Fellow
Department of Emergency Medicine
Wake Forest Baptist Health
Medical Center Blvd
Winston Salem, North Carolina

Anita A. Thomas, MD
Assistant Professor
Division of Emergency Medicine
Department of Pediatrics
University of Washington, Seattle Children's
    Hospital
Seattle, Washington

Sean Thompson, MD
Assistant Professor of Clinical Emergency
    Medicine
Assistant Professor of Clinical Pediatrics
Department of Emergency Medicine
Indiana University School of Medicine
Indianapolis, Indiana

Tseng-Che Tseng, MD
Emergency Medicine/Pediatrics Combined
    Resident PGY-3
Department of Emergency Medicine and
    Pediatrics
Louisiana State University Health Science
    Center
New Orleans, Louisiana

Brittany Tyson, MD
Resident Physician
Department of Emergency Medicine
Los Angeles County + University of Southern
    California Medical Center
Los Angeles, California

Matthew B. Underwood, MD, FACEP
Health Sciences Assistant Professor
Department of Emergency Medicine
University of California Riverside, School of
    Medicine
HCA Healthcare, Riverside Community Hospital
Riverside, California

Atim Uya, MD
Director, Point-of-Care Ultrasound
Associate Professor of Pediatrics
Department of Pediatrics
University of California-San Diego/Rady
    Children's Hospital
San Diego, California

Selina Varma, MD, MPH
Pediatric Emergency Medicine Fellow
Department of Pediatrics
Northwestern University Feinberg School of
    Medicine
Ann & Robert H. Lurie Children's Hospital
Chicago, Illinois

Tatyana Vayngortin, MD
Assistant Clinical Professor
Division of Emergency Medicine
Rady Children's Hospital San Diego
University of California, San Diego
San Diego, California

Adam E. Vella, MD, FAAP
Associate Chief Quality Officer
Associate Professor of Clinical Emergency
    Medicine and Pediatrics
Department of Emergency Medicine
New York-Presbyterian Hospital Weill Cornell
    Medical Center
New York, New York

Evan Verplancken, MD
Resident Physician
Department of Emergency Medicine
Medical University of South Carolina
Charleston, South Carolina

Robert Vezzetti, MD, FAAP, FACEP
Attending Physician, Pediatric Emergency
  Medicine
Associate Program Director, Pediatric
  Residency Program
Course Director, Pediatric Emergency
  Medicine Radiology, Pediatric Emergency
  Medicine Fellowship Program
Dell Children's Medical Center
Dell Medical School at the University of Texas–
  Austin
Austin, Texas

Brian Wagers, MD, FAAP
Physician Director of Pediatric and Maternal
  Quality and Safety
Riley Hospital for Children
Assistant Professor of Clinical Emergency
  Medicine and Pediatrics
Riley Hospital for Children and Indiana
  University School of Medicine
Indianapolis, Indiana

Emily Wagner, MD
Chief Resident
Emergency Medicine and Pediatrics Residency
  Program
Indiana School of Medicine
Indianapolis, Indiana

Jessica Wall, MD, MPH, MSCE, FAAP
Clinical Assistant Professor of Emergency
  Medicine and Pediatrics
Associate Pediatric Medical Director, Airlift
  Northwest
University of Washington, School of
  Medicine
Seattle, Washington

Dina Wallin, MD
Physician, Pediatric Emergency Care
Assistant Professor, Department of Emergency
  Medicine
UCSF Benioff Children's Hospital
San Francisco, California

Caroline Wang, MD
Pediatric Chief Resident
Department of Pediatrics
University of California, Davis
Sacramento, California

George Sam Wang, MD, FAAP, FAACT
Associate Professor of Pediatrics
Section of Emergency Medicine, Medical
  Toxicology
Department of Pediatrics
University of Colorado Anschutz Medical Campus
Children's Hospital Colorado
Aurora, Colorado

Yvette Wang, MD
Assistant Clinical Professor of Pediatrics
Department of Pediatrics, Division of
  Emergency Medicine
Rady Children's Hospital, San Diego
University of California, San Diego
San Diego, California

Crick Watkins, DO
Assistant Professor
Section of Pediatric Emergency Medicine
Department of Emergency Medicine
Wake Forest University School of Medicine
Winston-Salem, North Carolina

Rachel Weigert, MD
Pediatric Emergency Medicine Fellow
Department of Emergency Medicine
Children's Hospitals and Clinics of Minnesota
Minneapolis, Minnesota

Sarah N. Weihmiller, MD, FAAP
Attending Physician, Quality Assurance
  Committee Leader
Division of Pediatric Emergency Medicine
Department of Emergency Medicine
Levine Children's Hospital
Carolinas Medical Center, Atrium Health
Charlotte, North Carolina

Alexander Werne, MD
Resident, PGY-3
Department of Pediatrics
University of California, San Francisco
San Francisco, California

Heidi Werner, M.D., MSHPEd
Associate Professor
Department of Emergency Medicine
University of California School of Medicine,
  San Francisco
San Francisco, California

William White, MD, MA
Fellow, Pediatric Emergency Medicine and
  Emergency Ultrasound
Department of Emergency Medicine
Harbor–UCLA Medical Center
Torrance, California

Anne Whitehead, MD, FAAEM
Assistant Professor of Clinical Emergency
  Medicine and Pediatrics
Department of Emergency Medicine
Indiana University School of Medicine
Indianapolis, Indiana

Danielle Wickman, MD
Resident Physician
Department of Emergency Medicine
LAC+USC Medical Center
Los Angeles, California

Rachel Wiltjer, DO
Resident in Emergency Medicine/Pediatrics
  Program
Departments of Emergency Medicine and
  Pediatrics
University of Maryland Medical Center
Baltimore, Maryland

Dale P. Woolridge, MD, PhD
Block Director College of Medicine
  Curriculum: Digestion, Metabolism,
  Hormones (DMH)
Director of the Southern Arizona Children's
  Advocacy Center
Professor of Emergency Medicine, Pediatrics
  and Chemistry/Biochemistry
Department of Emergency Medicine
University of Arizona
Tucson, Arizona

Todd Wylie, MD
Associate Professor
Program Director, Pediatric Emergency
  Medicine Fellowship
Medical Director, Pediatric Emergency
  Department
Department of Emergency Medicine
University of Florida College of Medicine–
  Jacksonville
Jacksonville, Florida

Sheryl E. Yanger, MD
Physician, Pediatric Emergency Medicine
Ann & Robert H. Lurie Children's Hospital of
  Chicago
Assistant Professor of Pediatrics (Emergency
  Medicine)
Northwestern University Feinberg School of
  Medicine
Winfield, Illinois

Kelly D. Young, MD, MS
Health Sciences Clinical Professor of
  Pediatrics
David Geffen School of Medicine
  at UCLA
Pediatric Emergency Medicine Fellowship
  Program Director
Department of Emergency Medicine
Harbor–UCLA Medical Center
Torrance, California

Mark Zhang, MD
Resident Physician
Department of Emergency Medicine
Los Angeles County + USC Medical Center
Los Angeles, California

Elise Zimmerman, MD, MS
Assistant Clinical Professor of Pediatrics
Division of Emergency Medicine
Department of Pediatrics
Rady Children's Hospital San Diego
University of California, San Diego
San Diego, California

**Melissa E. Zukowski, MD, MPH, FACEP,
FAAP**
Medical Director, Emergency Department
Department of Emergency Medicine
The University of Arizona College of
  Medicine–Tucson
Banner University Medical Center–Tucson
Tucson, Arizona

PREFACE

Medicine is a humbling profession, and there are few examples where this is more apparent than caring for children in the emergency department. Clinicians manage a broad spectrum of patient complaints and acuities simultaneously with limited information and time. Crowded environments and a ubiquitous sense of urgency regardless of illness severity add to the challenge. Fortunately, most pediatric patients are not high risk, and very few are critically ill; however, many presenting conditions are *subtle*, and significant disease may be missed when a clinician is lulled into a false sense of security. While the majority of children are not seen in dedicated pediatric emergency departments and individual clinician's comfort in the care of children varies tremendously, it is still incumbent upon all of us to remain vigilant and strive for excellence. The pediatric examination can be difficult, and disease manifestation can be obscure. Thus, a solid understanding of the varying presentations of pediatric disease and what mistakes to avoid is the basis for "Avoiding Common Errors in Pediatric Emergency Medicine."

We believe that children deserve the highest quality of an initial emergency assessment and management regardless of where they present. This book has therefore been written with the broad range of medical providers caring for children in the emergency setting in mind. Chapters cover the breadth of medical topics relevant to emergency care of children in a succinct and accessible format easily referenced for guidance during patient care. It is our sincere hope that this collection of information will assist all providers in the appropriate identification and management of both the common conditions and also the subtle presentations of significant disease.

It would be our great error if we did not thank all who contributed as individuals or groups and to all the staff support toward the publication of this reference. We offer a special thank you to the authors and associate editors for time devoted in making their chapters cutting-edge, informative, and applicable to your care of children in the emergency setting. We thank the series editor, Dr. Lisa Marcucci, for allowing us the opportunity to create this piece of literature dedicated to our own specialty. We feel this will be a valuable addition to the series. We also want to thank the publisher and managing editors at Wolters Kluwer for their support in developing and publication of this work. On behalf of all the authors and editors, we would like to thank our source of inspiration: our students, residents, fellows, colleagues. You motivate us to pursue and disseminate knowledge for the benefit of pediatric patients everywhere. Thank you all!

Dale P. Woolridge, MD, PhD
Sean M. Fox, MD
James (Jim) Homme, MD
Aaron N. Leetch, MD
Timothy K. Ruttan, MD

CONTENTS

ENVIRONMENTAL/TOXICOLOGY   25

EAR NOSE THROAT   41

AIRWAY 105

CARDIOLOGY/DYSRHYTHMIA 122

■ ABDOMEN 141

GENITOURINARY AND RENAL 162

■ DERMATOLOGY 179

■ ENDOCRINE 191

▓ NEUROLOGY   203

■ HEMATOLOGY/ONCOLOGY   257

■ GENETICS/METABOLISM 273

172 Recognition and Management of Inborn Errors of Metabolism—
The Needle in the Haystack 273
James (Jim) Homme, MD

173 Have No Fear; an Inborn Error of Metabolism Is Here! Managing
Patients With Known Inborn Errors of Metabolism 275
James (Jim) Homme, MD

174 Be Aware of Abnormal Newborn Screens 277
Cree Kachelski, MD, FAAP and Jason (Jay) Homme, MD, FAAP

■ NEONATOLOGY 279

175 Umbilical Care: Do Not Confuse the Normal Granulation With
the Purulence of Omphalitis 279
Robert Peterson, MD

176 I Am So Hungry! Know the Right Questions to Ask About Feeding
Difficulty in the Neonate 280
Katina M. Summerford, MD and Rachel E. M. Cramton, MD

177 Is It Supposed to Look That Way?: Know What Is Normal
Postcircumcision So You Can Reassure Parents. 282
Alyssa Bernardi, DO and Rachel E. M. Cramton, MD

178 Skin and Bones, or Normal Growth: Identifying Failure to Thrive 284
Marci Macaraeg, MD and Rachel E. M. Cramton, MD

■ ALLERGY/IMMUNOLOGY 286

179 Anaphylaxis: It May Come as a Shock, but It Does Not Have
to End in Tragedy. 286
Lindsey Retterath, MD and Melissa E. Zukowski, MD, MPH, FACEP,FAAP

180 Primary Immunodeficiency: Know What to Expect When Cell
Lines Go Awry 287
Monica Hajirawala, MD and Julia Schweizer, MD, FAAP

■ COMMUNITY/LEGAL 290

181 Do Not Forget to Look for the Five W's of Cutaneous Injuries 290
Caroline Wang, MD and Julia N. Magana, MD

182 Do Not Miss Abusive Head Trauma! 291
Leah Sitler, MD and Julia N. Magana, MD

183 Broken Bones in Broken Homes: When to Get a Skeletal Survey 292
Lily Anne Jewett, MD and Julia N. Magana, MD

▪ APPLIED PRACTICE   302

▪ BEHAVIORAL HEALTH   310

▪ PHARMACY   313

THE CRASHING PATIENT

1

Overlooking the Basics and Focusing on Medications That Do Not Matter During Pediatric Codes

Michael S. Mitchell, MD and Crick Watkins, DO

The crashing pediatric patient can induce anxiety for providers and nursing alike, especially if encountered infrequently. Pediatric Advanced Life Support (PALS) guidelines should be followed when caring for a critically ill pediatric patient, and providers should be aware that these guidelines may not closely follow adult Advanced Cardiac Life Support (ACLS). "Kids are not little adults," nor should adult guidelines be followed when caring for pediatric patients. Below are some common pitfalls when caring for sick pediatric patients.

Weight

Accurate weights are an essential component of managing a critically-ill pediatric patient. All critical care medications are weight-based, thus small inaccuracies in estimated weight can significantly impact medication efficacy. Much literature has been devoted to the accuracy of guessing weights in pediatric patients and the conclusion remains the same: guessing weight based on perceived age is not accurate.

Length-based resuscitation tools, such as the Broselow tape, are more accurate if used correctly. Providers must follow the instructions very closely and ensure that the end of the tape is pulled up to the top of the child's head. Even these simple instructions can be misapplied, so careful interpretation of the tape is warranted. The Broselow tape demonstrates close agreement with actual weight but is least accurate when the child is over 25 kg, so if the child's length is near the end of the tape, assume that the weight may be less accurate. Also body habitus must be taken into account, as obesity levels remain high in American children. Some other weight estimation systems may outperform the Broselow tape; however, despite the chosen method, they all outperform guessing the weight. Do not guess the weight!

Suitable Cardiopulmonary Resuscitation

Given the limited cardiopulmonary reserve that is found in critically ill children, good, effective cardiopulmonary resuscitation (CPR) is essential. Chest compression depth should be 1/2-1/3 of total chest depth, and each compression should allow for full chest recoil. It is recommended to frequently switch team members performing CPR. Avoiding interruptions is paramount. This is especially true after performing defibrillation, in which a shock should immediately be followed by 2 minutes of high-quality CPR.

End-tidal CO_2 measurements ($ETCO_2$) may be beneficial when performing CPR. They can assist in ensuring the endotracheal tube is located in the trachea if the child is intubated. Furthermore, they also may help in guiding the efficacy of CPR. Prior guidelines suggested attempting to maintain an $ETCO_2$ above 15, which is consistent with good CPR; however, current guidelines challenge that number and state that while $ETCO_2$ measurements are recommended, there is no specific cutoff.

Medications Without Routine Benefit

Routine administration of several medications during pediatric codes is no longer recommended. These medications are calcium gluconate, sodium bicarbonate, and atropine.

1) Calcium gluconate: Calcium is not recommended for routine use with the exception of targeted therapy for documented hypocalcemia, calcium channel blocker overdose, hypermagnesemia, or hyperkalemia.
2) Sodium bicarbonate: It is not recommended for use in cardiac arrest as it has not shown routine benefit.
3) Atropine: No longer is atropine recommended as a peri-intubation agent to assist with rapid sequence intubation. It can be used if bradycardia is expected, such as with the use of succinylcholine.

KEY POINTS

- Use length-based resuscitation tool to determine weight; guessing is inaccurate and leads to errors in dosing resuscitation medications.
- Quality compressions are key with emphasis on few interruptions; $ETCO_2$ as a metric for quality.
- Calcium gluconate, sodium bicarbonate, and atropine are no longer routinely used in pediatric codes.

Suggested Readings

de Caen AR, Berg MD, Chameides L, et al. Part 12: Pediatric Advanced Life Support. 2015 American Heart Association guidelines update for cardiopulmonary resuscitation and emergency cardiovascular care. *Circulation*. 2015;132(suppl 2):S526-S542.
Wells M, Goldstein LN, Bentley A, et al. The accuracy of the Broselow tape as a weight estimation tool and a drug-dosing guide-a systematic review and meta-analysis. *Resuscitation*. 2017;121:9-33.

2

Placing Provider Comfort Over Family Presence

Michael S. Mitchell, MD and Sarah Bingham, MD

Pediatric trauma accounts for almost 30% of all emergency department visits annually with 12 000 deaths per year. These traumas occur mostly with family members present, thus, they are often the first to respond and initiate resuscitation. However, once the patient arrives to the hospital, family members are often left out of the trauma bay.

Providers have been resistant to implementing family-witnessed resuscitation (FWR) due to concerns for family disruption during the resuscitation. The most common myths related to family involvement will be outlined below with hopes of engaging all emergency department providers to invite families to be present for the resuscitation process. Notably, family presence during pediatric resuscitation is endorsed by the American Academy of Pediatrics.

Myth: Providers and Care Teams Are Hindered From Doing Their Jobs When Family Members Are Present During Resuscitation

Previous belief among physicians and care team members was that family members contributed to patient stress, slowed the team down, and potentially impacted a provider's decision-making ability.

Physicians envisioned emotional outbursts and potential physical harm from participating in their loved ones ongoing resuscitation. Initially, keeping family members out of the trauma bay was perceived as protecting the loved ones. However, research over the past 20 years has suggested otherwise.

Research supports that family member presence does not inhibit time-sensitive care nor does it interfere with the trauma team evaluation. Despite this evidence, inconsistent implementation of this practice remains. This may be due to lack of organization support, lack of educational opportunities, or concern for medical liability. Limited research has examined the medicolegal risks of this practice, but those studies suggest that there is no increased risk.

Finally, family members can be valuable allies in assisting the child's comfort and cooperation in traumatic resuscitation, further enabling the ability of the providers to seamlessly deliver the needed care. This point cannot be underestimated if the child undergoing resuscitation is alert and aware of the care being rendered. Family member presence will likely convey safety to the child and may lessen the child's stress, which can aid the team in a more thorough evaluation.

Myth: Family Members Are Emotionally Harmed by Being Present During the Resuscitation

"First, do no harm."

Historically, a large barrier to implementing FWR is the concern that witnessing such an event on their loved one could certainly introduce feelings of posttraumatic stress. At first glance, this concern seems valid. This family member just witnessed a traumatic event or critical illness with possible impending death of their loved one. Why would we introduce the added stress of witnessing the seemingly chaotic environment of a pediatric resuscitation?

Research suggests that the opposite is true, however. Many family members would choose to be present in the resuscitation if given the opportunity, but almost all at least want to be invited to attend. Further reinforcing the point, families who actually witnessed their child's trauma resuscitation would choose it again if faced with the same situation. Also research in prehospital care suggests that family members who witnessed their loved one's resuscitation, both adult and pediatric, have less symptoms of anxiety and depression afterward.

Potential benefits of being present include better understanding of care provided, sense of control, assisting in assisting in the grieving process grieving process, and providing closure if death should occur. Research supports that families had improved coping of their child's death, because they were present during the resuscitation.

KEY POINTS

- Family presence does not delay trauma evaluation and care.
- Families prefer to be at the bedside during resuscitation and can improve coping and grieving process.
- Barriers to involving family members are provider comfort, lack of resources, and lack of educational opportunities.

Suggested Readings

Jabre P, Belpomme V, Azoulay E, et al. Family presence during cardiopulmonary resuscitation. *N Engl J Med.* 2013;368(11):1008-1018.

Johnson C. A literature review examining the barriers to the implementation of family witnessed resuscitation in the emergency department. *Int Emerg Nurs.* 2017;30:31-35.

O'Connell KJ, Farah MM, Spamdorger P, Zorc JJ. Family presence during pediatric trauma team activation: an assessment of a structured program. *Pediatrics.* 2007;120(3):565-574.

3

Overlooking Opportunity to Help the Family by Saving Crucial Evidence

William E. Hauda II, MD, FACEP, FAAP

Only about 2% of all emergency department (ED) deaths occur in children. Unintentional injury remains the most common cause of death in the United States for persons aged 1-44 years of age. Homicide is the fourth most common cause in toddlers and school aged children, while suicide is the second most common for preadolescents and adolescents. Of the children with underlying medical problems, 3%-20% will die in an ED due to their underlying medical comorbidities.

Any death in the ED requires the ED physician to balance support of the family with making decisions about resuscitative efforts and possible forensic evidence. Family presence during the resuscitative efforts may seem challenging and difficult, but it assists in preparing the family for the expected outcome and does not lead to a disruption of care or delay in care. Communicating effectively and compassionately with the family during this traumatic time is difficult, requires training and tact, but skillfully conveying this "bad news" is a powerful therapeutic intervention. The presence of a social worker may assist the ED physician in preparing the family, delivering the "bad news," and referring the death to authorities for investigation if appropriate. A social worker may also be aware of prior investigations or concerns regarding the family which may heighten the suspicion of an unnatural death. Parents need to be treated with compassion and respect regardless of the suspicions of the health care providers. The parent or parents may have no knowledge that their child was injured as a result of another person's actions.

During resuscitation efforts, evidence may be found for accidental or inflicted injuries. Early involvement of a forensic nurse or forensic physician while the patient is still being treated in the ED can help with directing documentation of observed findings and procedures to avoid inadvertent destruction of evidence. ED physicians need to be aware that this evidence can be inadvertently altered or destroyed by resuscitative efforts such as by cleaning the skin for line placement, causing oral or dental injury during intubation, or leaving marks on the chest during chest compressions. DNA evidence can be inadvertently removed during cleaning of the genitals for urinary catheterization of a child who was sexually assaulted or when cleaning the hands or neck of a child who has physically assaulted or strangled. Forensic practitioners frequently train other providers during medical and nursing continuing education programs in preparation for the issues during the resuscitation of children.

Once death is pronounced, the emergency medicine practitioner must be willing to scrutinize the possible causes for death to determine if a medicolegal investigation may be appropriate. Many deaths of children will be investigated by an authority, as 70% of childhood maltreatment deaths occur in children under 3 years of age. It is important for ED physicians to know that each jurisdiction, often by county or state, has responsibility for the medicolegal investigation of death by a medical examiner or coroner. An autopsy may not occur in all cases of childhood death; this decision is often made by the investigating authority. Efforts should be made by the ED personnel to preserve evidence in cases being referred for investigation. Generally, the body should not be cleansed or altered after death if an investigating authority will be assuming jurisdiction in the death. Clothing, medications, and personal effects should be left with the deceased until a decision is made by the investigating authority. Therapeutic devices placed on the deceased should remain on the deceased to assist the investigating authority in determining the nature and cause of wounds and marks on the body. Organ and tissue donation are not prohibited by a medicolegal investigation, but local policies and practices will dictate which children are able to donate under specific circumstances of death.

KEY POINTS

- Childhood deaths in the ED commonly necessitate a medicolegal death investigation.
- Family presence during resuscitative efforts is beneficial for both the grieving family and the team of health care providers, but care should be taken upon death to preserve potential forensic information.
- Emergency medicine practitioners should be aware of local policies and procedures on the forensic documentation and preservation of evidence when a medicolegal death investigation will occur.

Suggested Readings

Bechtel K. Sudden unexpected infant death: differentiating natural from abusive causes in the emergency department. *Pediatr Emerg Care*. 2012;28(10):1085-1089.
O'Malley P, Barata I, Snow S, et al. Death of a child in the emergency department. *Ann Emerg Med*. 2014;64(1):e1-e17.

Epinephrine 1:10 000 vs 1:1000: Are You Prepared to Make Sense of This?

Samuel J. Spizman, MD, FAAP

Epinephrine is a critical medical intervention for cardiac arrest and multiple dysrhythmias that cause or can lead to cardiac arrest. It is also the primary treatment for anaphylaxis and hypotensive shock. In what seems like an intentionally confusing practice, it is prepared in two different concentrations—1:10 000 (0.01%) and 1:1000 (0.1%). Yet we base dosing on milligrams given per weight in kilograms. Clear as mud? Not really since considering the wrong dosing or the wrong route can be potentially harmful. Yet we must be sure to use the right dose and route for the indication!

First, it is important to understand what these numbers mean. Any listed ratio of a drug equates to the g/mL in that solution. Here is how the two concentrations compare:

1:10 000 = 1 g/10 000 mL or 1000 mg/10 000 mL. Cancelling out as many zeros as you can on both sides leaves you with **1 mg/10 mL**, 0.1 mg/1 mL, or 0.01 mg/0.1 mL.
The **1:1000** concentration is 10 times as concentrated, so the final ratio is **1 mg/1 mL**. Since this concentration is 1:1, it translates easily into 0.1 mg/0.1 mL, or 0.01 mg/0.01 mL.

Both drugs typically come in ampule form, with the 1:1000 in a 1 mL ampule and the 1:10 000 in a 10 mL ampule; in any event, each will have a total of 1 mg of epinephrine in the ampule.

The interventional dose of epinephrine for most conditions is 0.01 mg/kg for pediatric patients (or for low weight-for-age nonpediatric patients). While physicians often think in milligrams, nursing staff administering medications typically think and use milliliters of medication, so it is important to understand and be able to safely communicate appropriately. For this dosing regimen, you can now substitute the mg/kg dose with a mL/kg dose based on the concentration you are using:

For 1:10 000, this equates to 0.1 mL/kg/dose.
For 1:1000, this equates to 0.01 mL/kg/dose.

The 1:1000 concentration will therefore result in a very small volume, which is important when giving IM, such as for anaphylaxis.

When should the 1:10 000 concentration be used? Only when a very small volume could be problematic. Using a 20-kg child as an example, the volume per dose would be 2 mL for the 1:10 000 and 0.2 mL for the 1:1000 form. A volume of 0.2 mL barely makes it out of the hub when infused. For this reason, some sources recommend using the 1:10 000 form when giving epinephrine IV or IO. An alternative is to flush the line completely when using the 1:1000 concentration IV/IO to ensure complete administration.

Finally, some authors recommend a 10 times dose when giving epinephrine via endotracheal tube (ETT) due to decreased absorption and thus requiring higher doses. This would equal 20 mL of the 1:10 000 concentration and 2 mL of the 1:1000. So, when giving epinephrine via ETT (at a 10 times dose), use the more concentrated **1:1000** form.

Having just 1 concentration of epinephrine (1:1000) may prevent confusion between the two formulations. Yet this may require a dilution at the bedside creating a different chance for error. Fortunately, there may be sanity on the horizon with a movement to relabel this medication just like all other medications, as mg/mL. We can only hope.

KEY POINTS

- **The dose of epinephrine for arrest, dysrhythmia, shock, and anaphylaxis is 0.01 mg/kg/dose** (note: the mL/kg/dose changes with different concentrations).
- **The 1:1000 concentration can be used for all common emergent bolus dosing.**
- **Always use 1:1000 concentration (0.01 mL/kg/dose) for IM and 10 times ETT doses.**
- **If using 1:10 000 concentration for IV and IO doses, give 0.1 mL/kg/dose.**

Suggested Reading

Pediatric Advanced Support Provider Manual. American Heart Association; 2016.

IMAGING

Do Not Scan Head Trauma Based on Your "Gut"—Use Evidence-Based Guidelines!

Anna Schlechter, MD, FAAP

Pediatric emergency department visits for head trauma are a common occurrence, with ~60 000 such encounters annually. Computed tomography (CT) is the reference standard for emergently diagnosing traumatic brain injuries, but clinicians must be careful to use it when appropriate and not reflexively image all patients.

Despite the frequent occurrence of head injuries, clinically important traumatic brain injury (CiTBI) is a rare event. Furthermore, CT imaging of the head is associated with an increased lifetime risk of lethal malignancy. The estimated lifetime risk of lethal malignancy from a single head CT for a 1-year-old patient is 1 in 1000-1500 with risk decreasing to 1 in 5000 for a 10-year-old patient. Therefore, the risk of malignancy due to CT may prove higher than the risk of CiTBI in low-risk patients.

Among the various CT decision aids, the Pediatric Emergency Care Applied Research Network (PECARN)—Head Injury Prediction Rule has consistently been shown to have both extremely high sensitivity and relatively high specificity across several studies, and clinicians should consider using the tool to help guide imaging decisions.

For children younger than 2 years with a GCS of 15 without a severe mechanism of injury, who are acting normally per parental report, with no signs of altered mental status, no palpable skull fracture, no occipital, parietal, or temporal scalp hematoma, and no loss of consciousness of 5 seconds or more is recommended that no CT be obtained (<0.02% risk of CiTBI).

For children older than 2 years with a GCS of 15, and no other signs of altered mental status or basilar skull fracture, no history of loss of consciousness, no vomiting, no severe mechanism of injury, and no severe headache, it is also recommended that no CT be obtained (<0.05% risk of CiTBI).

In both patient groups, a severe mechanism is defined as a motor vehicle collision with patient ejection, death of another passenger, or rollover; pedestrian or bicyclist without helmet struck by a motorized vehicle; a fall of >3 ft (for those under 2 years) or 5 ft (for those over 2 years); or head struck by a high impact object.

In both age groups, patients who have a normal GCS and no signs of altered mental status, as well as no palpable skull fracture/signs of basilar skull fracture, it is recommended that the physician consider observation as opposed to an immediate CT. This consideration should be based on whether there are worsening symptoms and signs, parental preference, physician experience, multiple isolated findings or age <3 months. The younger age group is important to consider, as these are often difficult patients to examine and the risk of nonaccidental trauma may be higher. In addition, if the clinicians suspect nonaccidental trauma, these guidelines do not apply as they rely on a truthful and accurate historian.

By following these guidelines, it is estimated more than 50% of patients presenting to the emergency department with head trauma can be definitively spared a CT of the head. It is also important to note that isolated findings such as isolated loss of consciousness, isolated headache, and isolated vomiting also have a lower than 1% risk of CiTBI. Such patients should not automatically have head imaging performed, but rather risks and benefits should be weighed by the clinician with family involvement in the decision process.

KEY POINTS

- CT of the head without contrast is the reference standard for emergently diagnosing brain injuries in children.
- CT of the head is associated with an increased risk of lethal malignancy over the life of the patient.
- The PECARN Head Injury Prediction Rule in children with GCS scores >14 can be used to safely rule out the presence of CiTBI.
- In a low-risk patient, the risk of CT-induced malignancies is higher than the risk of CiTBI.

Suggested Readings

Babl FE, Borland ML, Phillips N, et al. Accuracy of PECARN, CATCH and CHALICE head injury decision rules in children: a prospective cohort study. *Lancet*. 2017;389(11087):2393-2402.

Easter JS, Bakes K, Dhaliwal J. Comparison of PECARN, CATCH and CHALICE rules for children with minor head injury: a prospective cohort study. *Ann Emerg Med*. 2014;64(2):145-152.

Kuppermann N, Holmes J, Dayan P, et al. Identification of children at very low risk of clinically-important brain injuries after head trauma: a prospective cohort study. *Lancet*. 2009;9696:1160-1170.

Mastrangelo M, Midulla F. Minor head trauma in the pediatric emergency department: decision making nodes. *Curr Pediatr Rev*. 2017;13(2):92-99.

Negative Scan—Positive Belly: Do Not Rely Solely on the CT Scan When Evaluating Children With Blunt Force Abdominal Trauma

Anna Schlechter, MD

Blunt abdominal trauma is the most common unrecognized fatal injury in pediatric trauma patients. Children have less intra-abdominal fat, the abdominal muscles are poorly developed, and abdominal organs are relatively larger compared to adult patients, which makes the risk of significant abdominal injury higher than in adults. The most common mechanism of blunt abdominal injury is motor vehicle collision. Bicycle injuries, falls, sports injuries, nonaccidental trauma, and pedestrians struck by motor vehicles are also frequent mechanisms of pediatric blunt abdominal trauma. Clinicians must be vigilant when identifying pediatric patients with abdominal injuries to provide appropriate care in the ED and not rely entirely on radiologic studies to exclude significant injury.

Primary and secondary surveys and appropriate history-taking should be the initial step in evaluation of the child with blunt abdominal trauma. A severe mechanism of injury, abdominal distention, abdominal tenderness, abdominal ecchymosis or abrasions, tachycardia, and low systolic blood pressures have all been shown to be significant risk factors for possible intra-abdominal injury. Frequently, gauging the presence of abdominal pain in a frightened and crying child is difficult. A child who has swallowed a significant amount of air from crying might also be perceived as having a distended stomach. As in adults, patients with altered mental status or a distracting injury may have unreliable abdominal examination findings.

Computed tomography (CT) scan of the abdomen and pelvis with intravenous contrast is the gold standard in imaging for abdominal injuries after blunt trauma in the hemodynamically stable pediatric patient. CT is sensitive and specific in detecting solid organ injuries and is relatively sensitive in detecting hollow-viscous injuries. However, CT should be performed judiciously, as it is estimated that the risk of a fatal cancer from radiation is 1 per 1000 pediatric CT scans in young children and 0.18% lifetime risk for abdominal CT in a 1-year-old child.

A patient who does not have any concerning findings on history or physical examination may be evaluated with bedside ultrasound FAST examination and/or laboratory tests such as complete blood count (CBC), liver function tests (LFTs), and urinalysis to further provide evidence that no abdominal injury is present. Serial abdominal examinations can also be employed in the stable patient with no concerning findings, with imaging or exploratory surgery performed should they develop. It is important to note that in contrast to adult patients, FAST in the hemodynamically stable pediatric trauma patient has not been shown to be sensitive in the detection of clinically significant injury.

While CT can be helpful in deciding which patients with blunt abdominal trauma have intra-abdominal trauma, it should not be considered to definitively exclude injury. In a meta-analysis of 2596 pediatric patients with blunt abdominal trauma, the overall rate of intra-abdominal injury after a negative abdominal CT scan was still 0.19% (95% CI 0.08-0.44). Another study of pediatric patients who received CT scans early in their clinical course showed the false negative rate of CT to be ~3.6% in blunt abdominal trauma patients with a seatbelt sign. Ultimately, the decision to proceed with operative management or admission should still be based on history, physical examination, and the hemodynamic status of the patient. Finally, an unstable patient should never have operative intervention delayed so that a CT scan may be obtained. Such patients should proceed immediately to the operating room for definitive management.

KEY POINTS

- CT of the abdomen and pelvis with contrast is the gold standard for diagnosing abdominal injury in the pediatric blunt abdominal trauma patient.
- CT of the abdomen and pelvis exposes a child to potentially harmful radiation and should only be performed if deemed necessary based on history and examination.
- A negative CT does not definitively rule out abdominal injury in a patient with worsening abdominal pain, evolving peritonitis, or unstable vital signs after blunt abdominal trauma.
- The unstable trauma patient should not have operative management delayed so that a CT can be obtained.

Suggested Readings

Chatoorgoon K, Brown RL, Garcia VF, et al. Role of computed tomography and clinical findings in pediatric blunt intestinal injury. *Pediatr Emerg Care*. 2012;28(12):1338-1342.

Hom J. The risk of intra-abdominal injuries in pediatric patients with stable blunt abdominal trauma and negative abdominal computed tomography. *Acad Emerg Med*. 2010;17(5):469-475.

Kopelman TR, Jamshidi R, Piere PG. Computed tomographic imaging in the pediatric patient with a seatbelt sign: still not good enough. *J Pediatr Surg*. 2018;53(2):357-361.

Schacherer N, Miller J, Petronis K. Pediatric blunt abdominal trauma in the emergency department: evidence-based management techniques. *Pediatr Emerg Med Pract*. 2014;11:1-24.

Appreciate Practice Differences in the Approach to Pediatric Nontraumatic Abdominal Pain

Paul Schunk, MD, FAAEM

Pediatric abdominal pain is a common presenting complaint to the emergency department (ED) and accounts for ~6% of all ED visits. CT utilization for nontraumatic pediatric abdominal pain (NTPAP) has become common in the ED, with rapidly increasing rates of use without a concurrent increase in relevant diagnosis or improvements in mortality. With ongoing and increasing concern about the potential dangers of radiation exposure in the pediatric population in addition to concerns about cost and ED length of stay, a prudent and conservative approach is recommended in many patients. Separate chapters evaluate non-CT modalities, and this chapter will highlight that clinicians must understand the clear indications and different modalities within CT use in NTPAP. Recognition of appropriate CT use will help to obtain the necessary diagnosis with causing delay or prolonged wait times in the ED.

Contrast Utility

Oral and rectal contrast is very rarely indicated in the evaluation of acute NTPAP in the pediatric patient. Oral contrast has been shown to increase the length of stay of patients without increasing the diagnostic yield of the study, including in cases of acute appendicitis. Oral contrast may be useful in postsurgical patients presenting with fever and concern for abdominal abscess or a leak from surgical anastomosis. Administration of rectal contrast should only be considered with specific consultation from specialists and is rarely indicated in the ED evaluation. Not only is it rarely needed, but this also adds a potentially uncomfortable and traumatizing experience to the pediatric patient. This is contrast to historical patterns, and ED clinicians should advocate for protocols to minimize unnecessary use of contrast in their facilities.

IV contrast is useful in the evaluation of masses, tumors, and infection and as a result is commonly administered in the Pediatric Emergency Department. A serum creatinine to evaluate renal function is often obtained during the evaluation of acute NTPAP, but it is not needed prior to CT with IV contrast in children unless the patient is a known renal transplant patient or has preexisting renal failure. This varies from typical practice in adult patients and can help to shorten the time until a study is performed and interpreted.

A prevalent false contraindication to the administration of iodinated IV contrast is a patient with a reported shellfish allergy. This myth has continued to be propagated even though there is no true data supporting it. The allergic component in shellfish is the protein tropomyosin and not the iodine. Iodine is an essential element that is needed for thyroid function, and true allergy would be rare. Contrast allergies are also not true IgE-mediated allergic reactions but rather are an anaphylactoid reaction. The contrast material acts directly to release histamine and other inflammatory components directly from mast cells. Premedication or pretreatment protocols for patients with contrast allergies should only be utilized in cases with previous diagnosed wheezing, bronchospasm, stridor, laryngeal edema, or anaphylaxis.

Conclusions

Most causes of NTPAP are better evaluated using imaging modalities other than CT. In patients with an acute abdomen CT can be utilized after other imaging modalities have failed to yield a diagnosis. In the well-appearing child with a benign abdominal examination, CT will rarely yield the diagnosis of the pain and potentially exposes the patient to unnecessary radiation. Evaluation of abdominal masses and suspected tumors is commonly evaluated by CT and is best done with the administration of IV contrast, which should not be delayed awaiting kidney function, or withheld due to a reported "iodine" or shellfish allergy.

KEY POINTS

- Most nontraumatic pediatric abdominal pain does not require CT as the initial imaging modality in the emergency department.
- Oral and rectal contrast is almost never indicated for CT scans of NTPAP.
- Shellfish allergy is not a contraindication to contrast administration.

Suggested Readings

Farrell CR, Bezinque AD, Tucker JM, et al. Acute appendicitis in childhood: oral contrast does not improve CT diagnosis. *Emerg Radiol.* 2018;25:257-263.

Shaw KN, Bachur RG. *Fleisher & Ludwig's Textbook of Pediatric Emergency Medicine.* Philadelphia, PA: Wolters Kluwer; 2016. Chapter 48.

Neuroimaging of Nontrauma Patients

Lekha Shah, MD, FAAP, FACEP

Parents commonly bring their children to the emergency department (ED) to be evaluated for headaches and first-time seizures and are anxious that these symptoms stem from serious pathology such as brain tumors. Despite a wealth of literature suggesting that cross-sectional imaging is not needed in most cases, rates of neuroimaging tripled from 1998 to 2008 (11.1% in 1998 to 31% in 2008) without finding a significant increase in clinically meaningful intracranial pathology. The disconnect between parental anxiety and clinician behavior with the rates of actual disease exposes children to unnecessary radiation and sedation risks and results in significant costs.

Who to Image

The decision who to image remains complex. Although clinical decision aids to identify worrisome risk factors such as the SSNOOPPPPY mnemonic have been proposed, they have not been prospectively validated and likely result in extraneous imaging (see Table 8.1). Clinical history and neurologic examination remain the best predictors of abnormal structural CNS pathology. Reasonable indications for imaging include consideration of predisposing risk factors (eg, first-time seizure in patients with neuro-cutaneous syndromes such as neurofibromatosis or tuberous sclerosis), worrisome headache history (progressively worsening headache, morning emesis, sudden-onset severe headache, altered mental status), and most importantly an abnormal neurologic examination. Abnormal neurologic examination encompasses the traditional neurologic exam elements (speech, alertness, motor, sensory, cerebellar, etc.) and the eye examination (papilledema and nystagmus). Neuroimaging is abnormal in <1% of patients with normal mental status and normal neurologic/eye examination, and this low rate of CNS pathology can be used to reassure worried parents in the context of thoughtful discussion.

Over-Testing

Clinician misperception also plays a role in over-testing. Since posterior fossa masses account for most childhood intracranial neoplasms, occipital headaches often prompt worried doctors to order MRI/CTs. However, recurrent occipital pattern headaches commonly result from primary headache

Table 8.1 ■ SSNOOPPPPY Mnemonic for Indications for Neuroimaging in Patients with Atraumatic Headache		
	Worrisome Risk Factors	Clinical Examples
S	Systemic symptoms	Fever, weight loss
S	Systemic disease	HIV, cancer
N	Neurologic signs/symptoms	Confusion, altered mental status, neurologic deficits, papilledema
O	Onset: sudden	Thunderclap headache
O	Occipital location	Occipital pain location
P	Pattern	Precipitated by Valsalva maneuver
P	Pattern	Positional
P	Pattern	Progressive
P	Parents	Lack of family history of migraine
Y	Years	Age <6 y

disorders (eg, migraines, tension, cluster headaches). Occipital headaches resulting from brain neoplasms almost always are associated with abnormal neurologic/eye findings. Of special note, Chiari I malformations have a typical pattern (transient headache worse with cough or Valsalva) that can be imaged on a nonemergent basis since they seldom result in herniation.

First-Time Seizures

Unprovoked (afebrile) first seizure in healthy children understandably triggers fear in parents who are anxious that their child may have epilepsy or a CNS tumor. Adults with first-time seizure, who often have concerning comorbid illness, frequently warrant emergent neuroimaging. However, neurologically intact children without risk factors have <1%-8% CNS pathology on imaging. Even fewer (<1%) children require urgent neurosurgical intervention. Of special note, benign rolandic epilepsy (BRE) is a fairly common pediatric seizure subtype in school-age children that uniquely occurs during sleep and awakening; most children outgrow this type of seizure and do not require neuroimaging. Most healthy patients with first-time seizure can be safely referred to an outpatient neurology clinic for outpatient evaluation.

Radiation

CT remains the most readily available neuroimaging for most ED physicians, but the radiation dose varies widely depending on the scanning protocol. Although the radiation dose of head CT using a pediatric protocol can be low (7 Grays), rates of malignancy linearly increase with accumulated radiation dose. Even when neuroimaging is warranted, outpatient MR is often preferred to CT in children who have returned to their baseline mental status.

KEY POINTS

- Neuroimaging is rarely needed in healthy children with a nonfocal neurologic examination and normal eye examination.
- If imaging is warranted, consider MRI in patients who have returned to their baseline mental status.
- Patiently reassure parents that brain tumor is exceedingly unlikely (<1%) if headaches or seizure are the sole presenting symptom.
- Recurrent occipital headaches are usually due to migraines. Imaging is not necessary.

Suggested Readings

Bear JJ, Gelfand AA, Goadsby PJ, et al. Occipital headaches and neuroimaging in children. *Neurology*. 2017;89:469-474.

Dayan PS, Lillis K, Bennett J, et al. Prevalence of and risk factors for intracranial anomalies in unprovoked seizures. *Pediatrics*. 2015;136:e351-e359.

Irwin SL, Gelfand AA. Occipital headaches and neuroimaging in children. *Curr Pain Headache Rep*. 2018;22:59.

Trofimova A, Vey B, Mullins ME, et al. Imaging of children with non-traumatic headaches. *AJR Am J Roentgenol*. 2018;210:8-17.

To CT or Not to CT: Develop Good Imaging Strategy

Stephanie G. Cohen, MD

Chest imaging is an essential tool for evaluating children with cough, chest pain, or dyspnea. These symptoms are nonspecific, and etiologies can range from community-acquired pneumonia to less common causes of airway foreign body and pulmonary embolism. Like any medical test, the imaging study is chosen based on weighing the pretest probability of finding evidence of treatable disease, potential danger of missed diagnosis with the financial and physical cost to the patient. Due to the risk of radiation-induced malignancy from medical imaging, the ALARA (as low as reasonably achievable) principle is recommended to reduce radiation exposure in children. The radiation exposure estimation of a chest CT is ~200 times that of a chest x-ray, so judicious use of imaging studies is obviously an important issue in caring for children with respiratory symptoms.

Imaging for Pneumonia

Initial imaging in children with cough and fever usually begins with *chest radiography* (CXR). CXR is usually sufficient for the evaluation of community-acquired or uncomplicated pneumonia. When an extensive consolidation or large pleural effusion is present, a "white out" may appear in the affected lung. Decubitus films can demonstrate layering of fluid but may fail to reveal a small pleural collection. CXR cannot reliably distinguish between pleural fluid and extensive consolidation, and further imaging with ultrasound or CT is sometimes indicated.

Chest ultrasound (US) is commonly performed to evaluate an infiltrate detected on CXR. US can detect even small effusions and can distinguish between pleural fluid and underlying lung consolidation. In addition to characterizing the nature of the pleural fluid, US can guide percutaneous drainage. *Chest computed tomography (CT)* has increased accuracy in assessing complications of infection such as necrosis, cavitation, abscess formation, and pleural complications; however, routine use is not generally recommended as it may not affect initial management. CT is most helpful in complicated or refractory cases that have poor clinical response, especially if surgical intervention is planned. CT imaging is also beneficial in patients with recurrent infections, atypical infections in the setting of immune compromise, or underlying congenital lung malformations.

Optimal technique for imaging complicated pneumonia in children is controversial. British Thoracic Society (BTS) guidelines recommend US to confirm the presence of pleural fluid and guide thoracentesis. CT guidance should be reserved for refractory cases or where US provides inadequate visualization.

Imaging for Pulmonary Embolism

Presenting signs and symptoms for pulmonary embolism (PE) are variable and may include chest pain, dyspnea, tachycardia, syncope, hypotension, or cardiac arrest. The evaluation for PE includes risk stratification to determine pretest probability and identify patients who require further imaging.

CT pulmonary angiography (CTPA) has high sensitivity and specificity and is the imaging study of choice for evaluation of PE. CT may also provide an alternative diagnosis when a PE is not present.

CTPA use has increased markedly in recent years. Despite more frequent testing, the overall incidence of the disease has not changed, which suggests a high degree of unnecessary testing. The role for multiorgan US (thoracic, cardiac, and leg vein) as a screening test in the evaluation of PE is under investigation. Used as stand-alone tests, these modalities have low sensitivity and cannot safely rule out PE. In combination, these applications have been shown to be more sensitive than single-organ ultrasonography. Multiorgan US may soon help select which patients require CTPA thereby reducing radiation exposure.

KEY POINTS

- CXR is recommended for evaluation of uncomplicated pneumonia.
- Chest US is recommended for detecting pleural effusion and guiding drainage.
- CT is not indicated for routine evaluation of pneumonia but plays a role in cases that do not respond to therapy.
- CTPA is the imaging study of choice for evaluation of PE.
- Multiorgan ultrasonography has potential as a screening test to select which patients need CTPA—Stay tuned.

Suggested Readings

Calder A, Owens CM. Imaging of parapneumonic pleural effusions and empyema in children. *Pediatr Radiol.* 2009;39:527-537.

Coley BD. Chest sonography in children: current indications, techniques, and imaging findings. *Radiol Clin North Am.* 2011;49:825-846.

Koenig S, Chandra S, Alaverdian A, et al. Ultrasound assessment of pulmonary embolism in patients receiving CT pulmonary angiography. *Chest.* 2014;145(4):818-823.

Kurian J, Levin TL, Han BK, et al. Comparison of ultrasound and CT in the evaluation of pneumonia complicated by parapneumonic effusion in children. *AJR Am J Roentgenol.* 2009;193:1648-1654.

Nazerian P, Vanni S, Volpicelli G, et al. Accuracy of point-of-care multiorgan ultrasonography for the diagnosis of pulmonary embolism. *Chest.* 2014;145(5):950-957.

Know the Options: Imaging Modalities for Pediatric Neck Masses

Naghma S. Khan, MD, FAAP, FACEP and Kina Le Goodman, MD, FAAP

Neck masses are a common presenting complaint in children, and diagnostic imaging is often necessary to narrow down the differential and distinguish between masses that require conservative therapy as opposed to elective or emergent surgical intervention. A stepwise approach that utilizes the least harmful imaging modality to help make a diagnosis and tailor intervention should be undertaken.

Soft Tissue Neck Radiographs

Soft tissue neck films are indicated when a deep neck infection is suspected or there are signs of airway obstruction. A true lateral view with the neck in extension with the image taken during inspiration is important to avoid false-positive results. In addition to the presence of a foreign body, a key finding is widening of the prevertebral space. At the level of C2-C3, the prevertebral space should be <1/3 to 1/2 the width of the adjacent vertebral body. At the level of C4-C7, the width should be equal to or less than the width of the vertebral body. Plain films are quick, cheap, easily available; have low radiation; and serve as a valuable screening tool.

Ultrasound of the Neck

For palpable neck masses, an ultrasound is the safest and least invasive choice and often provides valuable information. Sonographic penetration and resolution are better in children compared to adults because of the smaller neck size and less subcutaneous fat. Ultrasound images provide information about the location, shape, size, and vascularity of the neck mass and—most important—whether the mass is salivary tissue, a solitary mass/lymph node, or multiple nodes. Ultrasound helps distinguish lymphadenitis from suppurative lymph nodes or an abscess that needs incision and drainage. Combined with the physical examination, an ultrasound aids in deciding between outpatient vs inpatient antibiotic therapy, incision and drainage or the need for surgical intervention or biopsy. Serial ultrasounds may be required to follow progression or resolution of the neck mass. Point-of-care ultrasound by pediatric emergency physicians when compared to radiologists shows significant agreement ($\kappa = 0.71$; 95% confidence interval, 0.6-0.83) between the findings. If the mass is too large, too deep, or too irregular, cross-sectional imaging with a computerized tomography (CT) or magnetic resonance imaging (MRI) is indicated. While an ultrasound can differentiate between a solid tumor and benign neck masses, ultimately a CT or MRI is required to guide staging and management.

Computerized Tomography of Neck Masses

While a CT is the modality of choice for assessing neck masses in adults, it should be used judiciously in children due to the increased lifetime risk of cancer. However, when plain films or ultrasound do not provide sufficient information, a CT scan is indicated to guide diagnosis and management. A CT scan is also indicated when airway compromise or osseous involvement is suspected.

Magnetic Resonance Imaging of Neck Masses

An MRI with contrast is as effective as a CT scan, but it is more costly, less readily available, and may necessitate sedation in young children. Procedural sedation is contraindicated if there is a concern that the neck mass is compressing the airway. MRI is excellent for evaluation of a soft tissue neck mass, but CT is superior when there is a concern for bone involvement. If a vascular malformation is present in the head/neck region, an urgent MRI and MRA of the brain and neck is required to evaluate for an associated intracranial vascular anomaly like PHACE syndrome (posterior fossa, hemangioma, arterial, cardiac/aortic, and eye anomalies).

KEY POINTS

- Lateral neck films are helpful in diagnosing a retropharyngeal abscess.
- Ultrasound is the imaging of choice for most palpable neck masses.
- For congenital or neoplastic lesions, consider an MRI.
- When bony involvement is suspected, a CT is used for confirmation.

Suggested Readings

Bansal AG, et al. US of pediatric superficial masses of the head and neck. *Radiographics*. 2018;38(4):1239-1263.
Brown RE, Harave S. Diagnostic imaging of benign and malignant neck masses in children—a pictorial review. *Quant Imaging Med Surg*. 2016;6(5):591.
Friedman N, et al. Reliability of neck mass point-of-care ultrasound by pediatric emergency physicians. *J Ultrasound Med*. 2019;38(11):2893-2900.
Friedman ER, John SD. Imaging of pediatric neck masses. *Radiol Clin*. 2011;49(4):617-632.
Stern JS, et al. Imaging of pediatric head and neck masses. *Otolaryngol Clin North Am*. 2015;48(1):225-246.

11

Advanced Imaging—MRI in Children

Matthew Moake, MD, PhD

Increasing concerns about radiation exposure in children and increased availability of MRI imaging create new options for considering advanced imaging in pediatric patients. Clinicians must consider when MRI could be the most appropriate modality to provide a diagnosis.

MRI provides high-resolution cross-sectional imaging for evaluation of an ever-expanding list of disease processes. Outside of bony/calcified structures and acute bleeding such as in trauma where timeliness is of the essence and CT remains superior, MRI can now be used for almost all evaluations formerly reserved for CT. Limitations to the expanded use of MRI include availability and prolonged scan time, the latter of which has implications with pediatric patients.

Anatomic proportions, fat and water content of tissues, radiation sensitivity, and disease processes change as a child develops. These technical differences often necessitate size-specific coils and smaller slice thickness resulting in longer scan times compared to equivalent adult studies. Prolonged scan times are a major limiting factor for pediatric MRI, primarily due to behavioral intolerance limiting quality image acquisition. Solutions to this include optimizing behavioral tolerance, sedation, and focused MRI protocols that limit scan time.

In general, infants <3 months of age can tolerate standard MRI examination durations if fed immediately before and swaddled. Children <5 routinely require some level of moderate to deep sedation, which may necessitate need for an advanced airway with MRI compatible ventilators and monitors and is out of the scope of most ED practice. Children older than 10 can usually tolerate examinations with use of ear protection, child life specialists, and age-appropriate distraction techniques including toys, books, and audiovisual media. Children 6-10 are widely variable and must be individualized.

Age- and pathology-specific imaging protocols are essential to optimize sequence acquisition and minimize scan time. There is an expanding alphabet soup of MRI sequence acronyms, many of which are manufacturer-specific, that ultimately equate to faster sequences, improved image quality in the setting of motion degradation, and decreased need for IV contrast. Examples include DWI (diffusion-weighted imaging) and SSFSE (single-shot fast spin-echo) sequences for rapid assessment of major CNS territory stroke and ventricular size; SWI (susceptibility-weighted imaging) for evaluation of hemorrhage, calcification, and vascular structure; rapid single-shot sequences such as HASTE (half-Fourier acquisition single-shot turbo spin-echo) and RARE (rapid acquisition with relaxation enhancement) that can provide T2-weighted images in <1 second; and motion compensation techniques such as PROPELLER (periodically rotated overlapping parallel lines with enhanced reconstruction), which correct for in-plane rotation and translation artifacts.

Protocols incorporating these various sequences are institution specific, and discussion with the performing radiologist prior to acquisition allows protocol optimization as well as real-time interpretation to guide repeat or additional sequences as needed. Such clinically tailored protocols reduce scan time and avoid need for sedation with minimal loss of clinical information. The best example of this is "screening" or "fast" brain protocols, which can quickly (<10 minutes) evaluate for hydrocephalus, mass, hemorrhage, and infarct in a child of virtually any age without sedation, contrast, or radiation exposure. Such protocols may miss small focal lesions and are not appropriate for fine anatomic detail such as cranial nerve evaluation. More comprehensive study may subsequently be required, but this can often be done in an outpatient setting. Similarly, focused, rapid MRI protocols can be used to evaluate for appendicitis with similar performance metrics as CT while avoiding radiation and IV contrast.

KEY POINTS

- MRI is the gold standard for imaging of the CNS and soft tissue components of the musculoskeletal system but can be used for all parenchymal organs and soft tissues, with limitations being fine bony/calcified structures and the acute evaluation of trauma.
- Pediatric behavioral tolerance of MRI can be maximized with use of age-appropriate distraction techniques, child life specialists, and anxiolytic agents.
- New MRI sequences allow for faster acquisition, improved image quality in the setting of motion degradation, and decreased need for IV contrast.
- Clinically tailored imaging protocols, such as "fast-brain" studies can reduce scan time and avoid need for sedation and contrast with minimal loss of clinical information.

Suggested Readings

Courtier J, Rao AG, Anupindi SA. Advanced imaging techniques in pediatric body MRI. *Pediatr Radiol.* 2017;47: 522-533.

Darge K, Anupindi SA, Jaramillo D. MR imaging of the abdomen and pelvis in infants, children, and adolescents. *Radiology.* 2011;261(1):12-29.

Ho ML, Campeau NG, Ngo TD, et al. Pediatric brain MRI part 1: basic techniques. *Pediatr Radiol.* 2017;47: 534-543.

Riccabona M. *Pediatric Imaging Essentials: Radiography, Ultrasound, CT, and MRI in Neonates and Children.* Stuttgart, Germany: Georg Thieme Verlag KG; 2014.

Pediatric Lung POCUS: An Underutilized Tool for Pediatric Pneumonia

Erin Munns, MD

Millions of children around the world develop pneumonia every year, making it a major public health concern. The severity of the infection can range from an uncomfortable illness to a life-threatening disease. Most practitioners rely on a combination of history, clinical examination, and chest radiography to diagnose pneumonia. While widely used, chest radiography as an imaging modality has limitations. Although studies show it has a specificity of 98% in diagnosing pediatric pneumonia, it only has a sensitivity of 87%. This means that many cases of pediatric pneumonia would be missed if relying on chest radiography alone. Point-of-care ultrasound (POCUS) has been shown to be an excellent tool in the diagnosis of pediatric pneumonia and has superior diagnostic accuracy compared to chest radiography; however, lung POCUS remains an underutilized diagnostic modality.

Lung ultrasound is superior to chest radiography in diagnosis of early bacterial pneumonia and can also better visualize pneumonia in the retrocardiac space. Additionally, ultrasound spares children ionizing radiation and is often far less expensive than chest radiography. Perhaps equally if not more important, ultrasound technology can be lifesaving and readily available in resource limited settings. Moreover, it is a technique that is both easy to learn and straightforward to apply in the emergency department setting. A recent meta-analysis has shown that lung POCUS has a sensitivity of 96% and a specificity of 93% for the diagnosis of pediatric pneumonia when performed by emergency physician practitioners trained in POCUS.

Pediatric lung POCUS is performed by scanning through the lungs on the anterior, posterior, and midaxillary planes. Either a curvilinear or phased array probe can be used to ensure visualization of the bases of the lungs. The linear probe is best used to visualize the pleural lines. Pneumonia on lung ultrasound will appear as a segment of lung that has the appearance of liver tissue, commonly referred to as hepatization of the lung. This is due to an increased amount of density in the lung from fluid and inflammation. Multiple B lines signify the presence of fluid within the lung parenchyma. Visualization of three or more B lines within a lung segment may suggest a consolidation within the lung. When evaluating the pleural line, the "shred sign" (uneven pleura) can also assist in identifying the presence of pneumonia. A "spine sign" noted on imaging describes the phenomenon where the spine can be visualized above the diaphragm when scanning the thorax. Usually the spine cannot be seen above the diaphragm due to the fact that US waves do not move well through air. When there is increased fluid in the chest cavity, US waves can more easily move through the tissue, causing the spine to become apparent. In the context of pneumonia, the presence of a spine sign could reveal a pneumonia complicated by effusion.

Pneumonia is an important disease process for pediatric patients. The ability to swiftly make this diagnosis is vital for ensuring appropriate treatment of patients. The presence of hepatization of the lung, focal B lines, shred sign, and spine sign are sonographic signs that can help the sonographer diagnose pneumonia on POCUS imaging. Remember to consider the use of POCUS to diagnosis pneumonia in pediatric patients.

KEY POINTS

- Lung POCUS has a high sensitivity and specificity for diagnosing pediatric pneumonia.
- Lung POCUS can better diagnose early pneumonia and retrocardiac pneumonia.
- Proper technique should be utilized to ensure visualization of all lung fields.
- Emergency physicians are encouraged to become proficient in this ultrasound application.

Suggested Reading

Pereda M, Chavez M, Hooper-Miele C, et al. Lung ultrasound for the diagnosis of pneumonia in children: a meta-analysis. *Pediatrics*. 2015;135(4):714-722.

Do Not Apply the Adult FAST Criteria to Pediatric Trauma Patients

Anthony Arredondo, DO, FAAP

Trauma continues to be a major cause of morbidity and mortality among pediatric patients, and abdominal trauma accounts for 20%-30% of cases. Ultrasound has been identified as an imaging modality that can accurately identify as little as 100 mL of free fluid (FF) within the peritoneal cavity. As a result, the Focused Assessment with Sonography in Trauma, or the FAST examination, has become an integrated part of the ATLS (Advanced Trauma Life Support) algorithm for the care of an injured patient. Specific locations where FF can accumulate are in the subphrenic spaces, the hepatorenal recess (Morison's pouch), the splenorenal recess, the inferior aspect of the liver or spleen or kidney, and behind the bladder within the pelvis (rectovesicular pouch in males; rectouterine pouch of Douglas or posterior cul-de-sac in females). FAST has rapidly become an integral aspect of the adult trauma population, and clinicians have extrapolated this to the pediatric population; as a result, FAST has come in to widespread use.

Ultrasound allows the practitioner to safely and quickly identify FF at the bedside without exposing the patient to potentially harmful radiation. However, the majority of studies delineating the utility of ultrasound for detection of FF have focused on the adult population. The FAST examination remains of questionable utility in the pediatric population since there exists important differences between children and adults with respect to traumatic injuries. First, over one-third of pediatric solid organ injuries do not result in hemoperitoneum, and thus would result in a negative FAST examination. Second, the anatomy of a child differs from that of adults. Children have weaker abdominal muscles, the surface area of the abdomen represented by abdominal organs is larger in children, and children tend to have less adipose tissue, all of which lead to different injury patterns. Next, children tend to have physiologic FF within the peritoneum with studies citing a range of 1.5%-12% of children having physiologic fluid in the pelvis. The presence of physiologic FF in the pediatric abdomen can make the interpretation of the FAST examination challenging, as physiologic FF and pathologic FF can be indistinguishable immediately following a traumatic injury. Finally, the pelvis has been identified as the most sensitive single location for detection of FF in children, as opposed to the RUQ abdomen location in adults; clinicians who do not recognize this difference may not interpret examinations at the bedside correctly.

Since the pelvis is the most important location to interrogate in the pediatric FAST examination, ensuring that this region is scanned thoroughly is crucial. Urine within the bladder will create posterior acoustic enhancement, thereby making the ability to identify FF within the pelvis more challenging. An important rule of thumb is to decrease the gain while imaging the pelvis to ensure that fluid is not being masked by artifact.

KEY POINTS

- The pelvis is the most sensitive location for free intraperitoneal fluid among children.
- Children have an incidence of about 1.5%-12% of physiologic FF in the pelvis, with an estimated amount of 1 mL or less.
- The pediatric FAST examination is a good screening tool and a useful adjunct in the trauma setting; however, over one-third of solid organ injuries do not result in hemoperitoneum. Therefore, the absence of FF findings on FAST does not exclude an intra-abdominal injury.
- It is important to reduce the gain when scanning the pelvis, to ensure FF is not being masked by posterior acoustic enhancement.

Suggested Readings

Brenkert TE, Adams C, Vieira RL, Rempell RG. Peritoneal fluid localization on FAST examination in the pediatric trauma patient. *Am J Emerg Med.* 2017;35(10):1497-1499. http://doi.org/10.1016/j.ajem.2017.04.025

Jéquier S, Jéquier J-C, Hanquinet S. Intraperitoneal fluid in children: normal ultrasound findings depend on which scan head you use. *Pediatr Radiol.* 2003;33(2):86-91. http://doi.org/10.1007/s00247-002-0837-x

Ma OJ, Mateer JR. *Ma and Mateer's Emergency Ultrasound.* 3rd ed. New York, NY: McGraw-Hill; 2014.

Rathaus V, Grunebaum M, Konen O, et al. Minimal pelvic fluid in asymptomatic children: the value of the sonographic finding. *J Ultrasound Med.* 2003;22(1):13-17. http://www.ncbi.nlm.nih.gov/pubmed/12523605

Simanovsky N, Hiller N, Lubashevsky N, Rozovsky K. Ultrasonographic evaluation of the free intraperitoneal fluid in asymptomatic children. *Pediatr Radiol.* 2011;41(6):732-735. http://doi.org/10.1007/s00247-010-1927-9

Cardiac POCUS: Be Able to Distinguish Pericardial Effusions From Their Mimics

Daniel Slubowski, MD

Point-of-care ultrasound (POCUS) allows for rapid diagnosis of a pericardial effusion and cardiac tamponade. However, there are several other diagnoses that can be confused with pericardial effusions, which can lead to undue iatrogenic complications. Pericardial effusions appear anechoic, or dark, but can appear hyperechoic by the presence of other material such as fibrin or clots. In an asymptomatic patient, the pericardial space can accommodate ~20-50 mL of fluid. Physiologic pericardial fluid tends to be located anteriorly. Pericardial effusions, however, will be identified by the presence of >50 mL of fluid and tends to be dependent or circumferentially located. Pericardial effusions are best identified on subxiphoid and parasternal long views of the heart. Pericardial tamponade is the feared complication of a pericardial effusion and occurs when the heart is constricted by the surrounding fluid, resulting in compromised cardiac function. Cardiac tamponade can be identified sonographically by collapse of the right atrium or ventricle during diastole. Another finding consistent with cardiac tamponade is identifying an enlarged inferior vena cava (>2 cm) that collapses <50% during inspiration, signaling increased central venous pressure. Cardiac tamponade is an emergent condition that requires drainage of fluid by pericardiocentesis to restore normal cardiac function. Pericardiocentesis is a procedure that involves significant risks to the patient, thus distinguishing a pericardial effusion from other entities is one of the main indications to perform cardiac POCUS.

Pericardial Effusion vs Epicardial Fat

Epicardial fat is adipose tissue positioned between the myocardium and pericardium. Epicardial fat is a hypoechoic tissue density. This mimic is located exclusively anteriorly and will be visualized between the liver and myocardium on subxiphoid view. A key feature of epicardial fat compared to a pericardial effusion is that it normally disappears during diastole. To confirm the presence of epicardial fat, this finding is best visualized on parasternal views of the heart.

Pericardial Effusion vs Pleural Effusion

Pleural effusions are fluid collections located in the pleural space. Pericardial effusions can be difficult to distinguish from pleural effusions as these can look very similar on ultrasound. A key structure that can help distinguish pleural from pericardial effusion is the descending thoracic aorta. On parasternal long views of the heart, a pleural effusion will be noted posteriorly to the descending aorta, whereas pericardial effusions will be noted anteriorly. When visualizing a right-sided pleural effusion, the anechoic fluid collection will be noted next to the cardiac chambers and extending over the bare area of the liver in the subcostal views. Another possible finding that can confirm the presence of pleural effusions is visualization of a mobile and consolidated lung.

Pericardial Effusion vs Ascites

Ascites is another possible mimic of pericardial effusion. A collection of fluid located in the abdomen can appear anterior and to the right of the cardiac chambers on subxiphoid views of the heart. A key to distinguishing ascites from a pericardial effusion is identification of the falciform ligament in the subxiphoid view. This ligament attaches the liver to the anterior abdominal wall and denotes ascites if found deep to the liver in the echolucent space. If any doubt exists, the ultrasound examination can be extended to the abdomen and a focused assessment with sonography in trauma can be performed.

KEY POINTS

- Cardiac tamponade is a clinical diagnosis but can be aided by POCUS.
- Confirm your concerns of tamponade by looking for an enlarged, poorly collapsing vena cava and collapse of the right atrium or ventricle.
- Pericardial effusion should be confirmed by identification of pericardial fluid in several cardiac views. The descending thoracic aorta, the falciform ligament, and the lung are all structures that can assist in correctly diagnosing pericardial effusion and distinguishing pericardial effusion from its mimics.

Suggested Readings

Blaivas M, DeBehnke D, Phelan MB. Potential errors in the diagnosis of pericardial effusion on trauma ultrasound for penetrating injuries. *Acad Emerg Med.* 2000;7(11):1261-1266.

Blanco P, Volpicelli G. Common pitfalls in point-of-care ultrasound: a practical guide for emergency and critical care physicians. *Crit Ultrasound J.* 2016;8(1):15.

Cardello FP, Yoon DH, Halligan RE Jr, Richter H. The falciform ligament in the echocardiographic diagnosis of ascites. *J Am Soc Echocardiogr.* 2006;19(8):1074.e3-1074.e4.

Goodman A, Perera P, Mailhot T, Mandavia D. The role of bedside ultrasound in the diagnosis of pericardial effusion and cardiac tamponade. *J Emerg Trauma Shock.* 2012;5(1):72-75.

Scan First, Irradiate Second: The Error in Jumping to Computed Tomography

Robert Vezzetti, MD, FAAP, FACEP

Imaging can play an important role in the evaluation of the pediatric patient with a suspected nontraumatic abdominal surgical condition. The child's age and symptoms will guide diagnostic considerations and whether imaging is indicated. While not every child requires imaging, the appropriate test can lead to or exclude a diagnosis and impact patient treatment and disposition.

There are a variety of imaging modalities available to the clinician. The principle of ALARA (As Low As Reasonably Achievable) should always be considered when deciding to perform radiographic testing and every effort should be taken to reduce the amount of exposure to ionizing radiation. Historically, pediatric abdominal imaging was limited to plain radiography and computed tomography (CT). The former modality is useful to evaluate bowel gas patterns and the presence of free air; the latter is useful to evaluate bowel gas patterns, inflammatory or infectious processes, and abdominal/pelvic organs. Plain radiography, however, can be nonspecific and provides limited information about intra-abdominal contents. CT involves ionizing radiation exposure and necessitates intravenous (IV) placement and contrast utilization. While these modalities do have their place and are indicated in appropriate clinical settings, ultrasonography has emerged as an imaging modality that has excellent diagnostic accuracy and should be the test of choice when evaluating children for the most common pediatric surgical emergencies including appendicitis (sensitivity of greater than 90%, specificity of 40%-90%, positive predictive value of 98%, negative predictive value of 99%), intussusception (sensitivity of 98%, specificity of 98%, positive predictive value of 87%, negative predictive value of 99%), and pyloric stenosis (sensitivity of

100% and specificity of 100%). This imaging modality utilizes no ionizing radiation, is rapid, and requires no IV contrast. When malrotation is suspected, ultrasound may even be useful at evaluating bowel vessel orientation (sensitivity of 94%, specificity of 100%, positive predictive value of 100%, negative predictive value of 97%) and can be used in conjunction with other imaging modalities (such as an upper gastrointestinal series).

As with any test, there are limitations to the use of ultrasound technology that must be understood by clinicians. Ultrasonography is an operator-dependent imaging modality. To ensure the highest diagnostic accuracy, sonographers should be experienced in pediatric abdominal imaging, and the radiologist reading these studies should be comfortable with the interpretation of pediatric abdomen pathology. These may not be available in all general emergency department or urgent care settings, and in these cases, discussion with the nearest pediatric center is advised to determine if transfer is appropriate for the individual patient.

Many hospitals have institutional guidelines that include pediatric specific protocols, which can help guide the clinician in the diagnostic evaluation of the pediatric patient. As a general guideline, abdominal ultrasonography should be considered as the initial imaging modality for any child with concern for surgical abdominal condition. While IV contrast-enhanced CT remains a viable imaging option, this should be reserved for patients in whom ultrasound findings are equivocal or when there is evidence to suggest that CT might be a more appropriate test.

KEY POINTS

- Ultrasound is the preferred abdominal imaging modality for common abdominal surgical conditions in pediatric patients, including appendicitis, intussusception, and pyloric stenosis.
- Ultrasound is an operator-dependent imaging modality and thus diagnostic accuracy is highly dependent on the skill of the sonographers and radiologists interpreting the studies.
- Computed tomography should be reserved for patients in whom ultrasound is equivocal, ultrasound findings require further diagnostic study, or a complication is suspected.
- Always practice ALARA principles when choosing an imaging modality.

Suggested Readings

Kessler N, Cyteval C, Gallix B, et al. Appendicitis: evaluation of sensitivity, specificity, and predictive values of US, Doppler US, and laboratory findings. *Radiology*. 2004;23: 472-478.

Leeson K, Leeson B. Pediatric ultrasound: applications in the emergency department. *Emerg Med Clin North Am*. 2013;31:809-829.

Newman B, Callahan MJ. ALARA (as low as reasonably achievable) CT 2011—executive summary. *Pediatr Radiol*. 2011;41(suppl 2):453-455.

Sanchez TR, Corwin MT, Davoodian A, et al. Sonography of abdominal pain in children: appendicitis and its common mimics. *J Ultrasound Med*. 2016;35:627-635.

Swenson DW, Ayala RS, Sams C, et al. Practical imaging strategies for appendicitis in children. *AJR Am J Roentgenol*. 2018;211:909-911.

16

Skin and Soft Tissue Infections: Fifty Shades of Grayscale

Jason Gillon, MD, FAAP

Skin and soft tissue infections (SSTIs) are common in the pediatric population, and as a result, it is important to be able to distinguish cellulitis from abscesses because management may be quite different. Several studies have demonstrated poor-to-fair reliability of clinical examination alone to make this distinction. Point-of-care ultrasound (POCUS) is a well-validated imaging modality for the diagnosis of SSTIs and has been shown to change management in over 20% of SSTI cases. POCUS can help spare patients from unnecessary drainage procedures and identify patients who would benefit from drainage. Recent literature suggests that patients who have an abscess drained with POCUS guidance fail treatment at a significantly lower rate than those who have an abscess drained without the use of POCUS. POCUS for SSTI diagnosis requires minimal training, but there are certain pitfalls that need to be avoided.

SSTIs are best visualized with high-frequency linear probes (generally 5-20 MHz) as these provide excellent resolution at low depth. Ample use of ultrasound gel helps to both decrease the amount of pressure required to obtain quality images of these painful infections and also prevent signal dropout due to poor probe contact for convex abscesses. Clinicians can consider analgesia or anxiolytics as needed to facilitate the examination.

The most important question to answer regarding SSTIs is whether there is a drainable fluid collection. Cellulitis has an appearance that is classically described as cobblestoning, which represents fluid separation of fat lobules in the subcutaneous tissue. Abscesses, on the other hand, typically appear as anechoic or hypoechoic discrete and mostly ovoid structures.

While abscesses are typically anechoic to hypoechoic, they can be isoechoic and blend in with the surrounding tissue. In these cases, there are two important findings that can help make this diagnosis. The first is posterior acoustic enhancement, which is an increase in signal intensity seen at the inferior wall of the abscess since the fluid-filled abscess cavity transmits sound waves more effectively than the surrounding subcutaneous tissue. The second is called a "squish sign" or "swirl sign," which describes the movement of debris within the abscess cavity when the suspected abscess is compressed with the probe.

A final ultrasound tool that can be helpful to determine if a structure is an abscess is color Doppler. There is no vasculature within an abscess cavity and therefore it should not demonstrate flow with color Doppler. On the contrary, the walls of an abscess have increased blood flow as expected with inflammation and should demonstrate increased color signal compared to surrounding normal subcutaneous tissue. Color Doppler within a suspected abscess cavity should trigger consideration of alternative diagnoses such as lymph nodes or lymphatic malformations, vascular lesions, or tumors.

KEY POINTS

- In cases where clinical examination is equivocal, POCUS can effectively determine the presence of an abscess.
- Not all abscesses are anechoic or hypoechoic. It is important to use additional clues like posterior acoustic enhancement, squish/swirl sign, or color mode to make the diagnosis.

Suggested Readings

Gaspari RJ, Sanseverino A, Gleeson T. Abscess incision and drainage with or without ultrasonography: a randomized controlled trial. *Ann Emerg Med*. 2019;73(1):1-7.

Marin JR, Abo AM, Arroyo AC, et al. Pediatric emergency medicine point-of-care ultrasound: summary of the evidence. *Crit Ultrasound J*. 2016;8(1):16.

Sivitz AB, Lam SH, Ramirez-Schrempp D, et al. Effect of bedside ultrasound on management of pediatric soft-tissue infection. *J Emerg Med*. 2010;39(5):637-643.

Subramaniam S, Bober J, Chao J, et al. Point-of-care ultrasound for diagnosis of abscess in skin and soft tissue infections. *Acad Emerg Med*. 2016;23(11):1298-1306.

17

Errors to Avoid: Overlooking Potential for Lung Injury in Children Who Appear Well

Chad D. McCalla, MD and Ryan J. Reichert, MD

"You don't drown by falling in; you drown by staying there." While this is true, there has been increasing confusion over the past several years as to the mechanisms, classifications, and management of drownings. Here, we will put several of those misconceptions to rest and clarify management of asymptomatic patients involved in a drowning.

Drowning is defined as the process of experiencing respiratory impairment from submersion/immersion in a liquid medium. Previously used terms are outdated, and the terms fatal and nonfatal drowning event are now recommended.

The adage "an ounce of prevention is worth a pound of cure" holds true for drowning, and it has been estimated that 80% of drownings are preventable. When these prevention measures fail and a drowning occurs, the most important predictor of outcome is what happens at the scene. Studies have demonstrated that as little as 1-3 mL/kg of aspirated liquid can lead to surfactant washout leading to significant respiratory compromise. However, up to 93% of drowning victims who arrive at the emergency department with a pulse survive with a good outcome. This speaks to the importance of a rapid assessment of the patient's airway, breathing, and circulations (ABCs). Once ABCs have been assessed and initial stabilization has occurred, a good history and physical examination should be undertaken. Important historical points are duration of submersion (submersion times >10 minutes having poorer outcomes), water temperature (cold water drownings may have better outcomes than warm water), and what the patient was like when pulled from the water, that is, apneic, unresponsive, pulseless, etc.

If a child presents after an event and is symptomatic (ie, presenting with cough, wheezing, tachypnea, or respiratory distress), they should be stabilized and admitted for further management/observation. The larger challenge is what to do with an asymptomatic child or a child with mild symptoms. More recent literature suggests that not all these children necessarily need to be admitted and can potentially be discharged home after a 4- to 6-hour observation period. However, if they develop symptoms or have worsening of symptoms, then admission would be warranted. Recently, there have been many media stories concerning dry or secondary drowning in which a child was asymptomatic for numerous days after a mild submersion event but then decompensated and ultimately died. However, this phenomenon has largely been debunked in the drowning literature as these deaths have later been attributed to other causes and not to the drowning event. Therefore, a child that is asymptomatic or has resolved symptoms at the 6-hour mark can be safely discharged home with close outpatient follow-up.

Chest x-rays (CXRs) are often obtained; however, care should be taken in interpreting these as up to 60% of asymptomatic children may have an abnormal CXR, and 20% of symptomatic children may have normal films, suggesting that these are not a reliable indicator of clinical course. Many suggest only ordering these if the child's clinical status is deteriorating, or they are still symptomatic after 4-6 hours.

Laboratory workup is usually not indicated as most are normal and are of no clinical benefit. The amount of water needed to cause electrolyte disturbances is significant (up to 20 mL/kg) and far exceeds the amount of water actually aspirated.

Cervical spine injuries are rare in this population and cervical mobilization is often times overused, leading to increasing difficulties in airway management. For these reasons, the American Heart Association does not recommend use unless there are obvious signs of trauma, a high-risk mechanism (diving injury, boating accident, or significant fall), or a Glasgow Coma Score of <9. Because of this, routine cervical spine imaging is also not indicated.

Admission would be indicated for moderate/severe symptoms, or if during the observation period the child develops symptoms, or has persistent or worsening symptoms. Symptomatic patients may require oxygen supplementation with or without albuterol, aggressive fluid resuscitation, and even addition of pressors.

KEY POINTS

- Drowning classifications are dated and inaccurate.
- Prevention is key; education and safety measures to protect accidental entry and personal floatation devices are essential to protect children.
- Management is supportive and asymptomatic patients can be safely discharged after a 4- to 6-hour observation period without further imaging or laboratory testing.

Suggested Readings

Meyer RJ, et al. Childhood drowning. *Pediatr Rev.* 2006;27:163-169.

Schmidt AC, Sempsrott JR, Hawkins SC, Arastu AS, Cushing TA, Auerbach PS. Wilderness medical society practice guidelines for the prevention and treatment of drowning. *Wilderness Environ Med.* 2016;27(2):236-251. doi:10.1016/j.wem.2015.12.019.

Szpilman D, Sempsrott J, Webber J, et al. "Dry drowning" and other myths. *Cleve Clin J Med.* 2018;85(7):529-535. doi:10.3949/ccjm.85a.17070.

Tintinalli JE, Stapczynski J, Ma O, Yealy DM, Meckler GD, Cline DM, eds. *Tintinalli's Emergency Medicine: A Comprehensive Study Guide.* 8th ed. New York, NY: McGraw-Hill; 2016.

Not Aggressively Treating the Hypothermic Drowning Victim

Emily Rose, MD, FAAP, FAAEM, FACEP and Mark Zhang, MD

Drowning is the second leading cause of accidental death in children worldwide. While many children survive drowning events without subsequent sequelae, others can be neurologically devastated. The challenge is to successfully and adequately resuscitate potential survivors while ensuring an optimal neurological outcome.

Management

Resuscitation of the acutely drowned patient is primarily respiratory and supportive care. Surfactant washout from aspiration results in bronchospasm, pulmonary edema, shunting, and persistent hypoxia. Hypoxic insult may result in multiorgan system failure. Oxygen should be administered if hypoxia is present. Acute bronchospasm from pulmonary irritation may also require bronchodilators. While positive pressure ventilation assists ventilatory effort and oxygenation and may be helpful, intubation is indicated if unresponsive, apneic, or critically ill. Ventilator settings should follow lung protective strategies with tidal volumes of 5-6 mL/kg.

Active warming, intravenous fluid resuscitation, and vasopressors should be administered as indicated. Mild hypothermia (32°C-35°C) may be passively rewarmed with warm fluids/oxygen and passive external warming (removing wet clothing, blankets). Moderate hypothermia (28°C-32°C) will require both active external (heating blankets, forced air) and minimally invasive rewarming techniques (bladder lavage). Severely hypothermic patients (<28°C) require invasive warming techniques (peritoneal or thoracic lavage) and/or extracorporeal membrane oxygenation (ECMO). ECMO should be considered with circulatory compromise (systolic blood pressure [SBP] < 90 mm Hg or ventricular arrhythmias), core temperatures of < 28°C, and no obvious coexisting conditions (such as trauma). There is no benefit to prophylactic antibiotics or steroids after drowning events.

Potential underlying conditions or traumatic injury should be considered including nonaccidental causes or a spinal cord injury. Underlying cardiac arrhythmias (particularly prolonged QT syndrome), a seizure disorder, or other medical emergency may have triggered the drowning event.

Labs and imaging are not routinely indicated. However, both assist critical care in a child requiring resuscitation. Chest x-ray findings do not directly correlate with clinical severity. It requires ~11 mL/kg of aspirated material to impact volume status and double that amount to impact electrolytes; most drowning victims aspirate ~3-4 mL/kg of liquid (or may have laryngospasm and not aspirate any liquid). Hypoxic injury can cause insult to any organ, and sequelae includes multiorgan system failure and elevated intracranial pressure. These complications require supportive management.

Hypothermia

Hypothermia is neuroprotective *only* when the hypothermia occurs prior to the onset of ischemia. In most drowning incidents, a hypothermic patient simply correlates with a prolonged immersion time. Notably, there are many case reports of patients with severe hypothermia (core temperature as low as 13.7°C) who have survived with excellent neurologic outcome. Early mobilization of resources and initiation of ECMO in a hypothermic drowning patient is critical to optimal outcomes in the appropriate patient. Resuscitation of a hypothermic patient should continue until the patient is rewarmed to ~32°C and absence of cardiac motion confirmed by bedside ultrasound.

Length of Resuscitation

There is no single risk factor that reliably predicts outcome. The age and underlying health of the patient, circumstances of drowning, submersion time, water temperature, and time to initiation of cardiopulmonary resuscitation (CPR) all contribute to the ultimate outcome. There are multiple case reports of excellent outcomes despite prolonged submersion times. These cases all had significant hypothermia and utilized ECMO. Except for the hypothermic patient, prolonged resuscitation after drowning events typically results in a neurologically devastated survivor. In general, resuscitations for >30 minutes in warm water submersions, >60 minutes in ice-water submersions, or requiring three doses of epinephrine are unlikely to result in a good neurological outcome. Aggressively resuscitate the hypothermic patient as they are potentially salvageable with a good outcome if resuscitated well with the assistance of ECMO, particularly if early CPR was administered and hypoxia occurred prior to the onset of ischemic injury.

KEY POINTS

- Pulmonary resuscitation includes bronchodilation and positive pressure ventilation.
- Hypothermia is neuroprotective if it occurs prior to cerebral ischemia.
- ECMO should be considered early in the resuscitation of the severely hypothermic patient.

Suggested Readings

Brown DJ, Brugger H, Boyd J, et al. Accidental hypothermia. *N Engl J Med*. 2012;367:1930-1938.

Burke CR, Chan T, Brogan TV, et al. Extracorporeal life support for victims of drowning. *Resuscitation*. 2016;104:19-23.

Champigneulle B, Bellenfant-Zegdi F, Lebard C, et al. Extracorporeal life support (ECLS) for refractory cardiac arrest after drowning: an 11-year experience. *Resuscitation*. 2015;88:126-131.

Jenks CL, Raman L, Dalton HJ, et al. Pediatric extracorporeal membrane oxygenation. *Crit Care Clin*. 2017;33:825-841.

Main AB, Hooper AJ. Drowning and immersion injury. *Anaesth Inten Care Med*. 2017;8:401-403.

Drowning Prevention—Missing the Opportunity to Teach: Prevention When the Near-Miss Events Happen

Nicole Barbera, DO and Frederick Place, MD, FACEP, FAAP

In the United States, drowning is the number one cause of death among children 1-4 years of age and the third leading cause of death until age 19. The nomenclature has been updated so that the terms "drowning" and "near drowning" are synonymous with the only difference being the ultimate outcome. For every drowning fatality, four drowning victims will be cared for in the emergency department (ED). Survivors of a drowning event of any severity are at risk of being drowning victims in the future, and education in the ED can prevent this eventuality.

Drowning

Drowning is defined as submersion or immersion in a liquid that causes respiratory impairment; this includes both fatal events and nonfatal events (ie, near misses). A submersion event without respiratory symptoms is considered a water rescue. Drowning is a sequence of events, starting with water entering the mouth or airway, an initial struggle followed by brief laryngospasm and frequent swallowing, progressing to violent struggle, convulsive and spasmodic inspirations, continued pulmonary aspiration, and hypoxia leading loss of consciousness and ultimately death. In those who survive to reach the ED, water aspiration results in alveolar surfactant dysfunction and leads to pulmonary edema, decreased gas exchange, and central nervous system hypoxia. There is no such thing as "dry" or "delayed" drowning; children destined to become symptomatic will do so within 4-8 hours. While drowning victims may violently struggle, a key educational point for parents is that many drowning events in children are silent! Unlike the movies, drowning can occur without a single sound.

Prevention

The role of education in the ED creates a potential opportunity to prevent the next drowning event. The resources provided here can guide parental education.

The motto of the National Drowning Prevention Alliance (NDPA) is "drowning is preventable." The NDPA provides updated statistics, community events, and educational resources easily accessible online and emphasize these five points: (1) any amount of water, including in buckets and toilets, is a risk; (2) there is no alternative to direct adult supervision; (3) children who have had swimming lessons should not be thought of as "drownproof"; (4) toys and other enticing objects need to be removed from pools to reduce the attraction of kids toward the water; and (5) having a phone at poolside can be an essential lifeline. Safe Kids offers similar online information with checklists for different water exposure environments to ensure safety with information available in both English and Spanish. Similarly, the Consumer Product Safety Commission (CPSC) offers many detailed safety reports and how to help families install proper pool fencing and plan ahead to protect their children from drowning. All environments with water exposure create the potential for drowning events. The sights and sounds of drowning may not be what you expect. Not planning ahead is planning too late.

KEY SAFETY POINTS

- Most drownings occur in unsupervised pools, with a lack of fencing, mostly at home, with one or two parents who are out of sight for <5 minutes.
- Four-sided barrier fending with a latch-gate may be the single most effective preventative measure.
- Swim lessons are important; two-thirds of drowning victims cannot swim.
- The presence of lifeguards dramatically reduces the number of water rescues requiring medical attention.
- Having a responsible, sober adult who is dedicated to watching children at residential pools is also imperative.
- The beach is an especially dangerous location; children may swim or wade out beyond safe rescue distances, and rip tides may pose deadly risks to child and would-be rescuer alike.

KEY TEACHING POINTS

Do not stay silent! Take the opportunity to educate families of patients who present as a near miss. Reliable drowning prevention resources are easily accessible online.

- Never let a child swim alone, and never take your eyes of them.
- Life jackets and life preservers should be kept at the poolside and should be used for all open water and boating activities.
- Always keep a phone poolside, but do not let it be a distraction!
- A missing child could be a drowning child. Always look in the pool first.

Suggested Readings

CDC. National Center for Health Statistics. https://www.cdc.gov/injury/images/lc-charts/leading_causes_of_death_by_age_group_2017_1100w850h.jpg

National Drowning Prevention Alliance (NDPA). http://ndpa.org/

Newth CJL, Hammer J, Numa AH. 41: Drowning. *Kendig's Disorders of the Respiratory Tract in Children*, January 2019:634–638.e2. doi:10.1016/B978-0-323-44887-1.00041-9.

Safe Kids Worldwide. Water Safety At Home. https://www.safekids.org/watersafety?gclid=CjwKCAjwvuzkBRAh EiwA9E3FUu2qufcItVBvmT3FWDlIcYy-GjFbiFdB6lAaKvabJ5RIFlds_Sr53RoCulMQAvD_BwE

United States Consumer Product Safety Commission. https://www.cpsc.gov/safety-education/neighborhood-safety-network/toolkits/drowning-preventionaap.org/drowning

When Small Bites Matter: The Deadly Potential of a Pill

Ryan D. Brown, MD, FAAP and Mary Asal, MD, MPH, FAAP

Pediatric poisonings have a significant place in emergency medicine. The 2017 Annual Report of the American Association of Poison Control Centers reported 2 115 186 human exposures that year. Nearly 60% were children (≤19 years old) and 67% of those cases were three or younger. Table 20.1 shows this population's breakdown.

Emergency providers should have ingestions high on their differential for all mobile pediatric patients with altered mental status or unexplained symptoms. Most ingestions in ≤5-year-old children are accidental: from inadvertent overdosing, inappropriate/incorrect medication use by the caregiver, or self-ingestion of medications found by exploring children. Toddlers are naturally at highest risk due to their propensity for exploration and for placing found objects in their mouths. Children may ingest anything from beads to batteries; however, pills carry higher risk due to being easily mistaken for mints or candy.

In 1993, there were ~10 known medications that could kill a child from a single adult dose. That number increased to 27 in 2004 and has now doubled to over 50 medications.

Medications (not including chemotherapeutics) carrying single-dose mortality risk

Antidepressants	Quinidine	Morphine
Amitriptyline	Oral antihyperglycemics	Oxycodone
Desipramine	Chlorpropamide	Tramadol
Imipramine	Glimepiride	Antiplatelets/NOAC
Venlafaxine	Glipizide	Clopidogrel
Antipsychotics	Glyburide	Dabigatran
Chlorpromazine	Repaglinide	Prasugrel
Clozapine	Sitagliptin	Rivaroxaban
Loxapine	Multiple sclerosis drugs	Ticagrelor
Thioridazine	Dalfampridine	Calcium channel blockers
Ziprasidone	Fingolimod	Diltiazem
Antimalarials	Antiepileptics	Nifedipine
Chloroquine	Gabapentin	Verapamil
Hydroxychloroquine	Lamotrigine	Other
Quinine	Pregabalin	Camphor
Antiarrhythmics	Opioids	Imidazoline
Disopyramide	Buprenorphine	Methyl salicylate
Flecainide	Codeine	Podophyllin
Ivabradine	Fentanyl	Sildenafil
Procainamide	Hydrocodone	Theophylline
Propafenone	Methadone	

In 2017, there were 14 ingestion-related fatalities reported in the ≤5-year-old population, including 10 attributed to pharmaceuticals including: methadone, oxycodone, morphine, methadone, trazodone, nifedipine, quetiapine, and methamphetamine.

A concise history, high level of vigilance, and quick recognition of ingestion can help prevent long-term morbidity and mortality. Providers should remember **ABCD$_3$EF** (*Airway; Breathing; Circulation; Disability, Drugs, Decontamination; Electrocardiogram, Fever*) as a guide when managing ingestions.

Table 20.1 ■ Exposures by Pediatric Age Group

Toxic Exposures in Pediatric Populations, 2017

Age (y)	Exposures (N)	Exposures (%)
<1	107 126	8.5%
1	307 882	24.3%
2	296 003	23.4%
3	136 479	10.8%
4	67 258	5.3%
5	40 375	3.2%
Child 6-12	132 451	10.5%
Teen 13-19	171 303	13.5%
Total	1 265 052	

Modified from Gummin DD, Mowry JB, Spyker DA, et al. 2017 annual report of the American Association of Poison Control Centers' National Poison Data System: 35th annual report. *Clin Toxicol (Phila)*. 2018;56:1213-1415.

The National Poison Control Center (NPCC) is well equipped for toxidrome and pill recognition, medication information, and treatment algorithms. If further guidance and consultation are needed, specialized toxicologists are available.

Though many pediatric ingestions are accidental, they may reflect neglect or intentional abuse. The child's safety should be an utmost concern to providers, and the potential for abuse should be considered in each case. If a child is found to have ingested illegal substances, law enforcement and child protection services should be contacted.

Children of all ages are at risk of ingestion. Successful outcomes depend on provider vigilance in suspecting, intervening, and protecting the most vulnerable "one pill can kill" population.

KEY POINTS

- The number of medications that can kill a toddler with one dose is growing.
- Providers should always consider ingestion in their differential and intervene quickly.
- Maintain a low threshold to contact the Poison Control Center at **1-800-222-1222**.
- Be aware of signs of neglect and abuse with ingestions and report accordingly.

Suggested Readings

Bar-Oz B, Levichek Z, Koren G. Medications that can be fatal for a toddler with one tablet or teaspoonful: a 2004 update. *Paediatr Drugs*. 2004;6(2):123-126.

Calello D, Henretig F. Pediatric toxicology: specialized approach to the poisoned child. *Emerg Med Clin North Am*. 2014;32:29-52.

Gummin DD, Mowry JB, Spyker DA, et al. 2017 annual report of the American Association of Poison Control Centers' National Poison Data System: 35th annual report. *Clin Toxicol (Phila)*. 2018;56:1213-1415.

Koren G, Nachmani A. Drugs that can kill a toddler with one tablet or teaspoonful: a 2018 updated list. *Clin Drug Investig*. 2019;39:217-220.

Matteucci MJ. One pill can kill: assessing the potential for fatal poisonings in children. *Pediatr Ann*. 2005;34:12.

Activated Charcoal: Avoiding Worthless Usage of a Valuable Therapy

Jessica Kraynik Graham, MD and George Sam Wang, MD, FAAP, FAACT

Activated charcoal (AC) is a porous carbon product with a large surface area that is used for gastrointestinal (GI) decontamination in toxic ingestions. AC binds toxins on contact in the GI tract, which decreases absorption and mitigates systemic toxicity. The American Academy of Clinical Toxicology (AACT) does not recommend routine use of AC for poisoned patients. Rather, clinicians should use AC selectively on a case-to-case basis.

Indications

AC can be administered as single-dose activated charcoal (SDAC) or multiple-dose activated charcoal (MDAC), in which two or more doses are repeated over a period of time.

SDAC

SDAC should be considered for ingestions likely to cause severe toxicity or decompensation. Maximum benefits of SDAC are seen when given soon (<1 hour) after ingestion. Late administration can be considered for large ingestions, ingestions of modified release drugs, and ingestions of drug packets.
    Standard SDAC dosing is:

- 10-25 g or 0.5-1.0 g/kg for children up to 1 year old
- 25-50 g or 0.5-1.0 g/kg for children 1-12 years old
- 25-100 g for adolescents and adults

MDAC

MDAC should be considered for ingestions of drugs with delayed dissolution or prolonged release, or drugs that may recirculate into the GI tract (eg, enteroenteric, enterohepatic, and enterogastric). The AACT recommends MDAC for life-threatening ingestions of carbamazepine, dapsone, phenobarbital, quinine, or methylxanthines. MDAC is also frequently used in salicylate ingestions due to delayed dissolution and risk for serious toxicity. It may also be beneficial for ingestions of amitriptyline, dextropropoxyphene, digitoxin, digoxin, disopyramide, nadolol, phenylbutazone, phenytoin, piroxicam, and sotalol. MDAC varies in dose and frequency. Most commonly, it is first given as the standard SDAC dose, followed by 0.5 g/kg every 4-6 hours for up to 12-24 hours. If MDAC causes vomiting or is being given to a child <5 years old, smaller, more frequent dosing may be helpful.

Administration

AC is generally administered orally or via nasogastric tube (if intubated). AC has a strong sulfur smell and dark color, yet children will drink it if flavored; mixed with juice, soda, or chocolate milk; and given in a covered cup. Witty names such as "batman juice" may also encourage consumption. Antiemetics can be given beforehand for nausea/vomiting. Sorbitol-containing AC products increase risk of vomiting and electrolyte abnormalities and are contraindicated in children.

Contraindications

To decrease risk of aspiration, AC is contraindicated in patients with seizures or altered mental status and should never be forcibly administered. Caution is advised in nauseated or vomiting patients. Nasogastric tube administration is only recommended in intubated patients, as passage of an NG tube in awake patients may elicit emesis. AC is also contraindicated in GI obstruction, hydrocarbons, caustics (acids, alkalis), and in patients at risk for GI hemorrhage or perforation. AC does not bind metals (iron and lithium), salts (sodium, magnesium, potassium), or alcohols.

Adverse Effects

Adverse effects are rare when AC is used appropriately. Nausea and vomiting are most common and occur in 6%-26% of patients. Other reported side effects include abdominal fullness, headache, and diarrhea. Aspiration is uncommon but more likely in patients with altered sensorium, seizing, or vomiting. Serious aspiration events have occurred when AC was inadvertently administered directly into a patient's lungs (inappropriately placed NG tube, etc.). MDAC has been rarely linked to bowel obstruction.

KEY POINTS

- SDAC should be used selectively and is only indicated in recent ingestions in which a patient is likely to have severe toxic effects.
- MDAC is rarely recommended in children but can be considered for modified release medications and medications with GI reabsorption.
- SDAC is contraindicated in seizures, vomiting, and altered mental status and should not be given by NG unless a patient is intubated.
- To encourage young children to drink it, AC can be mixed with a flavored beverage or referred to with a creative name.

Suggested Readings

American Academy of Clinical Toxicology; European Association of Poisons Centres and Clinical Toxicologists. Position statement and practice guidelines on the use of multi-dose activated charcoal in the treatment of acute poisoning. *J Toxicol Clin Toxicol.* 1999;37(6):731-751. doi:10.1081/CLT-100102451.

American Academy of Clinical Toxicology; European Association of Poisons Centres and Clinical Toxicologists. Position paper: single-dose activated charcoal. *Clin Toxicol.* 2005;43(2):61-87. doi:10.1081/CLT-51867.

Juurlink DN. Activated charcoal for acute overdose: a reappraisal. *Br J Clin Pharmacol.* 2015;81:482-487. doi:10.1111/bcp.12793.

Lapus R. Activated charcoal for pediatric poisonings: the universal antidote? *Curr Opin Pediatr.* 2007;19:216-222.

Underestimating the Damage a Simple Laundry Detergent Pod Can Cause

David Muncy, DO and Craig T. Carter, DO

Laundry detergent pods are NOT candy!! While they look like fun afternoon snacks, they have been documented to cause pulmonary, central nervous system, ocular, integumentary, gastrointestinal (GI), and oropharyngeal injuries. These household toxic exposures, though, are not specific to only laundry pods. There are numerous other household chemicals that cause similar injuries. We use laundry detergent as an example. Laundry pods were developed to reduce environmental waste by increasing detergent concentration and reducing packaging. They have unsuspectingly become a pediatric chemical exposure risk with increasing exposures over the past 10 years. With the increased incidence of exposure—both accidental and intentional (think online "challenges" in the teen population)—to new formulations and packaging of household chemicals, it is important to recognize these common injuries and their treatments.

Like most of toxicology, treatment of laundry detergent pod and other household chemical exposures is symptomatic. Ingestions can cause a myriad of symptoms such as vomiting, respiratory distress, and neurologic depression. CNS depression for some ingestions can be profound. For severe exposures, if intubation is required, the assistance of video laryngoscopy/fiberoptics might be helpful to avoid exacerbating any mucosal membrane damage already present by an ingested product. Ingestions of hand sanitizer (isopropyl alcohol) can demonstrate significant CNS depression. Again, after patient stabilization, supportive care is the treatment. Regarding laundry pods, it is not clear as to what specific ingredient causes the GI injury as manufacturing companies are not particularly forthcoming with the chemical recipe of the pods. The pH of most laundry pods are around 8, which is not high enough to cause significant injury by itself. Via gas chromatography, it is believed that the surfactant components and solvents are what cause the GI and neurologic adverse effects. There are numerous case reports of significant CNS depression with laundry pod ingestion—so do not disregard CNS complaints by families even though the child may be well appearing. Other household products that can cause significant issues with ingestion include ethylene glycol (antifreeze), methanol (de-icing solutions/windshield washer fluid), mouthwashes (ethanol), and button batteries (alkali burns). For questions on button battery ingestion, the National Battery Ingestion Hotline may be able to offer additional answers. Depending on the location of the ingested/aspirated button battery, emergent removal may be needed.

Ocular exposure is another issue with household products. For laundry pods, it is the second largest cause of emergency department (ED) presentation and a frequent complaint, particularly in the 2- to 5-year age group. This is likely due to their increased mobility, exploration, and interpretation of these colorful small packets as toys or candy. For these patients, an alkali injury should be suspected and ocular pH measured. This should be investigated early as the pH can vary from neutral (7) up to 11. Copious irrigation to a neutral pH is the key with thorough eye examination. Consultation with ophthalmology and close follow-up are important.

For patients with skin/contact exposures, initial management in a stable patient consists of decontamination/removal from the offending agent. Removal of contaminated clothes may be all that is needed, but additional dilution of the contaminant may also be warranted. For pulmonary symptoms, respiratory support with oxygen or bronchodilators may help. Toxicologists and poison control centers are great resources as well.

Finally, use these ED experiences to educate the patients and families on home safety, emphasizing safe storage or optimal placement—out of the child's reach—of these household products. Prevent this from happening again. For adolescents who intentionally ingest these products, educate them on poor decision-making (eg, "Laundry Pod Challenge") but also assess whether this was an attempt of self-harm needing further evaluation. So, for fresh, "clean" breath, remember that toothpaste is a much better choice over laundry pods!

KEY POINTS

- Treat exposure to household chemical products symptomatically. Most are nontoxic, but symptoms can include respiratory distress, CNS depression, eye complaints, GI complaints, etc.
- Decontaminate if necessary. This may include dilution. Do not forget the eyes if needed.
- Laundry detergent pods are NOT candy. Do not eat them. Emphasize this to children who accidentally ingest or are exposed to them.
- Use these exposures as educational opportunities with patients and families and emphasize prevention and safety.

Suggested Readings

O'Donnell KA. Pediatric toxicology: household product ingestions. *Pediatr Ann*. 2017;46(12):e449-e453.

Yin S, Colvin J, Behrman A. Single-use laundry detergent pack exposures in children under 6 years: a prospective study at U.S. poison control centers. *J Emerg Med*. 2018;55(3):354-365.

23

Not Having a Plan to Safely and Effectively Cool Critically Ill Patients With Heat Stroke

Shad Baab, MD and James C. O'Neill, MD, FACEP

Heat illness produces a range of physiological derangements that are secondary to an elevated core temperature. The hyperthermia found in heat illness occurs as environmental exposure and endogenous heat production overwhelm the body's compensatory mechanisms. Predisposing factors include poor physical fitness, dehydration, lack of acclimatization, and substance use.

Heat is dissipated through evaporation, radiation, convection, and conduction, but evaporation secondary to sweating is by far the most effective. In environments with ambient humidity >75%, evaporative cooling is no longer effective. Radiation, convection, and conduction all require a temperature gradient between the skin and the surroundings and as such are not effective if the environment's temperature is greater than the patient.

Heat illness is most commonly categorized into heat exhaustion and heat stroke, although some classifications include heat injury as a third category between mild heat exhaustion and severe heat stroke. Clinically, heat exhaustion is characterized by core temperatures between 101 and 104, tachycardia, ataxia/syncope/collapse, weakness, cramping, headache, and dizziness. Generally, central nervous system dysfunction is not found in heat exhaustion, but mild, brief confusion may be present. Heat stroke characteristically includes a core temperature >104 and collapse with persistent CNS dysfunction (confusion, emotional lability, obtundation, coma, or seizures). Other end-organ damage is almost always also present. Morbidity and mortality are directly related to the length of time that the patient has an elevated temperature.

Heat illness—especially heat stroke—is a true medical emergency. There are multiple strategies for cooling therapy depending on the resources available. While some strategies are more effective than others, using the first available to begin treatment as soon as possible should be the initial goal of treatment.

As with any medical emergency, airway, breathing, and circulation must be addressed first. If heat illness is strongly suspected, then cooling therapy should begin immediately on arrival. If staffing/resources are limited, then cooling therapy should be prioritized over IV access and obtaining labs and should occur just after initial assessment assures there is adequate airway, breathing, and circulation.

The most effective cooling treatment is ice water immersion. Typically, ice water immersion can decrease core temperature 0.2°C per minute (0.4°F per minute). At this rate, most patients can be cooled adequately in 15-20 minutes. In patients who are unstable, particularly intubated or seizing patients, immersion therapy may not be feasible. Ice water immersion therapy is also limited by availability even in the hospital setting. If immersion is not practical or available, there are other less effective options:

Secondary options:

1) Ice packs to the neck, groin, and axilla.
2) Spraying tepid or room temperature water on the patient while continuously fanning the patient.
3) Covering the patient with cold, wet cloths and changing them out regularly (likely every 1-2 minutes).
4) Chilled IV fluid infusions.
5) Pharmacological (sedation and/or neuromuscular blockade) intervention to stop shivering. These can often be used in conjunction with each other and together can achieve cooling rates that approach that of cold water immersion.

Cooling efforts should be continued until the temperature reaches 100.4 and then the temperature should be closely monitored to assure that it does not begin to rise again.

After initial stabilization and cooling therapy, laboratory evaluation and treatment for common complications of heat illness should continue. Dehydration, rhabdomyolysis, disseminated intravascular coagulation, hyponatremic dehydration, cardiogenic shock, acute kidney injury, liver failure, and cerebral edema are all known to complicate heat illness. They can occur intercurrently or over the next 24 hours. As such, admission for all but the most minor cases of heat illness is recommended.

KEY POINTS

- Time is of the essence—morbidity and mortality are directly related to the duration of hyperpyrexia.
- Plan ahead—the most effective cooling requires equipment not commonly stocked in emergency departments (eg, immersion tank, large fans).
- Stop actively cooling once patient is 100.4, but continue to monitor for other complications.

Suggested Readings

Bouchama A, Dehbi M, Chaves-Carballo E. Cooling and hemodynamic management in heatstroke: practical recommendations. *Crit Care*. 2007;11:R54.
Bytomski JR, Squire DL. Heat illness in children. *Curr Sports Med Rep*. 2003;2:320.
Centers for Disease Control and Prevention (CDC). Heat illness among high school athletes—United States, 2005–2009. *MMWR Morb Mortal Wkly Rep*. 2010;59:1009.
McDermott BP, Casa DJ, Ganio MS, et al. Acute whole-body cooling for exercise-induced hyperthermia: a systematic review. *J Athl Train*. 2009;44:84.

Cold Illness: Be Prepared to Use All the Tricks for Aggressive Rewarming

Gena Cooper, MD, FAAP

Environmental cold exposure in children is unique and due to both physical and psychological features. Pediatric body habitus makes compensatory mechanisms problematic. Children have a higher surface area-to-volume ratio—meaning that heat loss is accelerated with minor temperature variations. This is why it is so important to keep babies warm. Neonates have very limited "insulating" subcutaneous fat, and infants have an extremely limited ability to shiver, so they struggle with heat production. Older children can use brown fat for heat production, but this also requires significant oxygenation and can result in a metabolic acidosis as well as hypoglycemia and hypocalcemia. For all these reasons, children have a unique disadvantage staying warm.

External signs of cold exposure are dependent on whether they are central vs peripheral. Central cold is called hypothermia and is defined as a core temperature <35°C and is further differentiated by core temperature readings. When able, children's symptoms start with shivering and vasoconstriction and progress to decreased cerebral blood flow, diuresis, cardiac irritability, and hypovolemia. Physical signs reflect these poorly perfused states. Cardiac irritability may be seen in these stages causing a classic Osborn wave EKG finding and may progress to ventricular fibrillation.

In severe hypothermia, children have muscle rigidity, loss of thermoregulation, decreased cardiac output, decreased cardiac conduction, and suspended cerebral activity. Children with severe hypothermia may appear dead, but there are numerous case reports of children resuscitated from hypothermic states with good neurologic outcomes—so do not give up easily.

Treatment of hypothermia follows a phased approach—dependent on the extent of hypothermia—with **passive, active external,** and **active internal** rewarming. Passive rewarming is removal from the cold environment and use of warm blankets. Active external rewarming includes forced air rewarming and radiant heat. In this setting, the torso should be warmed first. Active external rewarming is not ideal for severely hypothermic patients as it increases the risk of temperature afterdrop and subsequent cardiac dysrhythmias. Active internal rewarming may start with heated humidified oxygen and warm IV fluids but may progress to lavage of the pleura, bladder, stomach, or peritoneum with heated saline. Do not forget that extracorporeal membrane oxygenation (ECMO) may be used to raise the core temperature in severely cold children, especially those who are unresponsive. Studies have shown that nonasphyxial hypothermic cardiac arrest was associated with a higher incidence of return of spontaneous circulation (ROSC) with good neurologic outcomes.

While central cold is hypothermia, peripheral cold is most commonly called frostbite and is a description of frozen skin. Anatomic areas most frequently affected by frostbite are the digits, ears, nose, cheeks, and chin. Tissue destruction is thought to result from cell death with associated reperfusion inflammation made worse by thawing and refreezing.

Similar to thermal burns, there are degrees of frostbite. Superficial injury is described as first and second degree, ranging from normal skin to clear blisters to the possible need for tissue amputation. Deeper third-degree injury has initial cyanosis proximally with hemorrhagic blisters. These lesions will likely require tissue amputation and have functional sequelae. Fourth-degree lesions have initial cyanosis with hemorrhagic blisters and frequently result in amputation and are often associated with sepsis.

Like hypothermia, treatment of frostbite requires removing sources of cold first. Do not rewarm if there is any possibility of return to cold before definitive treatment. Do not rub or walk on frostbite as it causes friction injury to the digits. In a hospital, place the extremities in water heated to 37°C-39°C. After 15-30 minutes, digits should be thawed, and skin will be red or purple and soft to touch. Thrombolytics may be needed for severe injuries presenting within 24 hours, but this care would not be initiated in the ED. Finally, tetanus prophylaxis is recommended. Complications of cold exposure include amputation, long-term cold hypersensitivity, peripheral neuropathy, and functional limitations.

KEY POINTS

- Environmental cold affects young children profoundly and differently than adults.
- Hypothermia starts with core temperatures below 35°C. Treat with passive and active rewarming strategies.
- Cardiopulmonary bypass should be used early for unresponsive hypothermic patients.
- Treat frostbite (peripheral freezing) with a warm fluid bath in the ED. Digits are rewarmed when red or purple, and skin is soft.

Suggested Readings

Cushing TA, Harris NS. Hypothermia. In: *Auerbach's Wilderness Medicine*. 7th ed. Cambridge: Elsevier; 2014: 135–162.

Seeyave DM, Brown KM. Environmental emergencies, radiological emergencies, bites and stings. In: Bachur RG, Shaw KN, ed. *Textbook of Pediatric Emergency Medicine*. 7th ed. Philadelphia, PA: Wolters Kluwer; 2016: 1021–1025.

Rabies, It Is More Than Bats: Know Your High-Risk Cases

Adam Kochman, MD, FAAP, FACEP

Children used to fear "lions, tigers, and bears," but perhaps today's movies should instill the fear of "raccoons, bats, and skunks." Although the United States has only seen 23 reported cases of human rabies in the last decade, it remains a preventable disease responsible for thousands of deaths worldwide annually.

Rabies Virus

Rabies is a single-stranded RNA virus that replicates in the mammalian central nervous system (CNS) and is transmitted by direct contact. When the virus infects the host animal's salivary glands, it can be transmitted through a bite into the subcutaneous tissue and muscle of the susceptible host. The virus then replicates in the CNS spreading to virtually all tissues and organ systems and is almost uniformly fatal.

Clinically, rabies can present in two distinct forms: an encephalitic form (80% of cases) and a paralytic form (20% of cases). Both forms share a common prodrome for the first week characterized by nonspecific symptoms like fever, chills, malaise, vomiting, headache, and pain/paresthesia radiating from the wound site. The encephalitic form manifests as hyperthermia, hypersalivation, hydrophobia, pharyngeal spasms, and profound hyperactivity followed by paralysis, coma, and death. In paralytic rabies, an initial flaccid paralysis extending from the bite is followed by an ascending paralysis with fasciculations, loss of deep tendon reflexes, and complete quadriparesis.

Globally, the canine rabies virus variant accounts for over 98% of mortality from rabies virus. While this variant has been eliminated in the United States, raccoons, bats, and skunks remain important reservoirs. Foxes, coyotes, bobcats, and mongoose are other potential sources.

Postexposure Prophylaxis

Anyone bitten by one of the above-mentioned mammals requires immediate postexposure prophylaxis (PEP). Additionally, because certain species of bats carry a virus variant capable of replicating in the superficial dermis, PEP is recommended when contact with a bat is possible even without an identifiable wound (eg, someone sleeping in a room where a bat is found). For patients bitten by domestic animals such as dogs, cats, or ferrets where the risk is substantially lower in the United States, it is important to determine the vaccination status of the animal and whether the animal can be sequestered for observation. Animals will inevitably manifest symptoms and die within 10 days of viral infection of their salivary glands. Therefore, if the animal can be confined, PEP does not need to be immediately initiated. Any rabies symptomology should prompt euthanization of the animal and immediate initiation of PEP in the exposed patient. Rabies infection can be clinically excluded if the animal remains healthy during this 10-day period. Nonbite exposure from domestic animals as well as bites from rabbits and rodents (squirrels, mice, rats, and hamsters) rarely require PEP.

All bite wounds require local wound care (including tetanus and antibiotics as indicated) and should be irrigated thoroughly as virus may remain present at the local site. In the United States, concurrent usage of both passive and active prophylaxis is standard and should begin as soon as possible after exposure. Passive immunization is administered as 20 IU/kg of human rabies immunoglobulin (HRIG). Ideally, as much as possible of the HRIG should be administered at the site of the wound with the remainder administered IM at a separate site. Active immunization is administered as 1 mL of human rabies vaccine in immunocompetent individuals on the first day of PEP (day 0) as well as days 3, 7, and 14. In immunocompromised individuals, an additional dose of vaccine is administered on day 28. Patients having received the vaccination series previously require vaccine on days 0 and 3 only. No HRIG is indicated. In the event of uncertainty, contact your local health department.

KEY POINTS

- Rabies virus should be included in the differential diagnosis of any patient with unexplained, rapidly progressive encephalitis.
- PEP should be initiated immediately after exposure in anyone bitten by a high-risk animal, including raccoons, bats, skunks, and foxes. In domestic animals, PEP can be deferred pending observation for symptomology for 10 days.
- When in doubt with regard to prophylaxis treatment, consult your local health department or the CDC.

Suggested Readings

American Academy of Pediatrics. *Committee on Infectious Diseases*. Red Book. 31st ed; 2018:673-680.

Birhane MG, Cleaton JM, Monroe BP, et al. Rabies surveillance in the United States during 2015. *J Am Vet Med Assoc*. 2017;250:1117-1130.

Centers for Disease Control and Prevention. *Rabies*. https://www.cdc.gov/rabies/index.html. Accessed March 9, 2019.

Weber D. *Chapter 157: Rabies: Tintinalli's Emergency Medicine: A Comprehensive Study Guide*. 8th ed. New York: McGraw-Hill Education; 2016

Antivenom in Children Is Not Based on the Child's Weight

Joshua Siembieda, MD

Snake Bites

Pit vipers (Crotalinae) and coral snakes (Elapidae) are the two types of venomous snakes indigenous to the United States. The pit viper family includes rattlesnakes, copperheads, and cottonmouths. Rattlesnake bites are the most common snake bites in the United States and result in the most morbidity and mortality.

Crotalid Bites

Pit vipers have long, hollow fangs, which allow for a quick strike and envenomation of prey. About 75% of bites are envenomating bites, with the remaining 25% being "dry bites." Crotalid venom contains proteins that cause tissue damage and impair the coagulation cascade, resulting in edema and coagulopathy.

Nonspecific symptoms such as nausea and vomiting may be seen shortly after the bite. Within a few hours, there is usually pain and edema at the site of envenomation. Local wound care, analgesia, splinting, and elevation are recommended. Venom suction devices and tourniquets are not recommended.

Pediatric patients with normal labs, reassuring examination, and no signs of systemic toxicity should be observed for 8 hours. Lower extremity bites in children, however, are at risk for delayed toxicity and should be observed for at least 12 hours.

Patients with laboratory abnormalities (coagulopathy, thrombocytopenia) or progressive swelling should receive Crotalidae polyvalent immune Fab antivenom. The dose is the same for patients of all ages and sizes. Patients who are hemodynamically unstable or actively bleeding should receive 8-12 vials of antivenom. All others should receive 4-6 vials of antivenom. Reevaluate for signs of clinical and laboratory improvement at 1 hour. A repeat dose of antivenom should be given if labs are not improving or symptoms are progressing. Any patient receiving antivenom or who has a symptomatic bite should be admitted to the hospital.

Elapid Bites

Coral snakes have smaller teeth and fangs than the Crotalid family, necessitating a longer bite in order to envenomate prey. The characteristic color pattern of the snake can be remembered by the adage, "red on yellow kills a fellow; red on black, venom lack." The coral snake venom is a neurotoxin, which inhibits acetylcholine receptors, resulting in muscle weakness and paralysis. The Eastern coral snake and the Texas coral snake contain potent venom, whereas the Sonoran coral snake has not been associated with toxicity.

Initially, there may be minimal or no pain from the bite and symptoms can be nonspecific such as nausea, vomiting, and dizziness, after which neurotoxicity can be seen. The neurologic symptoms may present up to 12 hours after the bite and include bulbar weakness, descending paralysis, and respiratory failure.

Asymptomatic patients should be admitted and monitored for development of neurologic sequelae for 24 hours. North American coral snake antivenom should be given to patients with any neurologic symptoms. The dose is the same for patients of all ages and sizes. The initial dose is 3-5 vials, with severe cases requiring 10 or more vials. The current supply of North American coral snake antivenom is limited. Contact the local poison control center for assistance locating antivenom and for the most up-to-date information regarding the antivenom.

Scorpion Stings

The bark scorpion (*Centruroides sculpturatus*) is found in the Southwestern United States and is the only species capable of significant toxicity and mortality. The venom acts on sodium channels causing release of catecholamines and acetylcholine.

Symptoms range from localized pain at sting site to paresthesias, skeletal nerve and cranial nerve dysfunctions. There are often no obvious findings at the sting site; however, tachycardia, hypertension, hyperthermia, increased pulmonary secretions, and agitation are usually seen in severe envenomations. Opioid analgesics and benzodiazepines should be used to control systemic symptoms. The neurotoxic effects can progress rapidly to respiratory failure.

Centruroides antivenom is recommended for any patient with any signs of severe envenomation. For all patients, the initial dose is three vials intravenously over 10 minutes. Additional vials may be needed for persistent symptoms.

KEY POINTS

- Antivenom for severe pit viper, coral snake, and scorpion envenomations should be based on the clinical scenario, not the age or size of the patient.
- After a pit viper bite, observe all children with normal labs and reassuring examinations for at least 8 hours (at least 12 hours for lower extremity bites).
- After a coral snake bite, all asymptomatic patients should be admitted for close observation and monitoring for at least 24 hours.

Suggested Readings

Hessel M, McAninch S. Coral snake toxicity. *StatPearls*. Treasure Island, FL: StatPearls Publishing; February 2019 https://www.ncbi.nlm.nih.gov/books/NBK519031/.

Levine M. Pediatric envenomations: don't get bitten by an unclear plan of care. *Pediatr Emerg Med Pract*. 2014;11(8):6-11.

27

Otitis Externa: A Dive Into Swimmer's Ear

Peggy Gatsinos, MD, FAAP

Otitis externa (OE) is an inflammation of the external auditory canal that is most often infectious in etiology, and it is commonly known as swimmer's ear. Risk factors for development of OE include recent swimming, water exposure, or excessive cleaning or scratching of the ear canal. *Pseudomonas aeruginosa* is the most common pathogen that causes OE.

Patients will present most often with ear pain accompanied by pruritus of the ear canal. There may be discharge from the canal and less often a complaint of hearing loss. Patients will typically be afebrile as the infection is localized. On physical examination, the canal is erythematous, inflamed, and often edematous. The degree of edema can range from minimal to so severe that the canal appears almost fully occluded. Debris in the canal will be accompanied by varying amounts of discharge, causing an inability to visualize the tympanic membrane. Palpation of the tragus or pulling on the pinna often elicits pain.

Treatment is variable depending on the severity of the OE. Oral analgesics such as acetaminophen or ibuprofen can help ease discomfort. In mild cases where there is only pruritus and mild discomfort, treatment with an acetic acid 2% solution with a corticosteroid will likely be sufficient. The acetic acid solution helps return the auditory canal to an acidic pH, and the corticosteroid helps fight local inflammation. In moderate or severe cases where there is concern for bacterial infection, an acidic solution that combines antibiotics with corticosteroids (aminoglycoside/polymixin B/corticosteroid or a flouroquinolone/corticosteroid) is preferred. Removal of debris and discharge that has filled the canal with a cotton swab or mild suction prior to application of otic solutions can be helpful in allowing the topical agents to work more effectively by ensuring access to the entire ear canal. In a patient with severe OE where the edema is severe enough to prevent topical agents from getting into the canal, a wick should be placed after the ear canal is cleaned. This can be extremely painful for patients, so consider using appropriate analgesia or sedation as indicated. Patients should be advised to avoid swimming or getting water in the ear until the OE is resolved. Earplugs or a cotton ball dipped in petroleum jelly can be used to protect the affected ear during bathing.

Symptoms will usually resolve within a few days of onset of treatment. For most cases, a 7-day course of treatment is adequate for resolution of OE. If there is no improvement after initial therapy, a patient should be reevaluated to confirm that the diagnosis of OE is correct. Other considerations include fungal infections, otitis media with tympanic perforation and discharge, mastoiditis, chronic suppurative otitis media, contact dermatitis, and carcinoma of the external auditory canal.

A patient can take steps to prevent future recurrence of OE. After swimming, drying the canal with acetic acid 2% or diluted isopropyl alcohol can help prevent the canal from remaining moist for prolonged periods of time, thus decreasing the likelihood of development of OE. Additionally, patients should avoid causing trauma to the external auditory canal by either aggressively cleaning with a cotton swab or ear scratching.

42   Ear Nose Throat

KEY POINTS

- OE will typically present with ear pain, pruritus, canal edema, and discharge in the absence of fever.
- Treatment with acetic acid and a corticosteroid is adequate in mild OE. An antibiotic should be added in moderate to severe disease.
- Keeping the external auditory canals dry and avoiding local trauma are key to preventing future recurrence of OE.

Suggested Readings

Fleisher GR, Ludwig S. *Textbook of Pediatric Emergency Medicine*. 6th ed. Philadelphia, PA: Lippincott Williams &Wilkins; 2010.

Kliegman RM, Marcdante KJ, Jenson HB, et al. *Nelson Essentials of Pediatrics*. 5th ed. Philadelphia, PA: Elsevier Saunders; 2006.

Acute Otitis Media and Complications

Nehal Bhandari, MD, FAAP and Hannah Y. Lee, MD

Common Etiologies of Otitis Media

The most common bacterial pathogens known to cause acute otitis media (AOM) are *Streptococcus pneumoniae*, *Haemophilus influenzae*, and *Moraxella catarrhalis*. Respiratory viruses such as rhinovirus and respiratory syncytial virus also frequently cause AOM.

Diagnosis of Otitis Media

AOM should be suspected in children with acute onset of ear pain +/− fever. According to the American Academy of Pediatrics, AOM should be diagnosed in children who present with moderate to severe bulging of the tympanic membrane (TM) *or* new-onset otorrhea that is *not* due to acute otitis externa. Other considerations for diagnosis include children who present with mild bulging of the TM with either new-onset ear pain (<48 hours) or intense erythema of the TM. AOM should not be diagnosed unless a child has a middle ear effusion.

Of note, AOM must be differentiated from otitis media with effusion (OME). OME is a middle ear effusion without characteristic TM bulging/erythema, otorrhea, pain, or fever. Antibiotics are not recommended for OME.

Treatment of Acute Otitis Media

All children with severe AOM should be treated with antibiotics. Severe symptoms are defined as temperature ≥ 39°C in the last 48 hours, a child who appears toxic, or persistent otalgia for >48 hours. All children under 6 months with AOM should be treated with antibiotics regardless of the severity of the illness and regardless of laterality. Additionally, all children younger than 24 months with bilateral AOM should be treated with antibiotics. Observation is appropriate for children 6-23 months with unilateral AOM without severe symptoms. Observation is also appropriate for children older than 24 months with unilateral or bilateral AOM without severe symptoms. When considering observation, the clinician should have a joint discussion with the family to ensure that follow-up with a physician is possible within 48-72 hours. Lastly, if pain is present, pain medications should such as ibuprofen or acetaminophen are recommended.

Recommended first-line treatment for AOM is high-dose amoxicillin (90 mg/kg/d in 2 divided doses) for 10 days. Children who have taken amoxicillin in the last 30 days, have concurrent purulent conjunctivitis, or have failed amoxicillin should receive amoxicillin-clavulanate (90 mg/kg/d of amoxicillin in 2 divided doses). Alternative treatment for those with penicillin allergy or those that have failed amoxicillin-clavulanate is a third-generation cephalosporin such as cefdinir (14 mg/kg/d). Those who have failed the above treatments may be given ceftriaxone (50 mg/kg/d for 1-3 days). Children who continue to fail treatment should be referred to an ENT specialist. In general, use of macrolides such as azithromycin should be avoided due to increasing rates of resistance.

If the patient has AOM with otorrhea (presumed perforation of the TM) without any signs of acute otitis externa, the patient should be treated with oral amoxicillin. Children with AOM with tympanostomy tubes can be treated with topical antibiotics such as ofloxacin.

Complications of Otitis Media

The most common complication of AOM is OME. Patients with OME should followed closely by their pediatrician to monitor for signs of hearing loss or language delay. Other complications of AOM include TM perforation, mastoiditis, and chronic suppurative otitis media.

KEY POINTS

- AOM should only be diagnosed in patients with (1) the presence of a middle ear effusion and (2) characteristic signs and symptoms of middle ear infection (bulging or erythema of the TM, otorrhea without acute otitis externa, otalgia, +/− fever).
- Antibiotics should not be prescribed for OME.
- First-line treatment of AOM is high-dose amoxicillin (90 mg/kg/d in 2 divided doses for 10 days). When treating AOM, the provider should take into account age, severity of symptoms, laterality and assurance of follow-up.
- Patients should be referred to ENT with any signs of hearing loss or language delay.

Suggested Readings

Lieberthal AS, Carroll AE, Chonmaitree T, et al. The diagnosis and management of acute otitis media. *Pediatrics.* 2013;131(3):964-999.
Ren Y, Sethi RKV, Stankovic KM. Acute otitis media and associated complications in United States emergency departments. *Otol Neurotol. 2018;39(8):1005-1011.*

Don't Miss Hearing Loss—A Subtle Sign of Serious Pathology

Haig Setrakian, MD

Hearing loss is underreported by families and often goes undetected in the emergency department despite its relatively high prevalence. One in forty patients is affected by the age of 18, and special populations such as NICU graduates are at even higher risk. Unaddressed hearing loss in young children leads to significant challenges in social, intellectual, and academic development and may be the only observable sign of other serious pathology. Occasionally, acquired hearing loss can complicate preexisting disease. Though most children in the United States are screened, congenital hearing loss may be undetectable at birth and become more severe over time. Of the more than 500 genetic syndromes that affect hearing, most are not associated with obvious physical features.

Understanding the pathway for normal hearing will help identify causes of hearing loss. First, sound passes through the outer ear to the tympanic membrane (TM) to the ossicles to the cochlea. The cochlea translates vibration into an electrical signal that is conducted via the auditory nerve to the brain, which must interpret this signal in a meaningful way. Any problem getting the sound to the TM causes "conductive hearing loss" (CHL). Issues translating the sound from vibration to electrical impulse and relaying the sound to the brain result in "sensorineural hearing loss" (SNHL). Bedside techniques such as the Weber and Rinne test may narrow the differential to a conductive or a sensorineural problem. CHL and SNHL can coexist or be complicated by "central" hearing loss related to how the brain processes sound.

The most frequent cause of acquired hearing loss in children is otitis media (OM) with effusion. Patients may present after acute OM and visible signs of acute infection may have resolved. Ask about recent infection and use pneumatic otoscopy to evaluate for a persistent effusion. Cerumen impaction, otitis externa, and foreign bodies are also common causes of CHL.

Traumatic causes of hearing loss include blunt, penetrating, acoustic, and barotrauma. Temporal bone fractures or penetrating trauma to the inner ear may damage the TM, disrupting the ossicular chain, or the cochlea. Hearing loss suggests more severe injury in a child with head trauma and should prompt imaging. For suspected acoustic trauma, duration and intensity of noise exposure should be assessed. Infrequent, high-intensity sound, such as that produced by a gunshot, is often less damaging than relatively less intense but more frequent exposure to a common sound, such as loud music. Additionally, changes in atmospheric pressure as with air travel or scuba diving can cause barotrauma.

Bacterial meningitis is among the most historically significant causes of hearing loss in children. Vaccinations have contributed to a reduced incidence of bacterial meningitis and associated SNHL. Vaccination against measles, mumps, and rubella have had a similar effect on rates of both congenital and acquired hearing loss. A history of meningitis or gaps in immunization should not be overlooked. After asking about immunizations, remember to obtain a thorough medication history. Platinum-based chemotherapy, loop diuretics, aminoglycosides, and NSAIDs are amongst the drugs that can cause SNHL. Heavy metal exposure is also a known culprit and may disproportionately affect socially vulnerable populations exposed to higher rates of environmental contaminants such as lead.

If no source can be easily identified, more advanced diagnostic evaluation or referral is necessary. Hearing loss with multisystem involvement or focal neurologic deficits suggest malignant, inflammatory, or other proliferative disease and should prompt imaging. Traumatic causes of hearing loss such as temporal bone fractures are best visualized by computed tomography. Magnetic resonance imaging with contrast will visualize the brain, brainstem, and internal auditory canal. A laboratory evaluation is generally unhelpful unless directed towards a clinically suspected diagnosis such as Lyme titers or lead levels. For the remaining patients who are discharged home with unresolved symptoms, or an uncertain diagnosis, audiology and ENT referral should be provided.

KEY POINTS

- A normal newborn screening examination does not preclude congenital hearing loss.
- There is no single imaging or lab evaluation recommended for all patients with suspected hearing loss, but most should follow up with ENT and audiology.
- Patients suspected of hearing loss should have a thorough history with attention to predisposing conditions.

Suggested Readings

Gregg RB, Wiorek LS, Arvedson JC. *Pediatric audiology: a review*. Pediatr Rev. 2004;25(7):224-234.

Grindle CR. Pediatric hearing loss. *Pediatr Rev.* 2014;35(11):456-463.

Joint Committee on Infant Hearing. Year 2007 position statement: principles and guidelines for early hearing detection and intervention programs. *Pediatrics.* 2007;120(4):898-921.

Sokol JR, Martyn H. Hearing screening. *Pediatr Rev.* 2002;23(5):155-162.

Leaking the Information: Be Prepared to Manage Otorrhea

Selina Varma, MD, MPH

Otorrhea in children can be benign, such as from a retained jelly bean in an ear canal, or can be life threatening, such as from a cerebrospinal fluid (CSF) leak related to head trauma. Remember that common things are common but there are a few "don't miss" diagnoses to keep in mind.

Etiologies of Otorrhea

- **Otitis with a perforated tympanic membrane (TM)**
  This is more common in younger patients, and can present with pain, fever, tinnitus, vertigo, muffled hearing, and purulent drainage from the middle ear. It can be difficult to visualize the canal and TM due to copious purulent drainage, and this may require gentle cleaning with a cotton swab. The canal can be irritated by the drainage, but typically the canal itself is not damaged as the source is the middle ear. Potential complications include mastoiditis, intracranial extension of infection, and cholesteatoma or granuloma formation. Oral antibiotics as for otitis media are sufficient, but the addition of antibiotic with steroid drops is commonly used although not absolutely necessary.

- **Bacterial otitis externa (OE)**
  Commonly known as "swimmer's ear," OE is an inflammation of the external ear canal due to introduction of moisture with poor drainage. Gentle tugging on the pinna will often elicit significant pain. Upon visual inspection, flaky debris or granulation tissue and erythema can be visualized in the canal. Severe cases can be accompanied by preauricular adenopathy and tenderness to palpation. Treatment consists of keeping the canal clean and dry. Some patients benefit from placing an ear wick to minimize moisture and facilitate antibiotic penetration. Combination antibiotics with steroid drops are more beneficial than antibiotic drops alone. Antibiotics should include antipseudomonal coverage.

  Indications for otolaryngology referral include complications such as facial nerve paralysis or necrotizing/malignant OE, bacterial invasion of the skin, and subsequent spread to the cartilage, surrounding soft tissue, or base of the skull. Patients who are immunocompromised are more at risk for these complications. Keep a high index of suspicion for necrotizing otitis if the patient is endorsing pain with chewing, which is evidence of temporomandibular joint involvement, or facial nerve palsy.

- **Retained foreign body**
  Ear canal foreign bodies are common in toddlers and older children with autism spectrum disorder or developmental delay. Frequent objects include foods, toys, and expelled myringotomy tubes. If removal cannot be performed safely in the emergency department (ED) via otoscopy, referral to outpatient otolaryngology is warranted. The urgency of removal depends on the object, and most inorganic materials, with the exception of items such as button batteries can be deferred to outpatient removal if ED removal is challenging.

- **Trauma**
  Traumatic TM perforations present with a normal ear canal and serous or serosanguinous drainage. The most common cause is foreign object insertion, but acoustic barotrauma should be considered

as well. These can typically be discharged to follow-up with otolaryngology as an outpatient to ensure healing. In the setting of significant head trauma, hemotympanum or clear drainage is concerning for a temporal basilar skull fracture until proven otherwise.

■ **Tympanostomy tubes**
Otorrhea in the setting of recent tympanostomy tube placement is expected and can be managed with supportive care. Purulent, painful discharge with fevers is consistent with otitis in the setting of tympanostomy tubes. Treatment includes topical antibiotics with or without oral antibiotics, depending on the disease severity.

If symptoms do not improve within the first 48-72 hours of treatment, consider the following:

■ Fungal disease in purulent otitis media or externa unresponsive to standard antibacterial therapies.
■ Contact dermatitis in the setting of new cosmetics or otic cleaning solutions.
■ Immunodeficiencies may present with recurrent otitis, particularly if associated with other systemic illnesses.
■ Vasculitis, specifically granulomatosis with polyangiitis, may present with otorrhea; look for renal or pulmonary involvement as well.
■ Cholesteatoma can be a complication of scarring from recurrent infections. It is typically visualized in the inner ear behind an intact TM or can arise from the TM itself.

KEY POINTS

■ Most cases of otitis media with TM perforation can be managed with an oral antimicrobial alone.
■ Cranial nerve involvement in any child with otorrhea should prompt urgent otolaryngology consultation.
■ Have a high index of suspicion for complications of OE in patients who endorse pain with chewing or facial nerve paralysis.
■ Otorrhea in the setting of head trauma is indicative of a temporal basilar skull fracture until proven otherwise.
■ Otorrhea refractory to treatment should warrant suspicion for other possible diagnoses.

Suggested Readings

Beers SL, Abramo TJ. Otitis externa review. *Pediatr Emerg Care.* 2004;20(4):250-256.
Schmidt S. Otitis media. In: Hoffman RJ et al., eds. *Fleisher and Ludwig's 5-Minute Pediatric Emergency Medicine Consult.* Philadelphia, PA: Wolter Kluwer Health, Lippincott Williams & Wilkins; 2012;694-695.
Strother CG, Sadow K. Evaluation of otorrhea in children. In: Teach SJ, ed. *UpToDate*; 2018 https://www-upto-date-com./evaluation-of-otorrhea-ear-discharge-in-children.

Punching Up the Management of External Ear Trauma

Adrienne Smallwood, MD and Suzanne M. Schmidt, MD

The external ears of school-aged children are commonly injured due to the exposed location of the pinna. Injuries to the external ear can result in damage to the cartilage with necrosis, infection, and deformity, so recognition of these injuries and proper repair are imperative.

Auricular Laceration

The pinna, or auricle, of the ear is particularly vulnerable to laceration. Skin lacerations without involvement of cartilage can be closed with a single layer of simple interrupted 6.0 sutures. Significant cartilage lacerations should be repaired with absorbable sutures to avoid notching or cosmetic defect in healing. Prior to closure, copious irrigation of the wound and anesthesia with auricular block or local lidocaine without epinephrine should be performed. Exposed cartilage is at risk for infection or necrosis, so care must be taken in cleaning and closure. Indications for referral to a subspecialist include complex lacerations involving cartilage or extension into the external auditory canal, and avulsion of portions of the external ear.

Auricular Hematoma

A direct blow to the external ear may lead to bleeding between the cartilage and perichondrium, forming an auricular hematoma. The hematoma appears as an erythematous or purple tense swelling on the ear. When blood accumulates in the subperichondrial space, the cartilage is deprived of its blood supply. As a result, the cartilage may undergo necrosis, and disorganized healing, resulting in a deformed "cauliflower" ear, often seen in wrestlers or rugby players. Management involves evacuation of blood products and prevention of reaccumulation with a pressure dressing. Aspiration (only for small hematomas <48 hour old) or incision and drainage techniques may be used.

Aspiration Technique

1) Clean area with antiseptic solution.
2) Provide analgesia with local or auricular block.
3) Aspirate hematoma with an 18-gauge needle attached to a syringe. Milk the area of the hematoma to promote drainage.
4) Hold manual pressure, and then apply pressure dressing. For pressure dressing, place petroleum gauze in the external ear, molding to fill in the contours. Place 3-4 layers of cotton gauze behind the external ear and on top of the petroleum gauze on the pinna. Wrap the entire head with roll gauze to keep dressings in place.

Incision and Drainage Technique

1) Clean area with antiseptic solution.
2) Perform auricular block for anesthesia.
3) Make a small, curvilinear incision following the shape of the helix.
4) Evacuate hematoma using forceps to carefully open area and irrigate with sterile saline.
5) Consider placing mattress sutures or bolster to prevent reaccumulation of blood.
6) Apply pressure dressing as above.

Some experts recommend a 7- to -10-day course of antibiotics due to infection risk, preferably with pseudomonal coverage. Patients with an auricular hematoma require close follow-up in 24 hours to assess for reaccumulation. If reaccumulation occurs, surgical consultation and placement of a drain may be necessary.

Thermal Injuries

Burns to the external ear pose a risk for infection and necrosis of cartilage. Burn care includes topical antibiotics, frequent dressing changes, and close follow-up. Full-thickness burns may require subspecialty consultation for consideration of a skin graft. Special attention should be made to prevent pressure over the burned pinna, which can lead to necrosis.

Cold injury to the ear from frostbite should be managed with rewarming of the ear. This can be accomplished by submerging the pinna in warm saline, warm saline rinses, or warm compress application. Avoid rubbing the frostbitten area, as this can exacerbate tissue damage.

KEY POINTS

- Cartilage of the external ear has a tenuous blood supply and is at risk for necrosis, infection, and deformity after trauma.
- Consider subspecialty consultation for ear lacerations involving cartilage.
- Auricular hematomas should be completely evacuated and a pressure dressing applied, followed by close follow-up to prevent development of cauliflower ear.

Suggested Readings

Desai BK. Treatment of auricular hematoma. In: Ganti L, ed. *Atlas of Emergency Medicine Procedures*. New York, NY: Springer; 2016.

Martinez NJ, Friedman MJ. External ear procedures. In: King C, Henretig FM, eds. *Textbook of Pediatric Emergency Procedures*. 2nd ed. Philadelphia, PA: Lippincott Williams & Wilkins; 2008.

Niescierenko ML, Lee GS, et al. ENT trauma. In: Shaw KN et al., eds. *Fleisher & Ludwig's Textbook of pediatric emergency medicine*. 7th ed. Philadelphia, PA: Lippincott Williams & Wilkins; 2016:1142-1144.

Sarabahi S. Management of ear burns. *Indian J Burns*. 2012;20:11-17.

Do Not Miss Middle and Inner Ear Trauma: Not All Ear Drainage Is Infectious

Brian Wagers, MD, FAAP

"Knock-knock." "Who's there?" "Ken." "Ken who?" "Ken you hear me?" This is a joke my children love to tell at home, usually in the loudest possible voice. However, children with middle or inner ear trauma are at risk for not being able to participate naturally in such routine encounters. The anatomy and functions of the middle and inner ear are key to understanding injury patterns and pathology. Sound is transmitted from outside the ear to the tympanic membrane (TM), which then vibrates the malleus, incus, and stapes. These bones transmit sound waves to the cochlea, which converts them into electrical impulses interpreted by the brain.

Trauma to the middle and inner ear comes from many sources and manifests in varied ways that range from penetrating trauma to pressure-induced injuries. The most common type of injury is direct trauma from insertion of an object into the ear canal. Cotton-tipped swabs are most often the culprit, but the literature also reports digits, toys, keys, and many other objects as the cause of penetrating injury. Penetrating trauma can cause rupture of the TM, damage to the ossicles (fracture or disruption), injury to the cochlea or violation of all three. Penetrating trauma usually causes bloody otorrhea that obscures the TM and may require suctioning for visualization. TM rupture can also occur iatrogenically during cerumen disimpaction or removal of a foreign body. Sedation may be considered to avoid injury during such procedures. TM ruptures are usually treated with topical antimicrobials and heal within 2-3 weeks. During this time, patients should be reexamined for cholesteatoma formation, a cystlike structure containing skin cells and debris. If suspected, the patient should be referred to ENT for potential removal.

Barotrauma can also cause injury to the middle or inner ear. The eustachian tube serves to equalize pressure between the middle ear and the environment during times of pressure change. Ascent or descent during air travel or diving can cause a differential in pressure leading to trauma, particularly if eustachian tube dysfunction already exists. A direct blow to the outer ear can also transmit a large pressure wave or concussive injury to the middle and inner ear causing damage. If a large pressure differential between the middle or inner ear and the environment is not rectified, the middle ear mucosa swells, engorging and rupturing local blood vessels with subsequent leakage of blood into the middle ear cavity. Usually barotrauma will self-resolve within several weeks, but if persistent symptoms of vertigo, nausea, or hearing loss occur, an ENT should evaluate for the presence of a perilymph fistula or other serious sequelae. Cases that do not self-resolve may require insertion of pressure equalization tubes. If the cochlear membrane is disrupted, sensorineural hearing loss and vertigo are often permanent.

Prolonged exposure to sounds >85 decibels can also cause disruption of the hair cells of the cochlea resulting in permanent, sensorineural hearing loss. Injury is dose dependent in that prolonged exposure to loud noises can cause serious damage but short, extremely loud insults can also cause significant damage. For comparison, normal conversation is ~60 decibels and a lawn mower is 90 decibels. Ear protection is recommended to avoid such injury.

Fracture of the temporal bone can cause physical disruption of any of the structures of the middle or inner ear. This should be suspected when there is hemotympanum, clear or bloody otorrhea, or bruising overlying the mastoid process (Battle sign) in the setting of head trauma. Temporal bone fractures also place the patient at risk of facial nerve paralysis due to its course in the temporal bone. Always assess the function of the facial nerve if a temporal bone fracture is suspected or discovered and involve ENT in management.

Inflicted trauma or abuse should be considered in children with bruising to the outer ear or signs/symptoms of middle or inner ear trauma. Commonly, these children have bilateral injuries noted, though unilateral injury is usually left sided due to the predominance of right hand–dominant individuals in the population. Children <1 year of age commonly do injure the ear from falls as their mobility is limited (unless walking). Any infant with ear injury should be evaluated by a physician and the possibility of inflicted trauma and other injuries explored.

KEY POINTS

- Blood from the ear should be evaluated by a physician immediately.
- In head trauma, look for hemotypanum or cerebrospinal fluid otorrhea as signs of a temporal bone fracture.
- Have all patients with a perforated TM reevaluated for cholesteatoma after the TM has healed.
- All infants with middle or inner ear trauma should be evaluated for inflicted trauma.

Suggested Readings

Ameen ZS, Thiphalak C, Smith GA, et al. Pediatric cotton-tip applicator-related ear injury treated in United States emergency departments, 1990–2010. *J Pediatr*. 2017;186:124-130.

Kazahaya K, Handler S. Otolaryngologic trauma. In: Fleisher GR, Ludwig S, Henretig FM, eds. *Textbook of Pediatric Emergency Medicine*. 5th ed. Philadelphia, PA: Lippincott Williams & Wilkins; 2006:1498-1499.

Miyamoto R. Traumatic perforation of the tympanic membrane. *The Merck Manual* [Online]. https://www.merck-manuals.com/professional/ear,-nose,-and-throat-disorders/middle-ear-and-tympanic-membrane-disorders/traumatic-perforation-of-the-tympanic-membrane. .

Steele BD, Brennan PO. A prospective survey of patients with presumed accidental ear injury presenting to a paediatric accident and emergency department. *Emer Med J*. 2002;19(3):226-228.

Intranasal Foreign Bodies: Optimizing Chances of Successful Removal

Kristol Das, MD, FAAP and Priya Jain, MD, FAAP

History and Physical Examination

Children with nasal foreign bodies may present for this chief complaint, it may be incidentally noted on exam while in the emergency department (ED) for another concern, or it may be the source of another complaint such as recurrent epistaxis or purulent nasal discharge. Once a nasal foreign body has been identified, careful examination of the contralateral naris should follow.

Urgency of Removal

Nasal foreign bodies should be removed when they are identified due to the risk of aspiration. Foreign bodies that remain in the nose for an extended period of time may form a rhinolith, in which granulation tissue, calcium, and magnesium phosphate and carbonate make removal difficult. Alkali materials like batteries must be removed urgently as they can rapidly corrode and destroy nasal tissue.

Consultation

The ED provider should not attempt removal if the foreign body is impacted, if there is excessive bleeding, or if it is a large foreign body that entered the naris traumatically. Consider otolaryngology consultation after 1-2 failed attempts in the ED to minimize the risk of unintentional aspiration or additional trauma.

Removal Techniques

Choice of removal technique depends on tools available, the shape and texture of the object, and the degree of obstruction of the naris. To reduce the risk of iatrogenic complications, hands-free lighting, optimizing visualization of the object, and adequate techniques to soothe the child and limit movement are key. Consider procedural sedation if ideal body positioning cannot be achieved. Topical phenylephrine applied to the affected naris 5-10 minutes before removal attempt can control local inflammation and facilitate removal.

Mother's Kiss/Positive Pressure

The caregiver occludes the nonobstructed naris and blows into the patient's mouth. The caregiver must create an adequate seal around the patient's mouth. Success rates of this method range from 48.8% to 79%. This method may be a benign first approach as it typically produces little distress to the child. Alternatively, a male-male adapter attached to wall oxygen source, titrated to 10-15 L/min, and placed in the contralateral naris is an alternate source of positive pressure.

Forceps

Use direct visualization to retrieve the object. This technique is useful for foreign bodies with an edge or opening that can be grasped. This technique is not indicated for round foreign bodies.

Balloon Catheter

This technique applies to foreign bodies that partially obstruct the nasal cavity. An uninflated, lubricated catheter is advanced past the foreign body and subsequently inflated to 0.5-1 cc and then retracted out of the naris. A balloon catheter can also stabilize a foreign body from behind while it is removed with forceps.

Ear Curette/Right Angle
These tools are ideal for nongraspable round objects that partially obstruct the nasal canal. The instrument is passed behind the object, and the hook or loop is rotated to withdraw the object from the nose.

Suction
Place the end of the suction tubing directly onto the object. Apply suction and slowly withdraw the suction tubing.

Post Removal

It is imperative to reexamine the nasal cavity to evaluate for residual foreign bodies. In the event of mucosal trauma, consider saline, sterile water, or antibiotic ointment to the area.

Follow-up

Families should be counseled to return to care if they note foul-smelling or yellow-green discharge from the naris, which would be concerning for a nonvisualized retained foreign body. Families should also be educated on child-proofing the home to prevent repeat events. Patients with an embedded battery need otolaryngology follow-up to monitor for ongoing thermal burns and/or delayed septal perforation.

KEY POINTS

- Good visualization, lighting, and adequate techniques to soothe the child and limit movement are essential to successful removal.
- Have a variety of tools available before attempting extraction. Select the removal technique based on item shape, texture, and the degree of obstruction of the naris.
- Consider otolaryngology consultation after 1-2 failed attempts. This minimizes the risk of unintentional aspiration or additional trauma.

Suggested Readings

American Academy of Pediatrics. Foreign bodies of the ear, nose, airway, and esophagus. In: McInerny TK, Adam HM, Campbell DE, DeWitt TG, Foy JM, Kamat DM, eds. *American Academy of Pediatrics Textbook of Pediatric Care.* 2nd ed. Elk Grove Village, IL: American Academy of Pediatrics; 2017.

Kiger JR, Brenkert TE, Losek JD. Nasal foreign body removal in children. *Pediatr Emerg Care.* 2008;24(11):785-792. doi:10.1097/pec.0b013e31818c2cb9.

Loh WS, Leong J, HKK T. Hazardous foreign bodies: complications and management of button batteries in nose. *Ann Otol Rhinol Laryngol.* 2003;112(4):379-383. doi:10.1177/000348940311200415.

Blow by Blow on Nasal Trauma in Children

Anna G. Smith, MD, FAAP and Priya Jain, MD, FAAP

General Principles

Nasal trauma is a common injury in pediatric patients, and a few key principles will help distinguish the benign from the serious. While most nasal trauma may look worse than it actually is and management is straightforward, keep in mind the warning signs and how to manage serious and life-threatening complications. Nasal trauma may result from blunt or penetrating force due to play accidents, sports injuries, traffic accidents, or assault. When obtaining a history, determine the mechanism of injury and any comorbid conditions such as bleeding disorders, previous surgeries, or anatomic abnormalities. Physical examination should focus on identifying the presence of a nasal fracture, septal hematoma, cerebrospinal fluid (CSF) leak, and signs of associated ophthalmologic or serious head injury. Inspect for midface injuries to eyes, teeth, sinuses, and cervical spine, keeping in mind the risk of naso-orbit-ethmoid fractures. Edema and ecchymosis postinjury may be extensive and obscure the facial bones. At times, substantial mucosal and septal trauma can occur without outward signs of injury.

Nasal Fracture

Nasal fractures are less common in children due to soft, compliant cartilage, and deformities may not become obvious until swelling and ecchymosis have improved. Clinical findings associated with nasal fractures include epistaxis, nasal pain and deformity, septal deviation, hematoma, or mucosal injury. Radiography is not routinely indicated to evaluate nasal injuries or simple nasal fractures. Nasal cartilage injury may require specialized repair for optimal preservation of function and cosmesis. Treatment for simple nasal fractures is supportive care with pain management. Follow-up with otolaryngology or plastic surgery should occur to assess for deformity that would require surgical intervention. Compound nasal fractures or those associated with sinus fractures require antibiotic treatment.

Cerebrospinal Fluid Rhinorrhea

Clear watery rhinorrhea that occurs after nasal trauma is concerning for CSF leak, suggesting an underlying skull fracture resulting in a communicating intracranial injury. It is imperative to differentiate CSF leak from rhinorrhea. Using the halo test, nasal discharge is collected on filter paper. Any halo of clear fluid around blood is concerning for CSF. Glucose testing using glucose oxidase paper is subject to false-positive reactions and should be used cautiously. Beta-2-transferrin testing is the most specific test for CSF rhinorrhea, but results are seldom available in the emergency department. Computed tomography (CT) imaging can confirm an underlying skull fracture. If there is concern for CSF rhinorrhea, early consultation with otolaryngology and neurosurgery is prudent. In children with suspected CSF leak, admit for bed rest and elevation of head of bed to 30 degrees. Most CSF leaks heal spontaneously with rest and supportive care. Use of prophylactic antimicrobials is controversial.

Septal Hematoma

Septal hematomas form due to hemorrhage from an artery beneath the mucoperichondrium, separating it from the septal cartilage, robbing its blood supply. Hematomas can form up to 14 days after nasal trauma and are characterized by severe localized nasal pain with tenderness on palpation. They appear as an erythematous or violaceous bulge in the nasal cavity. The mass does not change in size when topical vasoconstrictor agents are applied and is fluctuant when probed. An adjacent fracture is likely. Consider otolaryngology consultation as septal hematomas require urgent incision and drainage with nasal packing or a pressure *dressing* to restore adequate blood supply to the septal cartilage. Long-term complications of persistent hematomas may include septal abscess formation, intracranial infection, cavernous sinus thrombosis, cartilage necrosis, and perforation resulting in a saddle nose deformity. Patients may require prolonged follow-up postinjury to monitor for signs of cartilage destruction and cosmetic changes.

KEY POINTS

- Nasal fractures may be difficult to detect shortly after trauma due to significant swelling. Nasal deformity persisting days after injury requires urgent subspecialty evaluation.
- Presence of CSF *rhinorrhea* suggests an associated skull fracture.
- Septal hematomas require urgent incision and drainage to avoid long-term complications.

Suggested Readings

Kazahava K. Otolaryngologic trauma. In: Fleisher GR, Ludwig S, eds. *Textbook of Pediatric Emergency Medicine*. 6th ed. Philadelphia, PA: Williams & Wilkins; 2010:1300-1301.

McConnell S, Drigalla D. Maxillofacia & neck trauma. In: Stone CK, Humphries RL, eds. *CURRENT Diagnosis and Treatment Pediatric Emergency Medicine*. New York, NY: McGraw-Hill Professional Publishing; 2015:232, 238.

Savage RR, Valvich C. Hematoma of the nasal septum. *Pediatr Rev.* 2006;27(12):478.

Stankovic C. Facial trauma. In: Hoffman RJ, Vincent JW, Richard JS, eds. *Fleisher and Ludwig's 5-Minute Pediatric Emergency Medicine Consult*. Philadelphia, PA: Wolters Kluwer Health; 2011:958-959.

Epistaxis: The Nose Knows How to Stop the Leak

Kimberly L. Norris, MD

Epistaxis is a common presenting complaint for children in the emergency department (ED) and most often occurs between the ages of 2 and 10 years. Most cases are the result of minor trauma, nasal irritation, desiccation of nasal mucosa or foreign body in the context of a rich, superficial vascular supply. Ninety percent of cases are anterior, typically unilateral, and oozing in nature. Bilateral epistaxis is concerning for a posterior bleed and often results in more profuse bleeding. Care should be taken to not only control active epistaxis and investigate abnormal bleeding, but also avoid excessive or unnecessary workup in the pediatric patient.

Close attention should be paid to history and physical examination. History of prolonged bleeding lasting longer than 30 minutes, spontaneous bleeding from other sites, onset before 2 years, or a family history of coagulopathy should prompt workup for a bleeding disorder. Examination should evaluate for bleeding vessels and evidence of foreign body, hemangiomas, telangiectasias, or uncommon tumors such as juvenile nasopharyngeal angiofibromas. Scant bleeding from the anterior nasal passages with blood in the posterior oropharynx should raise suspicion for a posterior source.

Laboratory and imaging studies are not routinely indicated. Clinical history concerning for bleeding disorder, use of anticoagulant therapy, or clinical evidence of severe blood loss may necessitate obtaining complete blood count, prothromin time, partial thromboplastin time, and screening for von Willebrand disease. Imaging should be reserved for patients with a history of significant facial trauma, suspicion for tumor, or history of recurrent/refractory epistaxis.

While epistaxis is a common complaint, outpatient management by patients and families is often fraught with misconceptions. During initial management of active bleeding in the ED, one should emphasize appropriate interventions, including sitting up and leaning slightly forward to prevent excessive swallowed blood, gentle evacuation of clots by blowing the nose, and constant, direct compression of the cartilaginous portion of the nose distal to nasal bones for 5-20 minutes.

Epistaxis refractory to direct pressure may require more extensive measures. Application of topical oxymetazoline or gauze soaked with epinephrine or phenylephrine result in vasoconstriction. Additional therapeutic adjuncts may include topical application of tranexamic acid (TXA) or the use of a gelatin sponge (Gelfoam) or collagen sponge (Surgicel) held to the site of bleeding. If epistaxis is persistent or severe, nasal cautery or packing may be required. Unilateral application of silver nitrate, rolling it over bleeding area for 5-10 seconds, is often effective; however, bilateral application should be avoided due to the risk of perforation of the nasal septum. Nasal packing may be achieved using commercial devices or ribbon gauze. Commercially available nasal tampons expand to tamponade bleeding. Alternatively, gauze impregnated with petroleum jelly may be placed in successive layers along the floor of the nose until the nasal cavity is fully packed. Packing may be held in place by tape and left for 3-5 days. Use of anterior nasal packing may be complicated by bacterial rhinosinusitis, toxic shock syndrome, or septal ulceration/perforation, so empiric antibiotic therapy should be considered. Posterior epistaxis is often refractory to the measures listed above, and posterior packs consisting of balloon catheters, endoscopic cauterization, or ligation of bleeding vessels by an otolaryngologist (ENT) may be necessary.

Education regarding appropriate home therapies should be discussed with patients and their families. Interventions may include use of cool-mist humidifiers, saline spray, and topical emollients such as petroleum jelly or antibiotic ointment. In addition, instructions regarding home management of acute bleeding should be reiterated, and patients with abnormal examination findings (eg, polyp, telangiectasia), severe/recurrent bleeding, or suspected posterior source should be referred for outpatient ENT evaluation.

KEY POINTS

- Anterior epistaxis is often unilateral and slow. Bilateral, brisk bleeding may indicate a posterior source.
- Laboratory tests and imaging are not routinely indicated.
- If bleeding persists despite direct pressure, use of topical vasoconstrictors or prothrombotic agents is indicated.
- Nasal cautery or packing may be considered for refractory bleeding.
- Emergent ENT consultation should be considered for posterior epistaxis or anterior epistaxis not responsive to noninvasive interventions.

Suggested Readings

Delgado EM, Nadel FM. Epistaxis. In: Bachur RG et al., eds. *Fleisher and Ludwig's Textbook of Pediatric Emergency Medicine*. 4th ed. Philadelphia, PA: Lippincott Williams & Wilkins; 2000.

Stallard TC. Emergency disorders of the ear, nose, sinuses, oropharynx, & mouth. In: Stone CK et al., eds. *CURRENT Diagnosis & Treatment: Emergency Medicine*. 8th ed. New York, NY: McGraw-Hill; 2017.

Yoon PJ et al. Ear, nose, & throat. In: Hay WW et al., eds. *Current Diagnosis & Treatment: Pediatrics*. 24th ed. New York, NY: McGraw-Hill; 2018.

Orbital Fractures: Be Careful to Avoid Getting Trapped

Amanda Price, MD

Orbital fractures are the third most common facial fracture in children and can lead to long-term visual and cosmetic complications if not identified and treated appropriately. In pediatrics, the prevalence is highest in adolescent males, which is frequently secondary to sports-related injuries.

Specific bone characteristics and sinus development create unique fracture patterns in children. The absence of frontal sinuses in young children leads to increased frequency of orbital roof fractures compared to adults, which can be associated with intracranial injury and supraorbital nerve damage. Frontal sinus pneumatization begins around age 7, which shifts predominance to orbital floor and medial wall fractures. These can cause muscle and soft tissue entrapment and injuries to the infraorbital nerve, lacrimal system, and medial canthal ligament.

The classic "blow-out" fracture of the orbital floor in an adult facial bone shatters and can have protrusion of orbital contents into the maxillary space. In children, bones are more elastic with a thick periosteum leading to a distinctive subtype known as the "trapdoor" fracture. Sudden pressure increase causes a portion of the orbital floor to temporarily displace and then spring back into place, increasing potential for inferior rectus entrapment within the fracture fragment and causing a high risk of tissue necrosis.

Clinical features include bony tenderness, ecchymosis, and swelling, with complaints of visual changes, often diplopia. Contrastingly, "trapdoor" fractures can present with diplopia or ocular motility loss without associated swelling or ecchymosis, coined the "white-eyed blowout fracture." Entrapment can lead to nausea/vomiting and bradycardia, secondary to the oculocardiac reflex. Nausea and vomiting have been shown to be highly predictive of entrapment in patients with orbital trauma.

All patients with orbital trauma must undergo a thorough ophthalmologic evaluation to assess for concomitant intraocular injury. Visual acuity loss may be an early sign of injury. Entrapment will classically lead to limited extraocular movement (unilateral loss of upward or lateral motility). In orbital floor fractures, the eye may have a sunken appearance (enophthalmos) as the globe is pushed further back into the orbit, or there may be orbital dystopia (an asymmetry in the horizontal level of the eyes). A tear-shaped pupil indicates an open globe, and proptosis or a new afferent pupillary defect suggests a retrobulbar hematoma. Supraorbital and infraorbital nerve regions should be assessed for decreased sensation. Fundoscopy, intraocular pressure (IOP), and—if possible—a slit lamp examination should also be performed.

The imaging modality of choice is computerized tomography (CT) with thin cuts of the orbits. This should be obtained in anyone with a clinically suspected orbital fracture. Plain film sensitivity is only about 50%, and ultrasound has a high false-negative rate for fracture. MRI can be considered if CT is negative for entrapment and clinical concern persists but is not recommended as initial imaging.

Emergency department management includes early stabilization of vision-threatening injuries and urgent subspecialty consultation for complex fractures. An open globe and retrobulbar hematomas are ophthalmologic emergencies, and lateral canthotomy may be indicated for the latter. Supportive treatment with the head of bed elevation, eye protection, pain control, and antiemetics can limit IOP spikes. Trapdoor fractures with nausea/vomiting or bradycardia require surgery within 12-24 hours of injury. Early surgical release of entrapment has shown better outcomes. Consider corticosteroids in patients with EOM limitation to reduce swelling. Uncomplicated orbital fractures need outpatient ophthalmology follow-up within 1 week, and discharge instructions should include sinus precautions and consider prophylactic antibiotics for fractures with sinus extension.

Many orbital fractures are uncomplicated and do not require surgical repair; if a thorough examination is performed and early subspecialty care is involved complications can often be mitigated.

KEY POINTS

- Orbital fractures necessitate a thorough eye examination and close ophthalmology follow-up.
- The trapdoor fracture is a hinged bony fragment that can entrap muscle and tissue with high risk of necrosis and is unique to the pediatric population.
- Keep a high index of suspicion for fracture in the patient with diplopia and/or limited EOM even in the absence of ecchymosis and swelling.
- Early surgical release of entrapment is associated with better outcomes.

Suggested Readings

Chung S, Langer P. Pediatric orbital blowout fractures. *Curr Opin Ophthalmol.* 2017;28:470-476.
Gerber B, et al. Orbital fractures in children: a review of outcomes. *Br J Oral Maxillofac Surg.* 2013;51:789-793.
Miller AF, et al. Epidemiology and predictors of orbital fractures in children. *Pediatr Emerg Care.* 2018;34:21-24.
Neuman MI. Facial trauma. In: Fleisher G, Henretig R, eds. *Textbook of Pediatric Emergency Medicine.* 6th ed. Philadelphia, PA: Lippincott Williams & Wilkins; 2005:1307-1315.

37

Not Using Absorbable Sutures for Children With Facial Lacerations

Emily Greenwald, MD and Nidhya Navanandan, MD

Lacerations are among the most common injuries in pediatric emergency care. Optimal cosmetic outcome is a key concern for patients and caregivers, as the possibility of a scar can be a major source of anxiety. An array of materials exists for closure of facial wounds, including steri-strips, tissue adhesives, and sutures. Decisions on appropriate closure technique and materials depend on numerous factors including the location, depth, and complexity of the wound. Here we advocate for the use of absorbable sutures for facial laceration repair and aim to dispel existing myths regarding their use for closure of facial wounds in children.

There are two main suture types: nonabsorbable and absorbable. The main difference between these suture types are in their strength and reactivity. Absorbable sutures provide an obvious benefit in eliminating a suture removal procedure and are thus especially beneficial for young children. Multiple studies now confirm that there is no difference in cosmetic outcome, dehiscence, or infection rates between wounds repaired by absorbable versus nonabsorbable sutures. Even a blinded randomized controlled trial in which outcome was assessed by plastic surgeons after laceration repair in the emergency department with nonabsorbable (nylon) versus absorbable sutures (plain gut) found no difference between long-term cosmetic outcome, rates of dehiscence, or infection between the groups. Other studies have demonstrated similar results as well as improved patient and caregiver satisfaction. A meta-analysis of randomized control trials (RTCs) comparing the two suture types also yielded similar results. Thus, current evidence convincingly supports use of absorbable sutures for closure of pediatric traumatic facial lacerations.

The choice of absorbable suture is also important in achieving optimal cosmetic outcomes. Strategies by suture type are detailed in Table 37.1.

Postrepair laceration care involves application of a topical antibiotic and nonadherent kid-proof dressing, keeping the wound dry for at least 12 hours postrepair and use of sunscreen to prevent postinflammatory hyperpigmentation.

In summary, the traditional belief that nonabsorbable sutures are superior to absorbable sutures for repair of facial lacerations is not evidence based. Absorbable sutures are equivalent to nonabsorbable sutures in terms of cosmetic outcome, rate of wound dehiscence, and infection. Absorbable sutures do not require suture removal, a clear advantage in pediatrics. Overall, absorbable sutures are a "go to" tool for pediatric facial lacerations.

Table 37.1 ■ Suture Characteristics

Suture Type	Size	Recommended Uses	Maintenance of Tensile Strength (Days)	Completely Dissolved (Days)	Tips/Tricks
Fast–absorbing gut	5-0 6-0	Superficial closure of all facial wounds	5-7	7	Smallest size minimizes scarring. For deeper lacerations, remove tension by closing deeper layers first. Pass suture through antibiotic ointment prior to use to improve pliability and breakage rate.
Polyglactin 910 (Vicryl)	5-0	Repair of deep dermal layers Decreasing tension Oral mucosal wounds (ie, vermillion border)	14-21	90	After deep layers are repaired using Vicryl, close superficial layer with fast-absorbing gut or tissue adhesive.
Nylon	5-0 6-0	No clear advantages over absorbable sutures	60	∞	Necessitates removal at 5-7 days

KEY POINTS

- Absorbable sutures, particularly fast–absorbing gut, are the preferred suture material for closure of pediatric facial lacerations.
- Absorbable sutures are similar to nonabsorbable sutures in terms of cosmetic outcome, infection rates, and wound dehiscence.
- Absorbable sutures improve patient and caregiver satisfaction.

Suggested Readings

Karounis H, Gouin S, Eisman H, et al. A randomized, controlled trial comparing long-term cosmetic outcomes of traumatic pediatric lacerations repaired with absorbable plain gut versus nonabsorbable nylon sutures. *Acad Emerg Med.* 2004;7:730-735.

Luck RP, Flood R, Eyal D, et al. Cosmetic outcomes of absorbable versus nonabsorbable sutures in pediatric facial lacerations. *Pediatr Emerg Care.* 2008;3:137-142.

Luck R, Tredway T, Gerard J, Eyal D, Krug L, Flood R. Comparison of cosmetic outcomes of absorbable versus nonabsorbable sutures in pediatric facial lacerations. *Pediatr Emerg Care.* 2013;29:691-695.

Navanandan N, Renna-Rodriguez M, DiStefano MC. Pearls in pediatric wound management. *Clin Pediatr Emerg Med.* 2017;18(1):53-61.

Xu B, Wang L, Chen C, et al. Absorbable versus nonabsorbable sutures for skin closure: a meta-analysis of randomized controlled trials. *Ann Plast Surg.* 2016;5:598-606.

38

Overlooking the Benefits of Regional Anesthesia in Children

Jonathan Orsborn, MD, FAAP

The face is the most common place for young patients to get a laceration, due to their top-heavy design and tendency to fall over. Many physicians who do not regularly practice pediatric medicine may have significant anxiety in dealing with these lacerations. With good pain control and distraction, there should be nothing to fear! For large lacerations, using local anesthetic only may bring you near the maximum anesthetic dose on a per kilogram basis, increasing likelihood of anesthetic related toxicity. Additionally, as cosmesis is extremely important on the face, local infiltration may significantly distort the laceration margins, making it more difficult to directly align the edges of the laceration to minimize the appearance of the scar.

One simple way to avoid these errors is to use targeted facial nerve blocks to anesthetize prior to repairing these facial lacerations. Three common facial blocks are supraorbital, infraorbital, and mental blocks.

The face is innervated by three branches of the trigeminal nerve (CN V) V1, V2, and V3. V1 supplies sensation to the forehead, V2 supplies sensation to the midface and upper lip, and V3 supplies sensation to the lower lip and chin. Each branch conveniently emerges from inside the skull along a vertical line from the middle third of the eyebrow to the lower mandible.

Technique

Each of these blocks requires only 1-2 cc local anesthetic to anesthetize the entire field, which will help keep you well below the maximum recommended anesthetic dose. If puncturing skin, the area should be cleaned with alcohol, and you should use a small needle, such as a 27 gauge. Additionally, before injecting anesthetic, it is important to gently pull back on the plunger to be sure there is no blood return before injecting. Once you inject, wait 5-10 minutes, and test the field before proceeding.

V1: This branch is easily accessible in the superior orbital fissure, palpated as an indentation over the medial third of the superior orbital ridge. The needle can be inserted a short distance; pull back to be sure you are not in a vessel and then inject 1-2 cc anesthetic.

V2: This branch is easily accessible via both the transcutaneous or intraoral route, although a small study found the intraoral route to be both less painful and more effective. The area you are attempting to access is over the maxilla, about 1 cm below center of lower eyelid. From the intraoral method, pinch lip and cheek, keeping one finger on the maxilla to keep you from entering the orbit and to help guide the needle tip position. After using viscous lidocaine or anesthetic spray to numb the gums at the puncture site, insert needle in the buccal fold, parallel to the face, about 1 cm towards the middle of the eye, just above the upper canine tooth. If you use a transcutaneous approach, find the area and directly inject.

V3: The mental nerve is easily accessible along the lower mandible and can be felt as an indentation called the mandibular foramen. It can also be accessed via an intraoral or transcutaneous method, although again, the intraoral approach was found to be more effective and less painful. Pinch the lower lip and insert the needle in the buccal fold around the lateral premolar about 0.5-1 cm towards the foramen, where you should be keeping a finger to guide the needle. For the transcutaneous approach, feel for the foramen, insert the needle from a medial position, and inject the anesthetic, being sure to not directly infiltrate the foramen to avoid nerve damage.

KEY POINTS

- Facial nerve blocks are an appropriate way to achieve anesthesia for facial wounds requiring closure.
- Facial nerve blocks often decrease volume of anesthetic used and can help preserve local landmarks.

Suggested Readings

Lynch MT, Syverud SA, et al. Comparison of intraoral and percutaneous approaches for infraorbital nerve block. *Acad Emerg Med.* 1994;1(6):514-519.

Moskovitz J, Sabatino F. Regional nerve blocks of the face. *Emerg Med Clin North Am.* 2013;31(2):517-527.

Salam G. Regional anesthesia for office procedures: part I. Head and neck surgeries. *Am Fam Physician.* 2004;69(3):585-590.

Syverud SA, Jenkins JM, et al. A comparative study of the percutaneous versus intraoral technique for mental nerve block. *Acad Emerg Med.* 1994;1(6):509-513.

Using Color of Rhinorrhea As a Justification for Giving Antibiotics

Mahnoosh Nik-Ahd, MD, MPH and Andrea Fang, MD

Diagnosis

Acute bacterial sinusitis is a clinical diagnosis, and there are no specific physical examination signs that are sensitive or specific for the diagnosis. Per the American Academy of Pediatrics, a diagnosis can be made in the following three scenarios:

1) At least 10 days of persistent upper respiratory infection (URI) symptoms without improvement
2) A URI after a period of initial improvement with new or worsening symptoms
3) Three consecutive days or more of severe URI symptoms (i.e. purulent nasal discharge with fever of at least 39°C)

Differentiating Bacterial Sinusitis From Viral URIs

Timing is key in distinguishing sinusitis from URIs. URIs generally last 5-7 days and peak by day 3-6. In URIs, fever and constitutional symptoms occur early and resolve within 1-2 days. Sinusitis is more prolonged, severe and/or waxing and waning. Sinusitis is also more often associated with sleep disturbance or green nasal discharge.

Treatment

The most common bacterial causes of sinusitis are *Streptococcus pneumoniae*, *Haemophilus influenzae*, and *Moraxella catarrhalis*. Uncomplicated cases can be treated with either high-dose amoxicillin or amoxicillin-clavulanate for 10-14 days. Sinusitis can also be observed for 3 days before starting treatment using shared decision-making with parents given symptoms can improve without treatment. Children with a mild penicillin allergy can be treated with a third-generation cephalosporin and clindamycin. Levofloxacin can be used in patients with a severe penicillin allergy.

Complications

Complications of sinusitis generally involve the eye or brain via local invasion or spread through the bloodstream. Suspicion of these complications should prompt diagnosis via a CT scan with contrast of the parasinuses and orbits or brain. An MRI can also be performed but is often less convenient to obtain.

Orbital complications of sinusitis include periorbital cellulitis, subperiosteal abscess, orbital cellulitis, orbital abscess, and cavernous sinus thrombosis. Cavernous sinus thrombosis can present with headache, photophobia, proptosis, periorbital edema, and/or cranial nerve deficits. Sinusitis is the leading cause of orbital cellulitis and can present with proptosis, and/or impaired extraocular motion. Mild periorbital cellulitis presents with swelling around the eye and can be managed as an outpatient. Otherwise, orbital complications should be admitted with consultation with otolaryngology, ophthalmology, and infectious disease.

Intracranial complications include subdural or epidural empyema, brain abscess, venous thrombosis, meningitis, and Pott puffy tumor (i.e. osteomyelitis of the frontal bone). Signs of intracranial complications include a severe headache, photophobia, seizures, or other focal neurologic findings and should be confirmed via a CT or MRI. These patients should be admitted with the appropriate consultations.

Empiric therapy for patients with orbital or cranial complications from sinusitis should cover the usual gram-negative culprits as well as *Staphylococcus aureus* and anaerobes (eg, ceftriaxone, vancomycin, and metronidazole).

KEY POINTS

- Sinusitis is a clinical diagnosis. Timing is key, and it should be considered if a presumptive URI is persistent, waxes and wanes, or is severe.
- First-line treatment is high-dose amoxicillin or amoxicillin-clavulanate for 10-14 days.
- Complications of sinusitis can involve the eye and brain and can present with eye swelling, proptosis, restricted/painful extraocular movements, severe headache, photophobia, seizures, or other focal neurologic findings.
- Any suspicion of orbital or cranial involvement should prompt confirmation via a CT or MRI with contrast and warrants admission with broad spectrum antibiotics and the appropriate consultations.

Suggested Readings

Chow AW, Benninger MS, Brook I, et al. Executive summary: IDSA clinical practice guideline for acute bacterial rhinosinusitis in children and adults. *Clin Infect Dis.* 2012;54(8):e72-e112.

Fang A, England J, Gausche-Hill M. Pediatric acute bacterial sinusitis: diagnostic and treatment dilemmas. *Pediatr Emerg Care.* 2015;31(11):789-797.

Shaikh N, Hoberman A, Kearney DH, et al. Signs and symptoms that differentiate acute sinusitis from viral upper respiratory tract infection. *Pediatr Infect Dis J.* 2013;32(10):1061-1065.

Smith MJ. Evidence for the diagnosis and treatment of acute uncomplicated sinusitis in children: a systematic review. *Pediatrics.* 2013;132(1):e284-e296.

Wald ER, Applegate KE, Bordley C, et al. Clinical practice guideline for the diagnosis and management of acute bacterial sinusitis in children aged 1 to 18 years. *Pediatrics.* 2013;132(1):e262-e280.

Basing Treatment of Strep Pharyngitis Solely on Centor Criteria

Crick Watkins, DO and Chad D. McCalla, MD

Group A Strep (GAS) pharyngitis is a common childhood infection, accounting for 20%-30% of acute throat infections in pediatric patients. Risk stratification tools, such as the Centor criteria or McIsaac modification, can be misleading and may result in missed diagnoses or unnecessary antibiotic prescriptions.

Background

Streptococcus pyogenes infections of the throat are more prevalent among children and adolescents than among adults. Signs and symptoms include fever, sore throat, pharyngeal erythema, tonsillar enlargement with or without exudate, palatal petechiae, tender cervical lymphadenopathy, vomiting, headaches, and upper abdominal pain. The infection is typically self-limited, lasting 3-5 days. Early antimicrobial treatment can reduce severity and duration of symptoms; however, treatment is more useful for:

- Preventing suppurative (ie, peritonsillar abscess, mastoiditis, lymphadenitis) and nonsuppurative (ie, acute rheumatic fever [ARF], post-streptococcal glomerulonephritis) complications
- Reducing transmission to others
- Reducing socioeconomic impacts of infection (ie, parental time off work, missed school)

Generally, children age 3 and younger should NOT be tested, because of low overall disease prevalence and low risk of developing ARF and other complications. Young children present differently and exudative pharyngitis is often absent, with mucopurulent rhinorrhea, excoriated nares, and diffuse lymphadenopathy being more common. You may consider testing in these patients to prevent transmission to at-risk household contacts.

Clinical Decision Rules

The Centor Criteria for GAS pharyngitis was designed for use in adults and assigns 1 point each for presence of fever (>38°C), absence of cough, tender and swollen anterior cervical lymphadenopathy (>1.5 cm), and/or tonsillar swelling and exudate. This system was modified by McIsaac to account for age-related disease prevalence and assigns an additional 1 point for patients age 3-14 years, 0 points for patients age 15-44 years, and −1 point for patients age >45 years.

Total scores of 0-1 are deemed low risk and likely of viral etiology; no further testing is needed. This is consistent with 2012 IDSA recommendations to avoid testing in patients with symptoms most consistent with an acute viral infection. It should be noted that even with a score of 1, rates of GAS infections can be as high as 14%; if suspicion remains high, testing may still be appropriate. Presumptive diagnoses in pediatric patients with scores of ≥4, on the other hand, should be strongly AVOIDED, as original and validation studies of these clinical decision rules (CDRs) found the rate of confirmed GAS infections among this subgroup is only 51%-57%, suggesting antibiotic treatment would be unnecessary in nearly half of these patients.

Testing

Testing should start with a rapid antigen detection test (RADT), which has a fairly low rate of false-positive results. RADT sensitivity ranges from 70% to 90%; therefore, negative tests should be followed by throat culture. The combined sensitivity and specificity of RADT and culture approaches 99% and 100%, respectively; no detection in both essentially eliminates GAS. Since antibiotic treatment should start within 9 days of symptom onset to prevent ARF, there is time to wait for culture results.

Treatment

Positive GAS detection, by RADT or culture, should be treated, and most antibiotic regimens require 10 days for eradication. Penicillin and its analogs (ie, amoxicillin) remain the treatment of choice given extremely low rates of resistance. Once-daily dosing with amoxicillin at 50 mg/kg (max of 1000 mg) is often easiest given its well-tolerated taste and low cost. If medication compliance is a concern, a one-time IM injection with benzathine penicillin G (600 000 units for <27 kg, 1.2 million units >27 kg) can be given. For patients with known allergies to penicillin without associated anaphylaxis, cephalexin is the antibiotic of choice. Acceptable alternatives in those with prior anaphylactic reactions include clindamycin, clarithromycin, or azithromycin (5-day course).

KEY POINTS

- CDRs can be unreliable; test for GAS if clinically suspected, unless obvious symptoms of viral etiology.
- Children 3 and younger do not need to be tested due to low disease prevalence and low risk of complications.
- Penicillin/amoxicillin is the drug of choice for treatment; cephalexin (no anaphylaxis), clindamycin, clarithromycin, or azithromycin if pen-allergic.

Suggested Readings

Fine AM, Nizet MD, Mandl MD. Large-scale validation of the Centor and McIsaac scores to predict group A streptococcal pharyngitis. *Arch Intern Med.* 2012;172(11):847-852.
Shulman ST, Bisno AL, Van Beneden C, et al. Clinical practice guidelines for the diagnosis and management of group A streptococcal pharyngitis: 2012 update by the Infectious Disease Society of America. *Clin Infect Dis.* 2012;55(10):e86-e102.

Neck Pain and Fever Does Not Always Mean Meningitis. Think of RPA. Retropharyngeal Abscess

Alison Gardner, MD, MS and Kimberly Myers, MD

Retropharyngeal abscesses are commonly diagnosed deep space neck infections. The most frequently diagnosed are young children, the most prevalent age is 5 years old with a slight predominance of boys. A retropharyngeal abscess often starts with an upper respiratory tract infection (URI). This URI then causes the lymph nodes in the retropharyngeal space to become suppurative. More rare causes include a risk for infection after pharyngeal trauma, such as a swallowed foreign body, or recent instrumentation in the setting of a medical procedure. In these instances, bacteria from the pharynx gets introduced directly into the retropharyngeal space. Since the retropharyngeal lymph nodes atrophy with age, infections in pubertal children and adults are rare.

Diagnosis can be difficult because a young child will be less able to participate in your history and examination. The most common presenting features of a retropharyngeal abscess are fever, neck pain, and dysphagia. The most common examination findings will be cervical lymphadenopathy and limited range of motion which can sometimes mimic meningismus. Although not a rule, experienced practitioners find the decreased range of motion in a retropharyngeal abscess is with neck extension as opposed to neck flexion, which is more limited in meningitis. Other examination findings could include tonsillar displacement, dysphonia, trismus, and in severe infections stridor. A CBC, strep swab, and blood culture could be useful in the workup. In unusual presentations tests like EBV, CMV or PPD could help in diagnosis as well.

Once retropharyngeal abscess enters the likely list of diagnoses, the next step is to obtain imaging to confirm your diagnosis. Lateral neck films may show possible gas or air fluid levels in the soft tissue of the prevertebral space as well as increased thickness of the prevertebral space, but use with caution as x-rays have a high false-positive rate. CT neck with contrast is the study of choice to determine if there is a definable abscess vs phlegmon and help determine management.

Treatment of a retropharyngeal abscess first requires an assessment of the airway to ensure that it is patent and stable. Interventions such as supplemental oxygen, airway adjuncts like nasal trumpet, and PPV if poorly ventilating should be considered. Intubation in this situation would be difficult given that there is likely to be a high degree of obstruction. The tissue of the airway will also be friable and attempts to intubate could cause trauma that would lead to uncontrolled rupture of the abscess. In summation, if there is need for intubation ensure that operative help is available if at all possible.

Retropharyngeal abscesses are typically polymicrobial in nature with the most common bacteria being *Streptococcus*, *Staphylococcus*, and respiratory anaerobes. If there is not a defined abscess, or if the abscess is small and not amenable to drainage, then admission for IV antibiotics will be undertaken. Antibiotics most commonly used would be Clindamycin, Ampicillin/Sulbactam, or Piperacillin/Tazobactam.

Complications of retropharyngeal abscess can be very serious. Due to the anatomy, there is the chance for extension to the diaphragm in the posterior retropharyngeal space which could lead to a mediastinitis. Obstruction of the airway is a risk, symptoms of obstruction should lead you to get surgery and anesthesia involved early, possibly deferring the examination until the OR. If untreated, the abscess will continue to grow and has been reported to cause atlantoaxial dislocation. The bacteria of the abscess can extend into the bony spine and lead to vertebral osteomyelitis. There is also the possibility of recurrence if there is inadequate drainage or failure of antibiotic therapy. Recurrence should be suspected if there is a resurgence of symptoms in a short interval from initial treatment.

KEY POINTS

- Consider the diagnosis of retropharyngeal abscess in the setting of a prepubertal child with fever and decreased range of motion of the neck, especially decreased extension.
- There is potential for airway compromise and the high likelihood that the airway will be difficult to secure so assess early and plan cautiously.
- While blood work may be obtained and can help to tailor therapy, CT with contrast is the gold standard of diagnosis.

Suggested Readings

Bochner RE, Gangar M, Belamarich PF. A clinical approach to tonsillitis, tonsillar hypertrophy, and peritonsillar and retropharyngeal abscesses. *Pediatr Rev.* 2017;38(2):81-92.

Grisaru-Soen G, Komisar O, Aizenstein O, et al. Retropharyngeal and parapharyngeal abscess in children—epidemiology, clinical features and treatment. *Int J Pediatr Otorhinolaryngol.* 2010;74(9):1016-1020.

Klein MR. Infections of the oropharynx. *Emerg Med Clin North Am.* 2019;37(1):69-80.

Oropharyngeal Puncture? Do Not Forget That There Is a Big Blood Vessel to Worry About

Rachel O'Brian, MD and Adam Kochman, MD, FAAP, FACEP

Oropharyngeal Trauma

Any parent who ever told their child not to run with toys in their mouth was spot on. Oropharyngeal trauma is often seen in the form of lacerations, impalements, and avulsions. There is a predominance in boys, typically <7 years old, with a history of running while holding an object in their mouth or hands. The most common culprits involved are toys, sticks, writing utensils, and toothbrushes. The greater proportion of right-handed children results in a higher incidence of left-sided injuries. While the injuries may initially appear minor, they warrant a high index of suspicion and a thorough clinical evaluation.

Complications

Although complication rates from intraoral wounds are low (4%–8%), an in-depth clinical assessment is necessary, because the consequences of a missed injury can be severe. The feared complications are secondary to damage of nearby anatomical structures in the posterior oropharynx. Injury to surrounding blood vessels, nerves, organs, and soft tissues can lead to mediastinitis, mediastinal or retropharyngeal abscesses, airway obstruction, and vascular injury.

Injury to the internal carotid artery (ICA) is perhaps the most feared complication and cannot be missed. Compression of the ICA between an object and the transverse processes of cervical vertebrae can cause intimal tears that predispose to thrombus formation. If the thrombus migrates to the cerebral vasculature, it can cause stroke and even death. This process can take hours to develop, so neurologic abnormalities may not manifest until up to 72 hours after the injury occurred.

Evaluation and Stabilization

Assuming ABCs are stable, a complete evaluation of the oropharynx is necessary to assess for bleeding, swelling, lacerations, and the presence of foreign bodies. These patients require evaluation for carotid bruits as well as assessment for abnormal neurologic findings. In the case of profuse bleeding or a pulsatile hematoma, the ED physician should make preparations for managing a difficult airway.

Diagnostic Imaging

How does one determine who should be imaged and what imaging modality should be utilized? While no clinical factors have proven to identify who is at highest risk for neurologic sequelae, children with lateral or deep penetrating oropharyngeal injuries may be more likely to have carotid injury. Plain radiography may be useful to visualize foreign bodies and subcutaneous air but is not helpful when evaluating for vessel abnormalities. Ultrasound findings do not correlate well with vessel injury and should not be used as a first-line imaging modality. Angiography is the gold standard to evaluate for carotid artery injury; however, given the significant associated risks (stroke, death, etc.), it is only utilized if a computed tomography angiography (CTA)/magnetic resonance angiography (MRA) is concerning for carotid injury, the patient's neurologic examination is grossly abnormal, or in cases of active hemorrhage. CTA is more commonly used because it is fast, widely available, and may avoid the need for anesthesia, but its sensitivity and specificity for detecting carotid artery injuries are slightly lower compared with MRA.

Management

Most oropharyngeal injuries are superficial and do not require repair. Antibiotics can be considered for large or contaminated lacerations and should cover oropharyngeal flora. Depending on the mechanism of the injury, tetanus status should be assessed. Similar to the lack of consensus on imaging guidelines, the period of observation of these patients is also up for debate. If there are any neurologic concerns, patients should be admitted to the hospital for serial neurologic checks, especially during the first 24–48 hours after the injury. Otherwise, low-risk patients are typically discharged home where they can continue to be monitored by parents or caregivers.

KEY POINTS

- Intraoral wounds can cause ICA injury leading to cerebral vascular thrombosis and severe neurologic sequelae.
- Lateral, posterior, and deep oropharyngeal wounds should raise more suspicion for carotid artery injury.
- Although carotid artery angiography is the gold standard, CTA/MRA are typically performed first given the high risks associated with CAA.
- Neurologic abnormalities may not develop until up to 72 hours after the injury, so it is important to counsel caregivers of patients discharged home about signs and symptoms of neurologic sequelae.

Suggested Readings

Brietzke SE, Jones DT. Pediatric oropharyngeal trauma: what is the role of CT scan? *Int J Pediatr Otorhinolaryngol.* 2005;69:669.

Soose RJ, Simons JP, Mandell DL. Evaluation and management of pediatric oropharyngeal trauma. *Arch Otolaryngol Head Neck Surg.* 2006;132:446.

Zonfrillo M, Roy A, Walsh S. Management of pediatric penetrating oropharyngeal trauma. *Pediatric Emergency Care.* 2008;24(3):172-175.

Not Believing the Parent Who Believes the Child Choked on Something

Collin Michels, MD and Andrea Fang, MD

Parents know their child best. Choking is the fourth leading cause of unintentional injury death in the United States, so when a parent believes their child choked on something, it is imperative to pursue further evaluation and management. Patients who aspirate tend to be younger than 3 years of age and can present on a spectrum from awake and talking to full cardiorespiratory arrest.

Upper Airway Obstruction

Pharyngeal foreign bodies are true medical emergencies that require immediate intervention as complete airway obstruction is most likely to occur at the time of aspiration.

Upper airway obstruction at the level of the larynx or trachea is not a diagnostic dilemma and should be met with prompt action. Patients will present with respiratory distress, changes in phonation, drooling, or stridor. In infants, if the patient is conscious but has signs and symptoms of complete upper airway obstruction and is not protecting their airway, then initiate five back blows followed by five chest compressions. In children, abdominal thrusts should be used for the same presentation. To do so, reach around the child's waist, place one closed fist just above the umbilicus, then place the other hand over the fist, and quickly pull up and back under the rib cage multiple times.

The most common cause of cardiac arrest in children is respiratory arrest. If a patient arrives in arrest or becomes unresponsive cardiopulmonary resuscitation should be initiated. If the arrest is secondary to aspiration, the priority is to secure the airway. Extraction should be made with McGill forceps, pick-ups, and the aid of a laryngoscope for improved visualization. If unsuccessful, intubate the child and advance the endotracheal tube deeply to push the foreign body into the right main bronchus. If unable to intubate a child, perform a needle cricothyrotomy with jet ventilation, if the child is <8 years old, or a surgical cricothyroidotomy to ventilate the patient below the obstruction.

Lower Airway Obstruction

In contrast to upper airway obstructions, foreign bodies in the lower respiratory tract can be difficult to diagnose. Patients present with common signs and symptoms that overlap many conditions including shortness of breath, wheezing, drooling, and cough. Bronchial foreign bodies are commonly misdiagnosed as asthma, croup, or pneumonia. When lower respiratory tract foreign bodies are not diagnosed, there can be significant complications including chronic cough, shortness of breath, frequent infections, and worsening respiratory distress. Classically, patients with a bronchial foreign body will have a cough, wheezing, or a focal decrease in breath sounds, but these are not reliable to rule out aspiration. With the child who you suspect or want to evaluate for a lower respiratory tract foreign body, imaging should be included in the work up. Two-view chest radiographs should be obtained to look for evidence of a foreign body. Signs including lung hyperinflation, atelectasis, and lung asymmetry may be seen even when no radiopaque foreign body is visualized. Even if imaging studies are nondiagnostic, clinicians should maintain a high index of suspicion for foreign body aspiration and consult otolaryngology or pulmonology for evaluation and bronchoscopy. Chest radiographs cannot rule out aspiration, and foreign body may only be visualized in up to 50% of aspiration cases. Children under 3 years of age are at higher risk for delayed, missed diagnosis of foreign body aspiration as they are unable to provide adequate history. Therefore, relying on the parent's and caregiver's history is vital.

KEY POINTS

- If the story fits for aspiration, bronchoscopy is indicated even with negative imaging studies.
- Think about foreign body aspiration in patients not responding to typical treatment.
- Reach for McGill forceps for complete upper airway obstruction.
- Secure the airway! If you cannot extract the aspirated foreign body from an arresting patient, right main stem intubation and needle or surgical cricothyroidotomy may be indicated.

Suggested Readings

Digoy GP. Diagnosis and management of upper aerodigestive tract foreign bodies. *Otolaryngol Clin N Am.* 2008;41:485.

Fox S. Delayed diagnosis of aspirated foreign body. https://pedemmorsels.com/delayed-diagnosis-aspirated-foreign-body/. Accessed July 16, 2014.

Rosbe KW, Burke K. Foreign bodies. In: Lalwani AK, ed. *Current Diagnosis & Treatment in Otolaryngology—Head & Neck Surgery.* 3rd ed. New York, NY: McGraw-Hill; 2012.

Soon AW, Schmidt S. Foreign body: ingestion and aspiration. In: Fleisher GR, Ludwig S, eds. *Fleisher & Ludwig's Textbook of Pediatric Emergency Medicine.* 7th ed. Philadelphia, PA: Lippincott Williams & Wilkins: 2015.

Do Not Treat Detergent Pods Like Any Other Type of Ingestion

Rajesh Sood, MD, FAAP and Minal Amin, MD, FAAEM

Laundry detergent pods represent a serious potential harm to children. Unlike traditional laundry detergent, highly concentrated pods can result in catastrophic injury and even death. Toddlers are particularly susceptible as they are more likely to place small objects in their mouths. Several cases of intentional ingestions by teenagers have also been documented. Packets may rupture and release an injurious substance into the oropharynx when ingested. Toxic effects from ingestion include central nervous system (CNS) depression, respiratory compromise, and mucosal injury. Emergency providers should be aware of these effects to assist with early recognition and prompt intervention in cases of known ingestion and in patients with altered mental status of unknown origin.

Introduced to the United States in 2010, detergent pods have become increasingly popular. Composed of highly concentrated laundry detergent encased in a water-soluble membrane, they are often bright and colorful and may appear harmless to children. Common routes of exposure include oral, ocular, and dermal. Compared with ingestion of traditional detergents, ingestions of laundry detergent pods are associated with worse clinical outcomes. The mechanism behind this difference is not well understood but may be related to compounds such as propylene glycol and ethoxylated alcohols that are present in higher amounts in detergent pods.

A sudden onset of lethargy with CNS depression can occur with ingestion of detergent pods. Apnea, hypoventilation, decreased cough, and decrease in gag reflexes can result. Rapid deterioration often requires urgent intubation and can last for several days. Patients who ingest detergent pods should be monitored closely for neurologic deterioration or seizures.

Mucosal injury occurs as the alkaline contents of detergent pods come into contact with the structures within the oropharynx. This results in edema of upper airway structures leading to obstruction and respiratory compromise. Additionally, sedation and decreased airway reflexes can lead to aspiration, further compromising respiratory function. Clinicians should monitor patients closely for signs of respiratory failure and be prepared for intubation. Racemic epinephrine and oral steroids may be useful in upper airway obstruction, and chest radiography should be used if aspiration pneumonia or esophageal perforation is suspected. Tracheal intubation should be considered for patients with a Glasgow coma score of <8.

Mucosal injury to oral and esophageal structures may result in dysphagia. Activated charcoal, neutralizing, or diluting substances should not be administered. Vomiting may be an initial symptom after ingestion and can be severe enough to cause metabolic derangements. Patients with a suspected pod ingestion should be made nothing by mouth (NPO) and placed on maintenance intravenous fluids with electrolyte abnormalities assessed regularly and corrected as needed. If oral mucosal injury or esophageal impaction is suspected, a gastrointestinal specialist should be consulted. The effects of ingestion may not be apparent until weeks later as inflammation and tissue reconstruction occur.

Ocular exposure to detergent pods can result in severe corneal abrasions or ocular burns. If ocular exposure is suspected, careful inspection and immediate decontamination should be performed to avoid prolonging chemical injury. Ocular pH and fluorescein staining to identify corneal abrasion should be performed. Immediate consultation with an ophthalmologist is indicated.

Providers should educate patients and families on the safe keeping of detergents around the house. Detergent pods should be kept in a secure container and out of sight of children. If ingestion is suspected, rapid assessment of ABCs and observation in the emergency room or hospital is warranted.

KEY POINTS

- Closely monitor GCS and respiratory status of patients with suspected ingestion due to risk of airway compromise.
- Make the patient NPO immediately and began IV fluid resuscitation especially if profound vomiting occurs.
- Avoid activated charcoal, neutralizing, or diluting substances.
- Educate patients and families about the risks of detergent pods and how to properly store in the household.

Suggested Readings

Health Hazards Associated with Laundry Detergent Pods—United States, May–June 2012. *Centers for Disease Control and Prevention.* Centers for Disease Control and Prevention; October 19, 2012. www.cdc.gov/mmwr/preview/mmwrhtml/mm6141a1.htm.

Shah LW. Ingestion of laundry detergent packets in children. *Critical Care Nurse.* 2016;36(4):70-75. doi:10.4037/ccn2016233.

Stromberg PE, et al. Airway compromise in children exposed to single-use laundry detergent pods: a poison center observational case series. *Am J Emerg Med.* 2015;33(3):349-351. doi:10.1016/j.ajem.2014.11.044.

Valdez AL, Casavant MJ. Pediatric exposure to laundry detergent pods. *Pediatrics.* 2014;134(6):1127-1135. doi:10.1542/peds.2014-0057d.

Not Appreciating "Recurrent Croup" to Be a Clinical Sign of Anatomic Airway Anomalies

Minal Amin, MD, FAAEM

Emergency physicians routinely manage the patient with stridor as if it is croup and, most of the time, treat it easily. While the most common cause of acute stridor and respiratory distress (with or without fever) is viral, some patients will have other important etiologies to consider. The spectrum of pediatric abnormalities that result in stridor is broad so it is important to maintain a high index of suspicion to correctly determine the cause.

Etiology: Is It Congenital, Infectious, or Traumatic?

The most common causes of stridor can be broken down into congenital, infectious, and traumatic causes.

Children with congenital anatomic obstruction of the trachea present with recurrent stridor and upper airway obstruction. In the neonate, choanal atresia, laryngeal webs, vocal cord paralysis, subglottic stenosis, tracheal stenosis, and tracheoesophageal fistulas may present with stridor, feeding difficulties, aspiration, or failure to thrive. In patients with a history of tracheoesophageal repair, tracheomalacia is a common complication.

Laryngomalacia is the most common cause of stridor in infants, and most will outgrow this by 18 months of age. It is usually managed expectantly and rarely surgically, but it may mask symptoms from another cause. Anatomical obstruction of the trachea is frequently the result of tracheal compression from an enlarged adjacent vessel. A double aortic arch, an aberrant pulmonary artery, and a dilated pulmonary artery from pulmonary valve atresia can all cause stridor. Although rare, a persistent right aortic arch or double aortic arch can result in a complete vascular ring and place pressure on both the trachea and esophagus, leading to stridor and dysphagia. When "croup" is recurrent in a pediatric patient older than 2 years of age, congenital or anatomical abnormalities must be considered.

Subglottic stenosis does not always present at birth and may be discovered when an infant has a viral illness in the first several months of life. Conversely, airway hemangiomas cause symptoms within the first few months of life due to their rapid growth but, fortunately, then recede after the first year of life. Other considerations include laryngeal clefts, webs, tracheal papillomas, and neoplasms that will require fiberoptic laryngoscopy or bronchoscopy to diagnose.

Of the self-limiting viral causes of laryngotracheobronchitis or "croup," most are due to parainfluenza virus and occur in the preschool population. Viral croup does not occur more than twice a year, usually in the fall and winter. Bacterial causes of stridor have declined dramatically due to vaccine introduction. Diphtheria, once a fatal cause of "pseudomembranous croup," has mostly been eradicated. Prior to the advent of the *Haemophilus influenzae* B (Hib) vaccine (early 1990s), epiglottitis was a major cause of morbidity and mortality in children. Epiglottitis caused by Hib typically presents with fever, stridor, and drooling. Sporadic cases are still reported due to vaccine noncompliance or atypical strains. Vaccine compliance should therefore no longer be assumed. Tonsillitis, either viral or bacterial, can result in inflamed, enlarged tonsils and can be an acute cause of stridor in young children. If large enough, a retropharyngeal abscess can also result in enough narrowing of the laryngeal space to cause stridor.

Traumatic causes of stridor include swallowed or aspirated foreign bodies, laryngeal fracture, and caustic ingestions (eg, detergent pod aspiration or ingestion). Although rare, simple nasogastric tube placement can also cause stridor even without known airway compromise.

Recommended initial evaluation includes focused history and examination, chest radiograph, and esophagrams for congenital abnormalities and clinical acumen for infectious etiologies. Appropriate referral for fiberoptic evaluation when subglottic abnormalities are suspected is reasonable to help avoid continuing to mislabel the patient as having "recurrent croup."

KEY POINTS

- Maintain a high index of suspicion for other etiologies of stridor.
  - In newborns, consider nasopharyngeal causes.
  - In infants, consider anatomic causes.
  - In older children, consider foreign bodies and traumatic/caustic causes.
- Persistent or recurrent stridor should precipitate a thorough diagnostic workup.
- For infants under 6 months of age or children older than 3 years of age, *recurrent* croup is a diagnosis of exclusion, especially when unresponsive to standard treatment.
- Remember to ask specifically about vaccine compliance.

Suggested Readings

Balfour-Lynn IM, Wright M. Acute infections that produce upper airway obstruction. In: Wilmott RW, Deterding R, Li A, Ratjen F, Sly P, Zar HJ, Bush A, eds. *Kendig's Disorders of the Respiratory Tract in Children*. 9th ed. Elsevier, Inc.; 2019:406-419.

Nayak G, Virk RS, Singh M, Singh M. Nasogastric tube syndrome: a diagnostic dilemma. *J Bronchology Interv Pulmonol*. 2018;25(4):343-345.

Stromberg PE, Burt MH, et al. Airway compromise in children exposed to single-use laundry detergent pods: a poison center observational case series. *Am J Emerg Med*. 2015;33:349-351.

Not Having a Strategy in Place to Manage the Patient With a Posttonsillectomy Hemorrhage

Mahnoosh Nik-Ahd, MD, MPH and Andrea Fang, MD

Primary posttonsillectomy bleeding is defined as bleeding that occurs in the first 24 hours after the tonsillectomy. It is often related to incomplete ligation or coagulation of blood vessels. Secondary bleeding accounts for nearly all bleeding posttonsillectomy patients and usually occurs 5-7 days after the procedure; however, patients can hemorrhage at any time. Secondary bleeding is generally due to clot and eschar sloughing.

Children >6 years old are at higher risk for requiring interventions to achieve hemostasis. Even minor bleeding that has resolved by the time of presentation to the emergency department (ED) can be a harbinger of a severe bleed within 24 hours. We must remain vigilant despite these patients' initial well appearance.

History

Focus on the volume of blood lost, bleeding duration, number of bleeding episodes, date of surgery, time of last oral intake, and whether it was a tonsillectomy or tonsillotomy. In addition, inquire if the patient has or is at risk for a bleeding disorder. Send testing when appropriate and consider giving von Willebrand factor, desmopressin, platelets, or fresh frozen plasma.

Initial Assessment

Posttonsillectomy hemorrhage can be severe and lead to significant complications including hematemesis, pulmonary aspiration, severe anemia, and hypovolemic shock. Focus on obtaining hemodynamic stability, protecting the airway, and controlling active bleeding during your initial assessment. If you see active bleeding, a clot, or oozing in the oropharynx, the patient likely requires operative management, and a pediatric otolaryngologist should be consulted.

Management

If the patient is hemodynamically stable, use a good light source to inspect for clot formation and oozing in the tonsillar fossa. If an object such as a tongue depressor is used, try to prevent further oral trauma and do not inducing coughing or touch the surgical site. In an older patient, consider having the patient sit and hold an age-appropriate Macintosh laryngoscope blade in his or her own mouth to move the tongue out of the way and provide a bright light source.

Active bleeding should be considered a surgical emergency, and operative management is the definitive treatment for life-threatening bleeds. Consult pediatric otolaryngology immediately. For life-threatening bleeds, activate your institution's massive transfusion protocol. Obtain intravenous (IV) or intraosseous (IO) access if necessary. Volume resuscitate with isotonic saline, and transfuse with blood products.

If there is active bleeding and the patient is awake, keep the patient upright and leaning forward or in the lateral decubitus position. If the patient is able to tolerate direct pressure without vomiting, then direct pressure techniques are the best initial steps. Use suction or gauze to remove any clot or blood and gain better visualization. Use Magill forceps with folded gauze soaked in epinephrine (1:10 000), lidocaine 1% with epinephrine (1:100 000), topical thrombin, or tranexamic acid.

In patients who develop altered mental status or whom cannot tolerate direct pressure techniques, consider sedation with ketamine and rapid sequence intubation with video laryngoscopy when available. Call for anesthesia in anticipation of a difficult airway. Additional large-bore suction catheters and a backup laryngeal mask airway (LMA) should be available. After intubation, use surgical packing that is bulky and radiopaque to maintain direct pressure on the bleeding tonsillar fossa until the patient can go to surgery.

KEY POINTS

- Posttonsillectomy bleeding can be a life-threatening surgical emergency. Most patients present 5-7 days post procedure.
- Even a minor bleed that has stopped can be a harbinger of a serious bleed in the next 24 hours. Observe or admit these patients.
- Focus your initial assessment on hemodynamic stability, the airway, and active bleeding. If any of these are concerning, consulting pediatric otolaryngology immediately, get access, volume resuscitate, and consider your institution's massive transfusion protocol.
- Attempt direct pressure techniques with Magill forceps and gauze soaked in a vasoconstricting or hemostatic agent.
- Anticipate a difficult airway—have an LMA and large-bore suction section ready; call for anesthesia.

Suggested Readings

Fields RG, Gencorelli FJ, Litman RS. Anesthetic management of the pediatric bleeding tonsil. *Pediatr Anesth.* 2010;20(11):982-986.

Isaacson G. Tonsillectomy care for the pediatrician. *Pediatrics.* 2012;130(2):324-334.

Peterson J, Losek JD. Post-tonsillectomy hemorrhage and pediatric emergency care. *Clin Pediatr.* 2004;43(5):445-448.

Sarny S, Ossimitz G, Habermann W, Stammberger H. Hemorrhage following tonsil surgery: a multicenter prospective study. *Laryngoscope.* 2011;121(12):2553-2560.

Wall JJ, Tay KY. Postoperative tonsillectomy hemorrhage. *Emerg Med Clin North Am.* 2018;36(2):415-426.

47

Attempting to Close Every Intraoral Laceration

Katie Rebillot, DO and Kelly D. Young, MD, MS

Intraoral lacerations in children occur mostly in a trauma, fall, or seizure. They occur more commonly in boys; the mean age of presentation is 4 years old. Primary complications include hemorrhage, airway obstruction, and tongue dysfunction. The most common tongue laceration location is the anterior dorsal tongue, followed by middle dorsal and anterior ventral. Posterior lacerations are uncommon and should prompt a search for other injuries and foreign bodies.

When assessing a patient with an oral laceration, address hemostasis and evaluate the airway promptly. Assess for foreign bodies that may obstruct the airway, such as teeth, tissue fragments, or Popsicle sticks. In the setting of trauma, explore the cranial, facial, and neck regions for associated injury. Following stabilization, an appropriate examination includes the tongue, sublingual space, buccal mucosa, soft/hard palates, posterior pharynx, and dentition. It is best to inspect the tongue at rest within the mouth, without protrusion or activity, as this is its usual state.

Many lingual lacerations do not require primary closure and will heal spontaneously due to the rich lingual artery vasculature, usually within 3-5 days. Spontaneous healing also decreases risk of infection or sedation complications. Repair, however, may help food manipulation, swallowing, and speech articulation. There are a few types of lacerations commonly accepted to benefit from primary closure. These include lacerations with persistent bleeding, tongue bisection, gaping wound at rest, wounds involving tongue margins, and lacerations larger than 2 cm. Young children may require procedural sedation, and risks and benefits of sedation vs spontaneous healing should be considered. Closure with 2-octyl cyanoacrylate (ie, Dermabond) has been reported as an alternative.

Two main approaches to analgesia are procedural sedation and local anesthesia. For simple lacerations, lidocaine 1% with epinephrine may be used with caution; significantly swollen tissue margins can be distorted with local infiltration. Another option is lidocaine 4% soaked gauze or topical paste directly applied to the laceration for 10 minutes. For complex lacerations requiring more time, regional blocks, such as inferior alveolar nerve block, which numbs the anterior two-thirds of the tongue, or lingual nerve block, and procedural sedation are options. To facilitate repair, keep the field dry with gauze or a suction catheter. Gauze pads placed in mucosal and sublingual spaces force tongue protrusion for better visualization and repair. A temporary suture is sometimes placed through the anterior tongue for an assistant to pull the tongue forward for better access. Closure with an absorbable suture material, such as 4.0 or 5.0 chromic gut, in simple interrupted pattern allows for easy healing and eliminates need for removal. Prophylactic antibiotics offer no proven benefits and are not recommended.

Intraoral lacerations elsewhere (gums, buccal mucosa) also often do not require repair, and indications for repair are similar to lingual (ie, widely gaping). Examine closely for salivary gland duct injury, and complications such as partial lingual amputation, fragmented dentition, and jaw fracture, which should prompt evaluation and management by the appropriate specialists. If foreign body or aspiration is suspected, securing definitive airway may be required. Special attention should be given to patients with bleeding disorders, in which a simple laceration can be life threatening. These patients should be managed concurrently with hematology and may require factor placement prior to repair, as well as aminocaproic acid or topical tranexamic acid.

All patients with simple intraoral lacerations, regardless of primary or secondary closure, should be discharged with instructions to follow a soft diet, and follow-up with primary care doctor in 5-7 days. Use of chlorhexidine rinses is recommended. For complex repairs or function loss, follow-up should be given to specialists or occupational therapy.

KEY POINTS

- Posterior lingual lacerations are uncommon and should elicit evaluation for concomitant injuries.
- Most tongue lacerations do not require repair, because the tongue is highly vascularized.
- Indications for repair include persistent bleeding, tongue bisection, gaping wound at rest, wounds involving tongue margins, and lacerations larger than 2 cm.
- Simple lacerations can be repaired with local anesthetic techniques; complex lacerations may warrant nerve blocks or procedural sedation.
- Chlorhexidine rinse for use as instructed should be considered for all intraoral lacerations.

Suggested Readings

Brown D, Jaffe J, Henson H. Advanced laceration management. *Emerg Med Clinics N Am.* 2007;25(1):83-99.
Das UM, Gadicherla P. Lacerated tongue injury in children. *Int J Clin Pediatr Dent.* 2008;1(1):39-41.
Kazzi MG, Silverberg M. Pediatric tongue laceration repair using 2-octyl cyanoacrylate (Dermabond®). *J Emerg Med.* 2013;45(6):846-848.
Seiler M, Massaro SL, Staubli G, et al. Tongue lacerations in children: to suture or not? *Swiss Med Wkly.* 2018;148:14683.

Thinking Ludwig Angina Only Happens in Adults

Jasmin England, MD, FAAP

Primary teeth typically first arrive after 6 months of life, while permanent teeth begin to erupt at after 6 years of age. Tooth enamel is hard and cannot regenerate. It overlies dentin, which can regenerate (Fig. 48.1). Dentin is pale yellow and protects the pink vascular pulp from caries or injury. The root uses the periodontal ligament to help attach it to the deeper alveolar bone. The submandibular lymph nodes are what drain dental infections.

Types of Dental-Associated Infections

Biofilms (plaque) are microorganisms encased in an extracellular matrix. *Streptococcus mutans* is associated with caries and is especially prevalent with frequent exposure to dietary sugars. **Dental caries** begin as a white chalky spot on the tooth (reversible) and progress to a brown-black discoloration (irreversible) that eventually results in the destruction of enamel and dentin, which is when this disease becomes painful or, at least, thermosensitive. It can progress to deeper infections such as pulpitis. Fluoride, good oral hygiene, and a low-sugar diet prevent caries formation. Dental caries can be managed as an outpatient by a dentist, though patients with exposed dentin, pulp, or root should have more expedited follow-up.

Periapical abscesses (associated with nonviable teeth) occur if pulpitis progresses into a pocket of localized pus appearing as a fluctuant mass over the adjacent gingiva. This is a clinical diagnosis. Incision and drainage is the definitive treatment after good anesthesia either by local bupivacaine or an appropriate nerve block. Antibiotics are not required for uncomplicated cases. Twenty-four-hour follow-up with a dentist is indicated.

Ludwig angina is a rapid spreading infection of the submandibular (specifically the sublingual and submylohyoid) space. It typically results from an infected 2nd or 3rd mandibular molar. While young children do not yet have their molars, it is incorrect to assume that they cannot develop Ludwig angina as it can develop from an inciting deep space neck infection. Ludwig angina has been reported

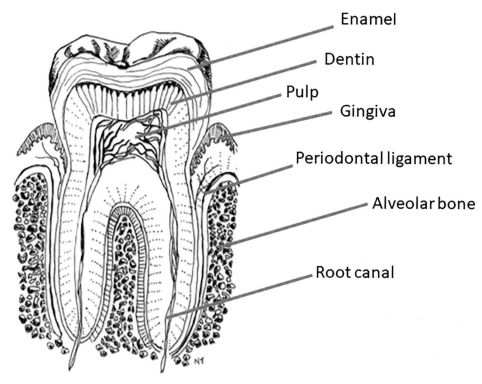

Enamel

Dentin

Pulp

Gingiva

Periodontal ligament

Alveolar bone

Root canal

FIGURE 48.1 Tooth Anatomy

in infants as young as 12 days old. It presents as a rapidly spreading cellulitis, typically without abscess formation. Subsequent posterior tongue displacement and spread to retropharyngeal space and can lead to asphyxia making the diagnosis a clinical emergency. Initial management includes consideration of an early intubation with possible nasotracheal intubation and early subspecialist consultation for a possible fiberoptic or surgical airway. Patients typically require a contrast computed tomography (CT) for evaluating the extent of infection, and they must all be admitted for intravenous antibiotics that cover gram-positive (ie, streptococcus mutans) and gram-negative anaerobic (ie, peptostreptococcus and *Capnocytophaga*) oral flora. Ampicillin-sulbactam or clindamycin would be appropriate first-line agents with the addition of vancomycin for sick patients.

Lemierre syndrome is another important consideration. It is a thrombophlebitis of the internal jugular vein from surrounding infected structures; a reported 4% originates from odontogenic infections. It is a difficult diagnosis especially as septic microemboli spread throughout the body, but it may begin with a swollen or painful neck, fevers, and headache. Similar imaging and admission for IV antibiotics is necessary as with Ludwig angina. A vascular surgeon needs to be involved if there is ongoing sepsis despite antibiotics.

KEY POINTS

- Patients with an infection of the pulp or root or a dental abscess should follow up with a dentist within 48 hours.
- Ludwig angina can occur in children, even though they lack molars.
- Submandibular swelling and tenderness suggestive of Ludwig angina is an airway emergency. It requires prompt consult with an otolaryngologist, broad-spectrum antibiotics, and inpatient admission.

Suggested Readings

DeAngelis AF, Barrowman R, Harrod R, Nastri AL. Review article: Maxillofacial emergencies: oral pain and odon-togenic infections. *Emerg Med Austral.* 2014;26(4):336-342. doi:10.1111/1742-6723.12266.

Nguyen DH, Martin JT. Common dental infections in the primary care setting. *Am Fam Physician.* 2008;77(6):797-802.

Pedigo R. Dental emergences: management strategies that improve outcomes. *Emerg Med Practice.* 2017;19:1-24.

Robertson DP, Keys W, Rautemaa-Richardson R, et al. Management of severe acute dental infections. *BMJ.* 2015;350:h1300.

Stephens MB, Wiedemer JP, Kushner GM. Dental problems in primary care. *Am Fam Physician.* 2018;98(11):654-660.

Overlooking Simple Strategies to Manage Pain Related to a Dry Socket

Jennifer K. Potter, MD and Sarah N. Weihmiller, MD, FAAP

Alveolar osteitis, commonly known as dry socket, is most frequently treated in dental offices; however, these patients may present to the pediatric emergency department after hours. It is an important dental complication that should not be overlooked by emergency medicine providers. To diagnose dry socket, there must be visible dislodgement of blood clot with bone exposure. Additionally, the pain must present between 1 and 3 days postextraction and occur at the site of extraction. Risk factors for dry socket include smoking, preexisting infection, traumatic extraction, and oral contraceptives.

Recognition of dry socket is key to appropriate treatment. The most common presentation in pediatrics is a patient who presents to the emergency department (ED) in severe pain. The pain occurs at the extraction site and is often described as throbbing, with radiation to the ear. It initially improves after leaving the dentist's office and then suddenly worsens. Dry socket is most common after third molar extractions and in patients >12 years old.

On physical examination, the extraction site will show a fully or partially dislodged clot and exposed alveolar bone. A foul odor may or may not be present. The diagnosis can be confirmed by irrigating the socket with warm saline; the pain will increase if dry socket is present. With severe dental pain, other etiologies to consider include foreign body, retained root tip, osteomyelitis, subperiosteal abscess, trismus, and osteonecrosis. If foreign body, retained root tip, or osteomyelitis are high on the differential, consider obtaining radiographs.

Treatment of dry socket in the ED should be focused on pain control, irrigation, and packing of the extraction site. First, provide optimal anesthesia with a dental block using a local anesthetic such as lidocaine without epinephrine. Next, irrigate the socket using a 60-cc irrigation syringe filled with warm saline to remove debris. Suction should be placed on low to prevent dislodging any remaining clot. The final step, packing the socket, is the key to providing pain relief. There are several commercially available products, including Dry Socket Paste and Dressol-X. Pastes last longer than ribbon gauze packing and are easier to apply. If these products are not available, packing materials can be created from items commonly found in the ED. Iodoform gauze can be soaked in 0.5% lidocaine, or Gelfoam sponges can be soaked in 160 mg of tranexamic acid (TXA). To secure the packing material, place a Gelfoam cap on top of the packing and have the patient bite down on a 2 × 2 gauze. In a calm patient with adequate analgesia, consider placing a figure-of-8 suture at the superior aspect of the socket over the Gelfoam cap to secure.

The disposition for patients with dry socket is home with close follow-up by the dentist. NSAIDs should provide adequate pain control; opioids are rarely necessary. Antibiotics for dry socket alone are neither supported nor refuted in the literature. Patients or their parents should be instructed to arrange immediate follow-up with the provider who extracted the tooth. Packing placed in the ED will need to be replaced every 24-48 hours, either in the office or the ED. The patient should be instructed to eat a soft diet and to avoid hot or cold substances, using straws, gargling, spitting, smoking, and manipulating the packing with their tongue.

KEY POINTS

- Occurs 1-3 days after extraction.
- Rare in patients <12 years old.
- Recognition is key; there is no consensus on prevention.
- Treatment includes analgesia, irrigation, and alveolar packing.

Suggested Readings

Beaudreau RW. Oral and dental emergencies. In: Tintinalli JE, Stapczynski J, Ma O, et al., eds. *Tintinalli's Emergency Medicine: A Comprehensive Study Guide*. 8th ed. New York, NY: McGraw-Hill; 2016. http://accessemergencymedicine.mhmedical.com.libproxy.lib.unc.edu/content.aspx? bookid=1658&sectioned=109444613. January 24, 2019.

Faizel S, et al. Comparison between neocone, alvogyl and zinc oxide packing for treatment of dry socket: a double-blind randomized control trial. *J Maxillofac Oral Surg*. 2015;14:312-320.

Mamoun J. Dry socket etiology, diagnosis, and clinical treatment techniques. *J Korean Assoc Oral Maxillofac Surg*. 2018;44:52-58.

Reichman EF. Post-extraction pain and dry socket (alveolar osteitis) management. In: Reichman EF, ed. *Reichman's Emergency Medicine Procedures*. 3rd ed. New York, NY: McGraw-Hill; 2019. http://accessemergencymedicine.mhmedical.com.libproxy.lib.unc.edu/content.aspx? bookid=2498&sectionid=201302787. Accessed January 24, 2019.

Dismissing Sialadenitis as a Simple Infection and Throwing Antibiotics at It

Zachary T. Burroughs, MD, FAAP

Anatomy and Physiology

The major salivary glands secrete saliva to facilitate taste, lubrication, and digestion of food. Saliva also provides tooth integrity and antibiotic properties. Three major pairs of salivary glands exist: parotid, submandibular, and sublingual. Saliva travels through the salivary glands via a network of ducts. Stensen duct (parotid gland) drains into the rear of the mouth near the second upper molar, and Wharton duct (submandibular gland) drains along the floor of the mouth near the frenulum of the tongue. The sublingual glands utilize multiple smaller ducts.

Sialadenitis

Sialadenitis is thought to be multifactorial in nature. A cycle of inflammation has been described of decreased salivary flow causing inflammation leading to ductal dysfunction and then increased mucinous saliva. Dehydration, infection, structural abnormalities, and immune factors are known predisposing factors. Bacterial and viral infections are more common in the parotid gland, while sialolithiasis is more common in the submandibular gland. Viral pathogens more commonly cause infectious sialadenitis than bacterial pathogens, with mumps historically being most common. Vaccination has led to a marked decline in mumps, but this still remains a cause in children. Systemic symptoms differentiate mumps from other causes of sialadenitis. A prodrome of fever, headache, and malaise is seen with subsequent development of sialadenitis. Other viral pathogens leading to sialadenitis include Epstein-Barr virus, parainfluenza virus, and HIV. Bilateral parotid gland involvement should lead one to strongly consider HIV as a cause. Bacterial pathogens causing sialadenitis include *Staphylococcus aureus*, *Streptococcus viridans*, *Haemophilus influenzae*, *Peptostreptococcus* species, *Streptococcus pneumoniae*, *Escherichia coli*, and *Bacteroides*. Sialadenitis due to sialolithiasis is uncommon in children and most often involves the submandibular gland. Other causes of sialadenitis include radiation and direct trauma.

Diagnosis

Acute sialadenitis presents with fever as well as swelling, pain, and erythema overlying the affected gland. Symptoms are typically unilateral. Patients often experience trismus and pain with mastication and swallowing. Erythema and edema are often present at the ductal opening of the affected gland, and purulence can sometimes be expressed. Diagnosis is typically clinical but can be assisted by ultrasound, computed tomography scan, or sialendoscopy in certain cases.

Chronic sialadenitis requires special consideration in the pediatric population as this can be associated with immune deficiencies and autoimmune disorders such as HIV, IgA deficiency, Sjögren syndrome, juvenile rheumatoid arthritis, sarcoidosis, and ulcerative colitis. In some cases, swelling or enlargement of the parotid gland can be due to a parotid mass such as adenomas, hemangiomas, and carcinomas.

Juvenile recurrent parotitis (JRP) is seen as a separate clinical entity and is thought to be second only to mumps as a cause of salivary disease in children worldwide. JRP is defined as recurrent episodes of inflammation and/or infection of the parotid gland without a definite etiology. JRP typically occurs between the ages of 3 and 6 and can be seen again at the onset of puberty. A slight male predominance has been seen with JRP. Diagnosis of JRP is clinical, and sialendoscopy is an effective means of diagnosis and management.

Management

Acute sialadenitis is managed with oral antibiotics, analgesics, hydration, sialogogues, and warm massages. Amoxicillin/clavulanate is first-line empiric therapy. For patients with a penicillin allergy, clindamycin may be used. In applicable cases, Gram stain and culture should be sent from purulent material expressed from the duct. Patients with systemic symptoms such as fever or leukocytosis may benefit from IV antibiotics. Surgical options for management include stone retrieval, lithotripsy, gland excision (less common), or sialendoscopy. Acute sialadenitis of JRP is self-limiting, but treatment is often as above for acute exacerbations. Newer evidence supports sialendoscopy as a means to reduce both acute exacerbations and in preventing future attacks on a long-term basis.

KEY POINTS

- Sialadenitis is often multifactorial, and antibiotics may not always be the answer.
- Viral and juvenile recurrent parotitis are the two most common etiologies of sialadenitis in children.
- Recurrent sialadenitis warrants referral to a specialist.

Suggested Readings

Francis CL, Larsen CG. Pediatric sialadenitis. *Otolaryngol Clin North Am.* 2014;47(5):763-778.
Orvidas LJ, Kasperbauer JL, Lewis JE, Olsen KD, Lesnick TG. Pediatric parotid masses. *Arch Otolaryngol Head Neck Surg.* 2000;126(2):177-184.
Patel A, Karlis V. Diagnosis and management of pediatric salivary gland infections. *Oral Maxillofac Surg Clin North Am.* 2009;21(3):345-352.
Ramakrishna J, Strychowsky J, Gupta M, Sommer DD. Sialendoscopy for the management of juvenile recurrent parotitis: a systematic review and meta-analysis. *Laryngoscope.* 2015;125(6):1472-1479.

Do Not Forget About the Secondary Teeth While Managing a Primary Tooth Injury

Moon O. Lee, MD, MPH, FACEP

Almost half of the emergency department visits for dental complaints in children <6 years old are associated with an injury. Trauma to the primary teeth must be taken care of in a timely fashion due to the time sensitive nature of injuries. Injuries to the primary teeth may affect the underlying permanent teeth buds that can lead to malformation or discoloration, impacted teeth, and eruption disturbances. Primary teeth begin to erupt by 6-10 months of age, and most will erupt by 3 years of age. The 20 primary teeth will then shed between 6 and 12 years of age.

Types of Dental Injuries

Understanding the types of dental injuries helps guide the care that needs to be provided.

- **Concussion** is a tooth that has tenderness to touch and has normal mobility.
- **Subluxation** is a tooth with increased mobility but is not displaced.
- **Extrusive luxation** is a partial displacement of the tooth out of the socket and can be excessively mobile.
- **Lateral luxation** is a displaced tooth and will be immobile.
- **Intrusive luxation** is a displaced tooth through the alveolar ridge and can impinge upon the permanent tooth bud.
- **Avulsion** is a tooth that is completely out of the socket.
- **Fractures** are classified based on the location and can involve the enamel, dentin, pulp, root, and/ or alveolar bone.

Diagnosis

In the emergency department, dental radiographs are not usually available. Some emergency departments are able to perform a panoramic dental radiograph (panorex). A panorex can provide information about injuries and the underlying permanent tooth buds. However, given the superficial nature of most dental injuries, the panorex is not crucial. Facial or chest radiographs should be obtained to locate a missing tooth fragment that may have been aspirated or displaced into the soft tissue. If there is clinical concern for an alveolar bone fracture, consider obtaining a facial CT. The face is one of the most frequently injured part of the body in child abuse cases and should be considered in assessing children with intraoral trauma.

Treatment

In the emergency department, treatment of primary teeth injuries is supportive care. Dental concussions, luxations, intrusions, and fractures without exposed pulp are managed conservatively with pain control, soft diet, and urgent dental follow-up. For primary teeth with extrusive luxation with increased mobility, you may consider extracting to tooth depending on the aspiration risk. Unlike permanent teeth, avulsed primary teeth should not be re-implanted back into the socket. Primary teeth with exposed dentin should repaired urgently by the dentist but do not need to be immediately covered in the emergency department. Dental fractures with exposed pulp should have a calcium hydroxide paste applied over the pulp, and the patient will need follow-up with a dentist within 24 hours.

Routine use of oral antibiotics is not recommended in most dental injuries. In contrast to permanent teeth, primary teeth should only be splinted when there is an alveolar bone fracture or intra-alveolar root fractures.

In addition to pain control, parents will need to be counseled to provide good oral hygiene to help healing. Patients should use a soft toothbrush and apply alcohol-free 0.1% chlorhexidine gluconate on the affected area with a cotton swab twice a day for a week. Patients should eat a soft diet for 10 days, and younger children should not use an oral pacifier.

KEY POINTS

- Primary teeth injuries can affect permanent teeth development, but the treatment for most is supportive care.
- Do not re-implant avulsed primary teeth.
- Good discharge instructions for parents to provide good oral hygiene will improve healing.

Suggested Readings

American Dental Association. https://www.ada.org/en/~/media/ADA_Foundation/GKAS/Files/GKAS-Primary-Tooth-Eruption-Chart

Da Silva Assunção LR, Ferelle A, Iwakura ML, et al. Effects on permanent teeth after luxation injuries to the primary predecessors: a study in children assisted at an emergency service. *Dent Traumatol.* 2009;25(2):165-170.

Fisher-Owens SA, Lukefahr JL, Tate AR; American Academy of Pediatrics, Section on Oral Health; Committee on Child Abuse and Neglect; American Academy of Pediatric Dentistry, Council on Clinical Affairs, Council on Scientific Affairs; Ad hoc Work Group on Child Abuse and Neglect. Oral and dental aspects of child abuse and neglect. *Pediatrics.* 2017;140(2).

Lewis C, Lynch H, Johnston B. Dental complaints in emergency departments: a national perspective. *Ann Emerg Med.* 2003;42(1):93-99.

Malmgren B, Andreasen JO, Flores MT, et al. Guidelines for the management of traumatic dental injuries: 3. Injuries in the primary dentition. *Pediatr Dent.* 2017;39(6):420-428.

Focusing on Only the Teeth When There Is Dental Trauma

Michael Hrdy, MD and Simone L. Lawson, MD, FAAP

Introduction

Dental trauma is a common reason for presentation to the pediatric emergency department (ED). Up to 20% of American adolescents will experience trauma to their permanent teeth. While it is hard to miss the dramatic appearance of a completely avulsed or fractured tooth, it is important to perform a thorough evaluation to ensure that additional, potentially serious, injuries are not overlooked.

First Things First (Primary Survey)

A patient with dental trauma is a trauma patient, and ATLS principles apply. Evaluate the patient fully before focusing on the dental trauma. There may be airway obstruction due to an aspirated tooth or sublingual hematoma due to maxillofacial trauma. Breathing and circulation are less likely to be impacted in oral-facial trauma but should be rapidly assessed before evaluating for additional injuries. Once the primary survey is complete, move on to catalogue the patient's injuries. We recommend starting outside the mouth and working toward the known dental injuries.

Extraoral Examination

A general physical examination will help reveal injuries that may not be as immediately apparent as the dental trauma. Nonaccidental trauma is a potential cause of dental trauma, and a thorough skin examination may reveal concerning bruising patterns. Perform a meticulous examination of the head and neck, as rates of mandibular and maxillofacial fracture in patients with dental trauma can be as high as 23%. Evaluate the skull, midface, periorbital area, and the mandible for bony step-offs, point tenderness, or crepitus. Look for signs of a basilar skull fracture. A cranial nerve examination can reveal neurologic as well as some orbital pathology. Record any abrasions, lacerations, or other soft tissue injuries. Given the traumatic mechanism, also consider the potential for cervical spine injury. The risk of C-spine injury is significantly higher in patients with mandibular fracture.

Oral Examination

Begin by having the patient attempt to open and close the mouth. Difficulties opening the mouth suggest damage to the mandible or temporomandibular joint (TMJ). Subjective change in teeth contact when biting (malocclusion) is 96% specific for mandibular fracture. The tongue blade test, where the patient clenches a tongue depressor between the molars of one side of the mouth while the examiner attempts to remove the stick, can also be used to evaluate for mandibular fracture. Inability to keep the stick in the mouth on either side is deemed a positive result. The incidence of mandibular fracture is lower in young children than in adolescents, but if there is concern for fracture, the recommended imaging includes x-rays, a Panorex, or a CT scan depending on availability and the patient's ability to cooperate with the required positioning.

Next, evaluate the intraoral soft tissues for lacerations and abrasions. All oral lacerations should be examined for foreign bodies such as retained tooth fragments. Palpate along the gumline, evaluating for alveolar ridge fractures indicated by mobility of multiple contiguous teeth. Prescribe antibiotics with oral flora coverage in the case of open mandibular fracture (concurrent gingival bleeding or laceration).

Account for and evaluate each tooth for injury. In patients presenting for dental injury, if one tooth is injured, it is likely that another tooth is injured as well. If a tooth is missing, consider chest x-ray to evaluate for aspiration. Visualization of the teeth may reveal hairline cracks in the enamel (infraction), uncomplicated fractures through the white enamel (Ellis class I) or yellow dentin (Ellis class II), or complicated fractures exposing the reddish pulp (Ellis class III). Compare each tooth to its neighbors, as there may be movement into or out of the socket. Percuss and palpate each tooth to evaluate for tenderness and increased mobility.

KEY POINTS

- If one tooth is injured, there is an excellent chance another tooth is injured too.
- Think outside the mouth! Dental injuries are often associated with facial and mandibular fractures as well as C-spine injury.
- Percuss and palpate each tooth to help identify difficult to detect intraoral injuries.
- The tongue blade test is sensitive to rule out mandibular fracture, a potential complication of dental injury in children.

Suggested Readings

Hall E, Hickey P, Nguyen-Tran T, Louie J. Dental trauma in a Pediatric Emergency Department Referral Center. *Pediatr Emerg Care.* 2016;32(12):823-826.
Murray JM. Mandible fractures and dental trauma. *Emerg Med Clin North Am.* 2013;31(2):553-573.
Subramanian K, Chogle SM. Medical and orofacial considerations in traumatic dental injuries. *Dent Clin N Am.* 2009;53(4):617-626.

53

Not Thoroughly Evaluating Facial Fractures

Ioannis Koutroulis, MD, PhD, MBA and Angelica W. DesPain, MD

With any facial trauma, it is important to inspect the mouth and oral cavity to assess for an injury to the maxilla and/or mandible. Obtain a computed tomography (CT) scan or panoramic radiograph (ie, Panorex) if there is suspicion for mandibular or maxillary fractures. Single view x-rays do not adequately visualize fractures given adjacent bones and the U-shape of the mandible.

Maxilla Fracture

Maxillary fractures may manifest as contusions over the cheekbone, malocclusion, or enophthalmos. Examine the maxilla by grasping and trying to move the upper central teeth or alveolar ridge anteriorly and posteriorly while stabilizing the forehead with the opposite hand. Lacerations, a gap, or step-offs in the palate may indicate a maxillary fracture. A laceration or step-off at the upper alveolar ridge suggests a midface fracture.

Most maxilla fractures require high-energy impact and are associated with concomitant injuries, including soft tissue lacerations, facial fractures, concussions, and other neurologic injuries. Test cranial nerve V as an injury to the nerve may occur from facial lacerations. Complex fractures of the midface are classified using the Le Fort system. Classic findings of raccoon eyes and midface mobility support the diagnosis of a Le Fort fracture but may not always be present. Do not assume bilateral facial symmetry or conclude the examination after finding an injury as other injuries may be missed.

Mandibular Fracture

Mandibular fractures can present with facial bruising, swelling, malocclusion, chin and tongue lacerations, jaw protrusion to one side, tooth fractures, temporomandibular pain, pain with mastication, numbness of the lower lip and chin, or ear pain. Palpate the mandibular symphysis, body, angle, and ramus externally and intraorally. Malocclusion is an indication of mandibular or maxillary displacement. Ask if the patient's bite feels normal. Inability to hold a tongue blade between occluded teeth on either side is suggestive of a mandibular fracture. Preauricular swelling and inability to fully close the mouth are consistent with a temporomandibular joint dislocation.

Depending on the mechanism of injury, mandibular fractures can occur in the symphysis, body, angle, ramus, or condyle. Falls and motor vehicle collisions, where force is directed against the chin, often result in fractures of the symphysis and condyles. Assaults often cause injuries to the body or angle at the point of impact. Unilateral condyle fractures will deviate the jaw toward the side of the fracture with mouth opening. Chin lacerations in children are often associated with condylar fractures. Since the growth center of the mandible is located in the area of the condyle, damage here can cause growth disturbances.

Management

All pediatric maxillary and mandibular fractures warrant dental or maxillofacial consultation. Most surgeons approach these pediatric fractures conservatively due to accelerated bone healing and osteogenic potential. Observation is adequate for nondisplaced or greenstick fractures. Minimally displaced fractures are treated with closed reduction and/or maxillomandibular fixation to avoid injuring permanent tooth buds and mandibular growth disturbances. Displaced fractures often require open reduction with internal fixation and should be treated within 2-4 days to achieve better results. Rapid healing in children may cause malunion if stabilization is delayed for more than 5 days. Delayed diagnoses increase the risk of malunion, nonunion, and malocclusion.

Reduce temporomandibular dislocations by applying downward traction to the posterior part of the mandible, and push the chin posteriorly to insert the condyle back into its fossa. Chin, tongue, gingival, oral mucosal, and palatal lacerations are often associated with maxilla and mandible injuries and vice versa. Carefully examine for maxilla and mandible fractures or temporomandibular dislocation whenever a facial laceration is present.

All open fractures and gingival lacerations require antibiotics; strongly consider prophylactic antibiotics that cover oral and sinus flora with all maxillary and mandibular fractures. Tetanus prophylaxis should be updated as indicated.

KEY POINTS

- Panorex or CT maxillofacial is recommended when there is a suspicion of maxilla and/or mandible fractures; single view x-rays are not sufficient.
- Carefully evaluate for lacerations associated with maxillary and mandibular fractures (eg, chin, tongue, gingiva, oral mucosa, palate) and vice versa!
- Perform the facial examination systematically; do not terminate examination after finding a single injury or assume facial symmetry.
- Refer to specialist early as rapid healing can cause malunion.

Suggested Readings

Haug RH, Foss J. Maxillofacial injuries in the pediatric patient. *Oral Surg Oral Med Oral Pathol Oral Radiol Endod.* 2000;90(2):126-134.

Morales JL, Skowronski PP, Thaller SR. Management of pediatric maxillary fractures. *J Craniofac Surg.* 2010;21(4):1226-1233.

Shaw KN, Bachur RG. *Fleischer and Ludwig's Textbook of Pediatric Emergency Medicine.* Philadelphia, PA: Lippincott Williams & Wilkins; 2016.

Put Down the Scalpel—A Thoughtful Approach to Neck Masses

Nicole Gerber, MD and Adam E. Vella, MD, FAAP

There are a variety of etiologies for neck masses, which can be divided into inflammatory, congenital, and neoplastic. It is important to remember the proximity to vital structures in the neck including carotid arteries, brachial plexus, and trachea when anticipating management.

Inflammatory

Cervical lymph node enlargement is a common neck mass and is most often reactive enlargement from a viral infection but may also be caused by bacterial infection. Reactive lymphadenopathy from a viral upper respiratory infection is usually characterized by nontender or minimally tender, mobile lymph nodes without overlying skin changes. One particular viral consideration is Epstein-Barr virus (EBV), which can cause pronounced lymphadenopathy. Monospot or serologic testing can be used to confirm the diagnosis. EBV is a self-limited illness; however, accurate diagnosis is helpful for prognosis as the symptoms may persist for weeks, and due to concomitant splenomegaly in some individuals, contact sports should be avoided to prevent splenic rupture.

Tender unilateral lymphadenitis with warmth or overlying skin changes may represent bacterial infection. Antibiotics are tailored toward the most likely infectious organisms—*Staphylococcus aureus* and group A strep. If there is an associated fluctuance, ultrasound should be utilized to evaluate for an abscess that would benefit from drainage, typically best done in consultation with a surgical subspecialist. If ill appearing, rapidly progressive or not responsive to oral antibiotics, the patient may require admission for IV antibiotics.

An accurate history is important as exposures may point to alternative bacterial causes of lymphadenitis. Cat scratch disease, caused by *Bartonella henselae*, is treated with azithromycin, and nontuberculous mycobacteria, suspected if there is a violaceous hue to the skin, is best treated by surgical excision.

Congenital Neck Masses

Congenital neck masses include branchial cleft cysts, which are found on the lateral neck, anterior to the sternocleidomastoid muscle, and midline thyroglossal duct cysts. Less common are neck hemangiomas, which may have important airway considerations.

The branchial cleft and thyroglossal duct cysts often present later in life when they become infected. Similar to other bacterial neck infections, ultrasound is a good first diagnostic modality to evaluate for the presence of a drainable collection, and treatment should be aimed at the most common skin/soft tissue organisms. Unlike typical bacterial lymphadenitis, the cyst must be surgically excised after infection has been controlled to prevent complications including reinfection. This may require further imaging for surgical planning and definitive diagnosis.

Hemangiomas of the neck are diagnosed clinically. They appear shortly after birth and undergo a period of growth followed by spontaneous regression. Some hemangiomas found in the beard distribution along the chin and neck will be associated with underlying subglottic hemangiomas, which have implications for airway management. Children often present with stridor that is mistaken for croup and may respond to initial croup management. In cases of recurrent "croup" without fevers, the possibility of a hemangioma should be taken into consideration.

Neoplastic

In adults, a higher suspicion for malignancy should be maintained, including for primary tonsil, tongue, and thyroid cancers as well as metastatic disease, typically from squamous cell carcinoma of the upper respiratory and digestive tracts. In younger patients, malignancy is less likely, although Hodgkin lymphoma should be considered in the adolescent patient. Hodgkin lymphoma classically presents with painless, rubbery, nonmobile lymphadenopathy with B symptoms including fever, weight loss, and night sweats. Lymphadenopathy may be accompanied by a mediastinal mass, which can remain asymptomatic even when quite large. Recumbent positioning may precipitate breathing difficulty, a key factor in the consideration of cross-sectional imaging. Due to their distal location, impingement on the airway will not be relieved by intubation. Caution should be taken to evaluate for a mediastinal mass prior to performing procedures in any patient in whom malignancy is suspected.

KEY POINTS

- Congenital neck masses often present when infected. Definitive treatment is surgical excision after treatment of the infection.
- What you see on the surface may be just a glimpse of what lies beneath. Consider the airway implications of cutaneous findings.
- Expanding neck masses can rapidly lead to airway compromise.

Suggested Readings

Badawy M. Pediatric neck masses. *Clin Ped Emergency Medicine*. 2010;11(2):73-80.

Geddes G, Butterly M, Patel S, et al. Pediatric neck masses. *Pediatr Rev*. 2013;34(3):115-124.

Meier J, Grimmer J. Evaluation and management of neck masses in children. *Am Fam Physician*. 2014;89(5):353-358.

Blunt Neck Trauma

Kara K. Seaton, MD, FAAP

Blunt neck trauma is relatively rare in pediatrics. When present, it may lead to critical injuries of the airway, esophagus, neck vasculature, or cervical spine. Clinicians should be cautious when assessing these injuries, as they may initially present with minimal symptoms yet progress rapidly. Children with significant neck trauma are also at high risk for maxillofacial, head, or thoracic trauma.

Pediatric-Specific Considerations

Compared to adults, children have relatively short necks with a mobile and pliable larynx positioned superiorly. This results in the larynx being partially protected by the mandibular arch attenuating the risk of fracture. However, the pediatric airway is substantially smaller than adolescents or adults whereby even a minor amount of edema or bleeding can lead to significant compromise. In addition, submucosal tissue is only loosely adherent to airway perichondrium increasing the risk of submucosal hematoma formation leading to obstruction.

Mechanisms of Injury

Motor vehicle accidents are the most common cause of blunt neck trauma in children. Other sources of injury occur from a "clothesline" mechanism associated with bikes, ATVs, snowmobiles, or jet skis and trauma from sports, falls, direct blows, or strangulation. Clinicians should consider nonaccidental trauma, especially in strangulation-type injuries or in infants and toddlers.

Airway Injuries

Assessing for airway injuries is of utmost importance in children with blunt trauma or significant force applied to the anterior neck. Injuries result from compression of the larynx against the spinal column or from rapid deceleration and shearing forces. Bruising to the anterior neck, crepitus, tracheal deviation, or palpable fractures suggest injury, although in some cases, there may be no external signs.

A wide spectrum of presentation of airway injuries occur, ranging from mild dysphonia or hoarse voice to stridor, aphonia, or respiratory distress. Other symptoms include dysphagia, hemoptysis, or neck pain. Children who have severe injuries may present with tachypnea, retractions, or inability to lay flat.

Non–Airway-Related Injuries

Pharyngeal and esophageal injuries also result from blunt neck trauma. The esophageal wall in pediatric patients is delicate and may be easily disrupted. Symptoms include dysphagia or odynophagia, hematemesis, tenderness or pain with palpation of the neck, or subcutaneous emphysema.

Vascular injuries are more common in penetrating trauma. However, such injuries should be carefully considered, especially in patients with concomitant cervical spine injuries, focal neurologic deficits, or altered level of consciousness. The most commonly injured vasculature in blunt neck trauma is the common carotid artery. The vertebral artery is rarely injured without associated cervical spine fracture.

Management of Blunt Neck Trauma

Patients who present to the ED with blunt neck trauma should be considered at risk for significant injury. Any respiratory symptoms must prompt rapid evaluation and stabilization of an anticipated difficult airway. Debate remains over the best method for airway control in such patients. Orotracheal intubation in the hands of an experienced physician is generally preferred with caution that this technique carries the risk of creating a false passage or inadvertently converting a partial to a full airway transection. With or without intubation, loss of the airway may occur. In these cases, emergent tracheostomy or cricothyroidotomy may be necessary.

In stable patients, it is reasonable to obtain imaging to delineate injury extent. Soft tissue lateral neck and chest x-rays can be done to reveal subcutaneous emphysema or pneumomediastinum. CT scan of the neck is the preferred modality for assessing blunt neck trauma, including fractures of the cartilaginous airway. Abnormalities on such imaging studies are an indication for laryngoscopy and/or esophagoscopy. Although there is a lack of evidenced-based data, it is generally advised that children with airway or oropharyngeal fractures should receive prophylactic antibiotics covering oropharyngeal flora. In patients with airway injury, transfer to a pediatric trauma center with an available otolaryngologist should be arranged promptly.

KEY POINTS

- Blunt neck trauma in children is rare but may lead to critical injuries of the airway, cervical spine, esophagus, or vasculature.
- Airway injuries may present with subtle signs but have the potential to rapidly progress.
- Pharyngeal and esophageal injuries may be difficult to diagnose.
- Consider rapid assessment and transport for children with blunt neck trauma exhibiting stridor, respiratory distress, crepitus, or dysphagia.

Suggested Readings

Franco K. Trauma, neck. In: Hoffman RJ, Wang VJ, Scarfone RJ, eds. *Fleisher and Ludwig's 5-minute Pediatric Emergency Medicine Consult*. Philadelphia, PA: Wolters Kluwer; 2012:968-969.

Losek JD, Tecklenburg FW, White DR. Blunt laryngeal trauma in children. *Pediatr Emerg Care*. 2008;24(6): 370-373.

Woodward GA, O'Mahony L. Neck trauma. In: Shaw KN, Baucher RG, eds. *Fleisher and Ludwig's Textbook or Pediatric Emergency Medicine*. 7th ed. Philadelphia, PA: Wolters Kluwer; 2016:1238-1279.

Penetrating Neck Trauma

Rachel Weigert, MD and Kelly R. Bergmann, MD

Background

Penetrating neck injury (PNI) in the pediatric population is relatively rare. Given the high risk of aerodigestive and neurovascular injury, such injuries need to be rapidly triaged and treated. Treatment of PNI has changed over time with a directed "zone" strategy that is utilized in some institutions, while others have progressed to a "no zone" approach that evaluates patients utilizing hard and soft signs.

Assessment

PNI is defined as an injury that passes through the platysma. All injuries need to be inspected and cautiously probed, to determine if the platysma is intact. Although zone of injury is not always used to determine intervention, it is still utilized in description of injury location. Zone 1 is from the clavicle to the cricothyroid membrane, zone 2 is from the cricothyroid membrane to the angle

Table 56.1 ■ Hard and Soft Signs of Penetrating Neck Injury	
Hard Signs	Soft Signs
Severe/uncontrolled hemorrhage	Minor hemorrhage
Large/expanding/pulsatile hematoma	Nonpulsatile, nonexpanding hematoma
Thrill/bruit	Proximity wounds
Shock; not responsive to IV fluids	Mild hypotension; responsive to IV fluids
Absent/decreased radial pulse	Dysphagia
Neurologic deficit concerning for stroke	Subcutaneous/mediastinal air
Air bubbling from wounds	Minor hemoptysis/hematemesis
Massive hemoptysis/hematemesis	Dysphonia
Respiratory distress	

of the mandible, and zone 3 is above the angle of the mandible. Zone 1 injuries carry a risk to mediastinal structures and pneumothorax and are managed as chest injuries. zone 3 can include significant vascular injuries and are challenging to intervene upon surgically. Injuries may appear to violate a single zone when in reality, with further evaluation through imaging or surgical exploration, actually cross multiple zones. As such, external zone identification may provide inadequate information regarding the extent of an injury. This is particularly true in infants and young children with compressed anatomy. Additional consideration of neck anatomy includes the anterior and posterior triangles divided by the sternocleidomastoid muscle with the anterior proving much more deadly if injured. Hard and soft signs of injury should be utilized to guide assessment and intervention (Table 56.1).

Management

The decision points for treatment of PNI include patient stability and symptoms. Clinical instability or hard signs of injury should result in immediate operative intervention. Stable symptomatic patients or those in which there is concern for occult injury should undergo computed tomography with angiography (CTA) imaging and close monitoring. Although treatment protocols vary by institution, stable and asymptomatic patients are typically monitored for at least 24 hours.

Following initial stabilization, all pediatric patients with PNI should be transferred to a level 1 trauma center, preferably with pediatric expertise. Penetrating debris should not be removed. Patients requiring an airway should undergo rapid sequence endotracheal intubation if possible, and bag/mask ventilation if an airway cannot be placed. Patients with zone 1 injuries should be frequently assessed for signs of tension pneumothorax including hypotension, tachypnea, subcutaneous emphysema, and unilateral breath sound reduction. Needle thoracostomy should be performed if there is concern for developing tension pneumothorax.

Surgical airway or jet ventilation may be required for significantly distorted anatomy or failed endotracheal intubation attempts with ongoing inadequate oxygenation and ventilation. Two points of access should be obtained, and pressure should be applied to bleeding wounds. The patient should be placed in Trendelenburg position to prevent air embolism if any bubbling/sucking wounds are present. As cervical spine injury is rare from low-velocity PNI, patients should only be placed in a cervical collar if their cervical spine cannot be cleared, and standard in-line precautions should be used during intubation.

Massive transfusion protocol should be activated for significant hemorrhage. Plain chest and neck radiographs should also be obtained if definitive imaging is delayed or unavailable.

KEY POINTS

- Modes of classifying PNI include zones, triangles, and hard/soft signs of injury.
- Unstable patients or those with hard signs should proceed directly to the OR, while stable symptomatic patients undergo a CTA. Stable and asymptomatic patients should be observed for 24 hours.
- Penetrating debris should not be removed, and pressure should be applied to bleeding wounds.
- Place the patient in Trendelenburg position to prevent air embolism if any bubbling/sucking wounds are present.

Suggested Readings

Ibraheem K, Khan M, Rhee P, et al. "No zone" approach in penetrating neck trauma reduces unnecessary computed tomography angiography and negative explorations. *J Surg Res*. 2018;221:113-120.

Stone ME Jr, Farber BA, Olorunfemi O, et al. Penetrating neck trauma in children: an uncommon entity described using the National Trauma Data Bank. *J Trauma Acute Care Surg*. 2016;80(4):604-609.

Tessler RA, Nguyen H, Newton C, Betts J. Pediatric penetrating neck trauma: hard signs of injury and selective neck exploration. *J Trauma Acute Care Surg*. 2017;82(6):989-994.

Torticollis: Maybe a Twist but Hopefully Never a Shout

Amber M. Morse, MD, FAAP and Heather A. Heaton, MD, FACEP

Torticollis, also known as "twisted neck" or "wryneck," is a common presenting complaint to the emergency department (ED). Patients have neck stiffness and/or neck pain and hold their head in a characteristic position. In most cases of torticollis, there is shortening or spasm of the sternocleidomastoid (SCM) muscle causing the head to tilt toward the shortened muscle, ipsilaterally, and the chin to be rotated away from the muscle, toward the contralateral side. Torticollis arises from both congenital and acquired processes (Table 57.1) and the differential is broad but can be pared down with a thorough history and physical.

Congenital Torticollis

Usually present by 1 month of age, congenital muscular torticollis is thought to arise from birth trauma or intrauterine malposition such as breech presentation. Infants will have one of three presentations: SCM mass, muscular, or postural. Diagnosis is mainly clinical, although ultrasonography (US) can be used to identify the SCM mass type and radiographs of the cervical spine can rule out congenital bony abnormalities seen in syndromes such as Klippel-Feil. Treatment involves manual stretching techniques and positioning during feeding and play to stretch the affected SCM.

Acquired Torticollis

Most patients who present with torticollis will have benign, self-limiting conditions causing their symptoms. However, there are life-threatening causes of torticollis.

Trauma

Torticollis caused by cervical spine injuries are uncommon and usually the result of high-energy mechanisms such as motor vehicle accidents and falls. In the setting of trauma, cervical spinal motion restriction should be initiated and radiographs obtained to rule out fractures and subluxation. Computed tomography (CT) may be used as an adjunct to better identify bony abnormalities while magnetic reso-

Table 57.1 ■ Causes of Torticollis	
Congenital	Acquired
Congenital muscular torticollis	**Trauma**
SCM mass type	Cervical spine fracture
Muscular type	Atlantoaxial rotary subluxation
Postural type	Atlantoaxial dislocation
Skeletal malformations	Subdural/epidural spinal hematoma
Klippel-Feil syndrome	Muscular spasm/contusion of the neck
Sprengel deformity	**Ocular**
Atlantoaxial instability	Strabismus
Down syndrome	Cranial nerve/extraocular muscle palsies
Morquio syndrome	Refractive errors
Marfan syndrome	**Neurologic**
	Posterior fossa tumors
	Brachial nerve palsies
	Arnold-Chiari malformation
	Syringomyelia
	Infectious
	Retropharyngeal abscess
	Lemierre syndrome
	Cervical adenitis
	Cervical osteomyelitis/discitis
	Inflammatory
	Grisel syndrome
	Juvenile idiopathic arthritis
	Miscellaneous
	Benign paroxysmal torticollis
	Cervical dystonia
	Spasmus nutans
	Sandifer syndrome
	Drug-induced torticollis/dystonia

nance imaging (MRI) more clearly highlights ligamentous and spinal cord injuries. Depending on the injury, treatment will often require immobilization, analgesics, and/or surgical consultation.

Neurologic

Space-occupying lesions such as astrocytomas arising in the posterior fossa may cause torticollis as a compensatory mechanism for diplopia or through irritation of the spinal accessory nerve via cerebellar tonsillar herniation. The patient will likely have other signs of increased intracranial pressure or neurologic deficits that will necessitate a workup including CT or MRI. Treatment is directed at the underlying lesion.

Infectious

Infections of the neck may cause torticollis as an early presenting sign. Two such entities to be aware of are retropharyngeal abscess and suppurative jugular thrombophlebitis (Lemierre syndrome). Retropharyngeal abscess, most commonly seen in ages 2-4 years, creates limited motion of the neck, sometimes presenting as torticollis, along with fever, dysphagia, drooling, and respiratory distress. Lemierre syndrome causes fever, respiratory distress, and localized neck pain sometimes with features of torticollis due to SCM irritation and inflammation. Both of these infections are diagnosed via CT of the neck with contrast and are treated with proper antimicrobial therapy.

KEY POINTS

- Torticollis presents with head tilt toward (ipsilateral) the affected SCM and chin rotation away (contralateral) to the SCM.
- Most causes of torticollis are benign and self-limited.
- Life-threatening cases of torticollis are often due to trauma, tumors, or infectious processes.
- Patient history and a thorough physical examination will often lead the practitioner to the diagnosis. US, CT, and MRI are supportive adjuncts.

Suggested Readings

Do TT. Congenital muscular torticollis: current concepts and review of treatment. *Curr Opin Pediatr.* 2006;18: 26-29.

Hague S, Bilal Shafi B, Kaleem M. Imaging of torticollis in children. *Radiographics.* 2012;32:557-571.

Tomczak KK, Rosman NP. Torticollis. *J Child Neurol.* 2012;28:365-378.

Tzimenatos L, Vance C, Kupperman N. Neck stiffness. In: Shaw KN, Bachur RG, eds. *Fleisher & Ludwig's Textbook of Pediatric Emergency Medicine.* 7th ed. Philadelphia, PA: Wolters Kluwer; 2016:303-311.

Atlantoaxial Rotatory Subluxation (AARS): When Children Truly Look Like Little Birds

Heather A. Heaton, MD, FACEP and Amber M. Morse, MD, FAAP

Etiology

Given increased laxity of joints and ligaments, with more mobility in facet joints of the cervical spine, increased synovium, and the disproportionally larger head of a child, children are susceptible to atlantoaxial rotatory subluxation (AARS). More commonly occurring in children under 13 years of age, AARS occurs due to a variety of etiologies (Table 58.1).

Presentation

Children presenting with AARS may present to the emergency department (ED) acutely following an inciting event or several weeks later. The classic description of a child with AARS is "cock-robin," or with the head titled and neck slightly flexed, with the child's chin pointing to the side contralateral to the subluxation. Oftentimes, these patients will have persistent torticollis and decreased range of motion of the neck, but no neurological deficits. On occasion, AARS is associated with cervical myelopathy or occipital neuralgia, but these findings are less common.

Table 58.1 ■ Atlantoaxial Rotary Subluxation Etiologies	
Etiology	**Examples**
Trauma	• Motor vehicle accidents • Falls • Neck manipulation • Bumping the head
Infection	• Retropharyngeal abscess • Upper respiratory infection • Otitis media
Congenital anomalies of C1-C2 joint	• Incomplete or complete occipitalization of C1
Developmental syndromes	• Down syndrome • Achondroplasia • Spondyloepiphyseal dysplasia • Larsen syndrome • Klippel-Feil syndrome • Morquio syndrome

Diagnosis

The typical diagnosis of a patient with AARS includes common findings on the child's physical examination, including palpable deviation of the C2 spinous process, sternocleidomastoid muscle spasms of the ipsilateral side (opposite of muscular torticollis), inability to rotate the head past midline, and/or a bulge in the posterior pharynx wall indicative of anterior displacement of the C1 arch.

Definitive diagnosis is made by radiological studies. Plain radiographs can be used, but computed tomography (CT) is preferred. CT scan provides the ability to reformat and reconstruct, allowing for better ability to identify subtle cervical spine fractures when evaluating these patients. Magnetic resonance imaging (MRI) can be used as well; while subpar in bony resolution to CT, MRI has better soft tissue resolution and might be helpful when the ligaments need closer evaluation than CT provides. Classification of AARS is typically based on a system developed by Fielding and Hawkins in 1977 (Table 58.2).

Treatment

Most cases of AARS resolve with conservative management. Cervical traction, followed by immobilization and use of anti-inflammatory medications are common practice. If the dislocation is long standing

Table 58.2 ■ Classification of Atlantoaxial Rotatory Subluxation	
Type I	• Most common type • Rotatory fixation without anterior subluxation • Odontoid process acts as the pivot point
Type II	• Second most common • Ligamentous disruption of the transverse ligament • Articular mass acts as the pivot point • 3-5 mm of anterior displacement of anterior arch of C1 in relation to the odontoid
Type III	• More than 5 mm of anterior displacement of the C1 arch with associated disruption of the transverse and alar ligaments
Type IV	• Least common • Rotatory fixation with posterior displacement • Associated with fractures or congenital anomalies of the odontoid process

or unstable, surgical fusion may be required. Surgery is also indicated when there is an unstable or significant structural deformity present or neurological symptoms exist.

KEY POINTS

- AARS occurs most commonly in children under age 13.
- Patients typically present with the "cock-robin" appearance.
- Conservative management with traction, immobilization, and anti-inflammatory medications will resolve the majority of these cases.
- Long standing or unstable cases may require surgical fusion.

Suggested Readings

Harma A, Firat Y. Grisel syndrome: nontraumatic atlantoaxial rotatory subluxation. *J Craniofac Surg*. 2008;19:1119-1121.

Kinon MD, Nasser, R, Nakhla J, et al. Atlantoaxial rotatory subluxation: a review for the pediatric emergency physician. *Pediatr Emerg Care*. 2016;32(10):710-716.

Pang D, Li V. Atlantoaxial rotatory fixation: part 3-a prospective study of the clinical manifestation, diagnosis, management, and outcome of children with atlantoaxial rotatory fixation. *Neurosurgery*. 2005;57:954-972.

Subach BR, McLaughlin MR, Albright AL, et al. Current management of pediatric atlantoaxial rotatory subluxation. *Spine (Phila Pa 1976)*. 1998;23:2174-2179.

Managing Pediatric Eye Injuries: You Will Shoot Your Eye Out, Kid!

Kathleen M. Smith, MD, MPH

Ocular trauma accounts for 8%-12% of all childhood injuries and remains the leading cause of blindness among U.S. children. Physical examination of an injured eye in a child may be challenging but should include external examination, visual acuity, pupillary reactions, ocular motility, visual fields, slitlamp exam, intraocular pressure (IOP), fluorescein staining, and fundoscopy.

Orbital Fractures

Orbital fractures, most commonly seen in the orbital floor or medial wall due to thinner bones in these areas, are usually caused by blunt trauma. Signs and symptoms of an orbital fracture include periorbital ecchymoses; hypoesthesia in the lower eyelid, cheek, and upper lip; restricted extraocular movements; diplopia; pain with ocular movement; nausea; and vomiting. Computed tomography (CT) scan is the preferred imaging modality. Up to 25% of pediatric patients with orbital fractures have an associated ocular injury.

Ruptured Globe

Children are at higher risk for open globe injuries than adults and usually have a poorer prognosis. Clinical findings of a tear drop pupil, extrusion of vitreous, marked decrease in visual acuity, relative afferent pupillary defect, 360-degree subconjunctival hemorrhage, and enophthalmos are warning signs that a child has an open globe injury. Children with open globe injuries should have an eye shield placed and receive analgesic and antiemetic medications. Therapeutic or diagnostic eyedrops, ocular ultrasound, and IOP testing are contraindicated.

Anterior Chamber Injuries

Injuries to the anterior chamber include corneal abrasions, foreign bodies, hyphema, and traumatic iritis. Corneal abrasions are common in children, typically presenting with severe eye pain, photophobia, and/or a foreign body sensation and are a common etiology of irritability in an afebrile infant. Patients with corneal abrasions usually have immediate relief with anesthetic eyedrops, a staining defect on fluorescein examination, and normal visual acuity and pupillary reactions. Most corneal foreign bodies may be removed with a moistened cotton swab after the child receives an ocular anesthetic. Embedded foreign bodies may require ophthalmologic consultation. Treatment includes artificial tears or antibiotic drops/ointment and cyclopentolate 1% to relieve ciliary spasm. Eye patches are not indicated.

Blunt trauma to the anterior chamber may initially result in a hyphema and/or traumatic iritis 24 to 72 hours later. Clinical findings of hyphema include photophobia, visual impairment and blood in the anterior chamber. Signs and symptoms of traumatic iritis include eye pain, photophobia, visual impairment, ciliary flush and miosis of the injured eye. The diagnosis is made by slit lamp exam. Cyclopentolate !% and steroid eye drops are recommended after ophthalmologic consultation.

Posterior Chamber Injuries

Injuries to the posterior chamber include vitreous hemorrhage and retinal detachment. Point-of-care ocular ultrasound is an excellent imaging modality for detection of these injuries. Pediatric traumatic vitreous hemorrhage is associated with a retinal tear or detachment, abusive head injury in infants and young children, and accidental subdural or subarachnoid hemorrhages. Symptoms include decreased or hazy vision, black spots, or cobwebs. The optic disc, retina, and vessels may be partially or completely obscured on fundoscopic examination. Red reflex may be absent with large vitreous hemorrhages. A CT of the head should be considered in patients with traumatic vitreous hemorrhage. Retinal detachment results in partial or complete vision loss. Patients often complain of light flashes, floaters, and a loss of peripheral or central vision. When history, physical examination, or point-of-care ultrasound (POCUS) are suggestive of vitreous hemorrhage or retinal detachment, the emergency clinician should arrange for urgent ophthalmologic consultation.

Retrobulbar Hemorrhage

Retrobulbar hemorrhage in children is associated with blunt trauma to the eye. A rapid increase in intraorbital pressure results in orbital compartment syndrome (OCS) with ischemia of the optic nerve. Key physical examination findings include marked decrease in visual acuity, afferent pupillary defect, proptosis, restricted extraocular movements, periorbital ecchymoses, increased IOP, and diffuse subconjunctival hemorrhage. OCS is a true ophthalmologic emergency that requires lateral canthotomy and cantholysis to decompress the orbit within 60 minutes of the injury. Once the orbit is decompressed, ophthalmologic consultation and orbital CT imaging is indicated. Elevation of the head of the bed, rest, analgesics, and antiemetics are adjuncts in management of retrobulbar hemorrhage.

KEY POINTS

- In patients with a high likelihood of open globe injury avoid any diagnostic or therapeutic intervention that may place pressure on the eyeball.
- Time is vision: for patients with OCS, a lateral canthotomy and cantholysis should be performed within 60 minutes of injury to preserve vision.
- CT of the orbits without contrast is the preferred imaging modality for patients with serious traumatic eye injuries.

Suggested Readings

Bagheri N, Wajda BN. *The Wills Eye Manual: Office and Emergency Room Diagnosis and Treatment of Eye Disease.* 7th ed. Philadelphia, PA: Lippincott Williams & Wilkins; 2016.

Salvin JH. Systematic approach to pediatric ocular trauma. *Curr Opin Ophthalmol.* 2007;18:366-372.

Shaw KN, Bachur RG. *Fleisher and Ludwig's Textbook of Pediatric Emergency Medicine.* 7th ed. Philadelphia, PA: Lippincott Williams & Wilkins; 2016.

Be Prepared to Manage Eye Lacerations

Nicholas Pokrajac, MD

The emergency department is often the first point of physician contact for patients with an eye laceration. Thus, emergency physicians require an understanding of eye anatomy and of injuries associated with lacerations to avoid potential long-term negative cosmetic and functional outcomes. Common etiologies in children include animal bites, accidental impacts with sharp objects, and ball sports. Associated ocular injuries also occur in approximately two-thirds of patients with eyelid lacerations. Eye lacerations can be classified as either simple (superficial lacerations of the lid) or complex (lacerations that are full thickness, involve the lid margin, or involve the canalicular system).

Examination

The goal of a physical examination in a patient with an eye laceration is to (1) identify signs of a complex laceration and (2) identify signs of surrounding injury (Tables 60.1 and 60.2). Pediatric patients may require sedation for adequate examination depending on age. If a complicated laceration or globe injury is strongly suspected, it may be preferable to place an eye shield and allow full examination and repair under anesthesia or sedation in coordination with a pediatric specialist. Indications for computed tomography (CT) imaging of the orbits include suspected globe injury, high-speed projectile injury, and findings concerning for orbital fractures or ocular entrapment.

Treatment

Eyelid lacerations ideally should be repaired within 24 hours of injury. Emergency providers should consult pediatric ophthalmology or oculoplastic specialists in patients with complex lacerations or lacerations with associated globe injury. Complications of inadequate repair include poor cosmetic outcome, excessive tearing, chronic eye irritation, entropion, and ectropion. In most pediatric patients, absorbable sutures such as 6-0 fast absorbing gut or Vicryl Rapide is preferable for repair to eliminate need for removal. Use of tissue adhesives is problematic due to the proximity to the globe and difficulty controlling unwanted spread to surrounding structures. Systemic antibiotic prophylaxis is unnecessary for simple lacerations unless the wound is contaminated, involves the globe, or is the result of an animal bite.

Table 60.1 ■ Signs of Complex Eye Lacerations
Prolapsed orbital fat
Involvement of lid margin
Deep lacerations involving muscle, tarsal plate, or canthal ligaments
Lacerations involving medial one-third of the lid (canalicular system)
Substantial tissue loss

Table 60.2 ■ Selected Associated Injuries and Their Physical Examination Findings	
Injury	Physical Examination Findings
Orbital fracture	Significant periorbital edema, ecchymosis
Corneal abrasion, laceration	Corneal fluorescein uptake
Ocular foreign body	Visualized foreign body, multiple linear/vertical abrasions
Traumatic hyphema	Blood visualized in anterior chamber
Globe rupture	Seidel sign, teardrop pupil, herniated iris

KEY POINTS

- Eyelid lacerations require a thorough evaluation for injuries of surrounding structures.
- If a pediatric patient's age or level of cooperation limits an examination, sedation in coordination with a pediatric ophthalmologist may be required.
- In general, complex lacerations should be repaired by an ophthalmologic specialist.

Suggested Readings

Chang EL, Rubin PA. Management of complex eyelid lacerations. *International Ophthalmology Clinics.* 2002;42(3): 187-201.

Knoop KJ, Dennis WR. Ophthalmologic procedures. In: Roberts JR, Custalow CB, Thomsen TW, eds. *Roberts and Hedges' Clinical Procedures in Emergency Medicine and Acute Care.* 7th ed. Philadelphia, PA: Elsevier; 2018: 1295-1338.

Weaver CS, Knoop KJ. Ophthalmic trauma. In: Knoop KJ, Stack LB, Storrow AB, Thurman J, eds. *The Atlas of Emergency Medicine.* 4th ed. New York: McGraw-Hill Education; 2016:96-97.

Be Prepared to Care for the Other Pediatric Red Eye: Hyphema

Mylinh Thi Nguyen, MD

A hyphema is characterized by blood in the anterior chamber. It is most commonly caused by blunt or penetrating injury to the eye. Blood, which is heavier than aqueous fluid, usually settles out in the inferior portion of the anterior chamber. The blood may be microscopic identified only by slitlamp examination (microhyphema).

Blunt force to the eye results in an instantaneous increase in intraocular pressure resulting in tearing of the vessels of the ciliary body or iris. In penetrating trauma, bleeding comes from the damaged iris. Spontaneous hyphemas occur in patients with hemoglobinopathies, diabetes mellitus, juvenile xanthogranuloma, inherited or secondary clotting disorders (thrombocytopenia, hemophilia, von Willebrand disease, medications), iris melanoma, retinoblastoma, and other tumors of the eye. Patients with sickle cell disease or trait are at increased risk for complications of a hyphema including increased intraocular pressure, optic atrophy, and secondary hemorrhage, placing them at a higher risk of permanent vision loss.

Although they may seem relatively innocuous, hyphemas are serious injuries with potential complications of loss of vision, re-bleeding, glaucoma, and blood staining of the cornea and require close ophthalmologic evaluation and follow-up.

Signs and Symptoms

Acute loss of vision and eye pain are common presenting complaints in patients with a hyphema. Other symptoms are photophobia, decreased visual acuity, anisocoria, elevated intraocular pressure, and corneal blood staining.

Diagnostic Evaluation

Goals of initial assessment include recognition and characterization of the hyphema and identification of associated orbital and ocular injuries. All patients with hyphema warrant prompt evaluation by an ophthalmologist. Slitlamp examination can be used to detect microhyphema and to measure directly the distance (mm) between the inferior limbus and the top the erythrocyte layer. Macroscopic hyphemas are graded by the height of the blood in the anterior chamber (AC) with a direct correlation between grading and prognosis. Grade 1, <1/3 of the AC; grade 2, 1/3 to 1/2 of the AC; grade 3: 1/2 to nearly the entire AC; and grade 4, fills the entire AC.

Treatment

Treatment of a hyphema is directed at minimizing complications such as re-bleeding, glaucoma, and corneal staining. The eye should be shielded and the patient placed on bed rest with the head elevated 30-45 degrees. This position helps allow blood within the anterior chamber to settle inferiorly, allowing clearance of the visual axis, improvement of vision, and a better view for the ophthalmologic examination. After an open globe is excluded, cycloplegic agents are used to immobilize the iris along with topical or systemic steroids to minimize intraocular inflammation. Antiemetics should be considered in nauseated patients to decrease increases in intraocular pressure from retching and vomiting. Agents that may promote bleeding such as nonsteroidal anti-inflammatories and aspirin should be avoided. The majority of hyphemas resolve over 4-5 days with observation and activity reduction. Patients with sickle cell trait or disease are at higher risk of acute loss of vision secondary to elevated intraocular pressure or optic nerve infarction and may require more aggressive intervention. Any individual with a traumatic hyphema should have lifelong monitoring for development of glaucoma.

KEY POINTS

- Hyphema is blood in the anterior chamber.
- Hyphemas are serious injuries with potential complications including vision loss, re-bleeding, glaucoma, and corneal staining, necessitating ophthalmologic evaluation of all patients.
- Evaluate for associated injuries such as orbital fractures and open globe.
- Treatment includes placing an eye shield, elevating the head of the bed to 30-45 degrees, pain control, antiemetics, cycloplegics, and steroids.
- Goals of treatment are to minimize threat to vision loss.

Suggested Readings

Fleisher GR, Ludwig S, Henretig FM. *Textbook of Pediatric Emergency Medicine*. 6th ed. Philadelphia, PA: Lippincott Williams & Wilkins; 2010:1456-1457.

Gharaibeh A, Savage HI, Scherer RW, Goldberg MF, Lindsley K. Medical interventions for traumatic hyphema. *Cochrane Database Syst Rev*. 2019;1:CD005431.

Hyphema and microhyphema. In: Ehlers JP, Shah CP, eds. *The Wills Eye Manual: Office and Emergency Room Diagnosis and Treatment of Eye Disease*. 5th ed. Philadelphia, PA: Lippincott Williams & Wilkins; 2008:19.

SooHoo JR, Davies BW, Braverman RS, Enzenauer RW, McCourt EA. Pediatric traumatic hyphema: a review of 138 consecutive cases. *J AAPOS*. 2013;17(6):565-567.

Trief D, Adebona OT, Turalba AV, Shah AS. The pediatric traumatic hyphema. *Int Ophthalmol Clin*. 2013 Fall;53(4):43-57.

Pediatric Vision Loss

Nicky Amin, MD

Vision loss ranges from decreased acuity to blindness, affecting one or both eyes. Pathology occurs anywhere along the visual pathway. It is useful to categorize location of defect into visual media, retinal, or neuro-optic pathway pathology.

Visual Media Pathology

Infectious causes are common and may present with decreased visual acuity or loss. Examples include conjunctivitis, keratitis (HSV or contact lens related), and iritis. Additionally, open globe injuries, chemical burns, hyphema, vitreous haemorrhage, and glaucoma may all present with some degree of vision loss.

Retinal Pathology

Detachment and tears: While incidence of retinal detachment (RD) in pediatrics is low, they require urgent ophthalmologic evaluation. Symptoms include flashing light (photopsia), hazy vision, black spots, floaters, or "curtain vision" with partial or complete vision loss. RD can be traumatic vs nontraumatic.

Traumatic RD is typically unilateral, presents acutely following significant head injury, and is associated with vitreous and intracranial hemorrhages. Nonaccidental trauma must always be considered. The retina, optic disc, and retinal vessels may be obscured if vitreous hemorrhage is present and the red reflex may be lost.

Nontraumatic RD can be unilateral or bilateral and causes include myopia, congenital abnormalities, and nonhereditary anomalies. Congenital anomalies may cause subluxation of the lens due to defective collagen synthesis or extracellular matrix proteins, weakening the structure of the vitreous.

Central Retinal Artery Occlusion (CRAO)

This condition is a rare, emergent condition in pediatrics as occlusion time directly correlates to degree of vision impairment. This presents as sudden, painless, but severe monocular vision loss. Vascular occlusion typically occurs secondary to embolization. Pediatric causes include trauma, hypercoagulable state, vasculitis, or sickle cell disease. Clinical findings may include limited visual acuity, afferent pupillary defect, and a white retina secondary to intracellular edema with "cherry spot" at the fovea.

Central Retinal Vein Occlusion (CRVO)

This condition similarly occurs secondary to thrombus occlusion of the central retinal vein causing disc edema, dilated veins, and retinal hemorrhages. Cotton wool spots may also be seen.

Tumors

Retinoblastoma is the most common primary intraocular malignancy in children presenting in children <5 years old with leukocoria, with or without strabismus and a loss of the red reflex. Unilateral disease occurs in 75% of cases.

Hemangiomas are the most common childhood tumor and occur secondary to uncontrolled vascular endothelial proliferation. Though benign and self-limiting, their location can pose a threat to a child's vision through obstruction of the visual axis, mechanical ptosis, strabismus, and astigmatism, all of which can lead to amblyopia.

Neuro-optic Pathology

Optic Neuritis

This is a rare, inflammatory demyelinating disorder of the optic nerve generally related to post-infectious cause. Symptoms include decreased vision, impaired color vision, and painful ocular movement. Bilateral involvement is common. Infectious causes include syphilis, tuberculosis, varicella-zoster virus, and Epstein Barr virus. Neuroimaging with MRI is essential in evaluation to differentiate from other disorders that can present similarly.

Orbital Cellulitis vs Periorbital Cellulitis

Differentiation of orbital from periorbital (preseptal) cellulitis is crucial, as the treatment, pathogenesis, and sequelae are different. Infections can travel indirectly through the valveless venous drainage or spread into the paranasal sinuses via the thin lamina papyracea. This can lead to a myriad of infections including subperiosteal abscesses, osteitis, orbital abscess, and orbital cellulitis. Clinical findings of orbital cellulitis include proptosis, diminished visual acuity, chemosis, papilledema, pain with extraocular movements, erythema, and periorbital edema.

Periorbital cellulitis is common and clinically may present with fever, erythema, induration, tenderness, and warmth *over* the periorbital tissues. If clinical differentiation cannot be made, a CT scan and consultation with ophthalmology should occur. Treatment of orbital cellulitis requires IV antibiotics, ensuring coverage of *Streptococcus pneumoniae*, nontypable *Haemophilus influenzae*, Group A *Streptococcus*, *Staphylococcus aureus*, and anaerobes. Periorbital cellulitis can often be treated with oral antistaphylococcal and streptococcal agents.

Idiopathic Intracranial Hypertension

This condition leads to optic nerve compression secondary to increased intracranial pressure via CSF production. Commonly found in obese female patients present with headache, vision alteration, and papilledema. Lumbar puncture is both diagnostic and therapeutic though these patients are at risk for permanent vision loss.

Migraines

Complex migraines can lead to transient monocular or bilateral vision loss by affecting the visual sensory or ocular motor pathways by causing neuronal depression. Patients generally complain of acute onset vision loss accompanied by flashes, sparks, or the appearance of a bright light (photopsia). Visual loss is usually temporary; however, permanent loss of vision has been reported.

KEY POINTS

- Vision loss in pediatrics is a medical emergency and should include ophthalmologic consultation.
- Lesions occur anywhere along the visual media, retinal, and neuro-optic pathways.
- A multidisciplinary team is often required to prevent permanent visual loss.

Suggested Readings

Naradzay J, Barish RA. Approach to ophthalmologic emergencies. *Med Clin North Am*. 2006;90:305-328.
Prentiss KA, Dorfman DH. Pediatric ophthalmology in the emergency department. *Emerg Med Clin North Am*. 2008;26:181-198.

63

Be Prepared to Manage Eye Burns—Chemical, UV, Thermal

Ashley L. Flannery, DO, FACEP, FAAEM

Eye burns are an ocular emergency with the potential for long-term visual disturbances drastically impacting a child's quality of life. Burns occur as the result of chemical, thermal, or ultraviolet (UV) sources. The risk to young children is much higher than previously estimated. Extent of injury correlates with type, volume, and temperature of substance and length of exposure. The general approach to a patient with an ocular burn should include removal from source, identification of material, and assessment and removal of potential foreign bodies. Emergency provider should assess visual acuity, stain the eye with fluorescein, and measure ocular pressures.

Chemical burns are common, most frequent in children 1-2 years of age. The chemical can be in liquid, solid, or gaseous form and causes damage to the surface epithelium, cornea, and anterior segment of the eye.

Injury occurs within minutes of exposure. Alkaline materials cause a liquefactive necrosis that damages the deeper structures of the eye. Acidic substances cause a coagulation necrosis and tend to be more superficial and less severe than alkali exposure. The exception is hydrofluoric acid, which behaves similar to an alkali. Common sources are listed in Table 63.1.

After a chemical exposure, immediate irrigation of the eye is critical. In the prehospital setting, simple tap water may be used. In a health care facility, normal saline or Ringer lactate are appropriate. A scleral lens with tubing may be used to facilitate irrigation. Historically, 2 L or 30 minutes of irrigation were recommended. Currently, guidelines indicate irrigation until the eye returns to a normal pH. Treatment should also include pain management with both topical and systemic analgesia and ophthalmology consultation.

Thermal injuries are the result of a hot liquid, object, or flame contacting the eye. UV burns begin after unprotected exposure to UV radiation. Sun exposure at high altitudes can damage the corneal epithelium causing superficial punctate keratitis. Visualization is easily accomplished with fluorescein staining or slitlamp examination with a characteristic appearance of tiny circular islands of epithelial erosion often widespread across the cornea. Prolonged exposure to UV light can result in cataracts and retinal burns.

After both thermal and UV burns, the child will frequently report severe pain and vision loss. Symptoms may be delayed up to 1-2 days. The child should be removed from the source of exposure and eyes irrigated and any foreign bodies removed. Topical and systemic analgesia along with cool compresses are paramount to alleviate pain. Artificial tears or ointment are initiated to prevent the formation of adhesions. Cycloplegic drops are indicated for UV keratitis. Ophthalmologic consultation should be obtained.

The key to prevention of these injuries is public education about the dangers of eye burns and best practices for safe storage of chemicals. If an exposure occurs, immediate irrigation should be taught prior to medical evaluation as damage develops within minutes. Medical professionals should perform careful eye examinations, including fluorescein staining and everting the lids to look for foreign bodies. It is important to maintain a high index of suspicion for potential burns.

Table 63.1 ■ Common Products Causing Alkali and Acidic Chemical Burns	
Acidic	Alkali
Bleach	Lime
Vinegar	Plaster
Toilet cleaner	Oven and drain cleaner
Glass polisher, rust remover	Ammonia
Battery fluid	Fireworks
Pool cleaner	Airbag chemicals

KEY POINTS

- Eye burns are an ocular emergency and result from chemical, UV, and thermal exposure.
- Removal from offending source and immediate irrigation with tap water, Ringer lactate, or normal saline are the first steps in effective treatment.
- Prevention should be discussed with parents and caretakers, including safe storage of chemicals, eye protection, and immediate management steps if exposure occurs.

Suggested Readings

Eslani M, et al. The ocular surface chemical burns. *J Ophthalmol*. 2014;2014:196827.

Haring RS, et al. Epidemiologic trends of chemical ocular burns in the United States. *JAMA Ophthalmol*. 2016;134(10):1119-1124.

Ratnapalan S, Lopamudra D. Causes of eye burns in children. *Pediatr Emerg Care*. 2011;27(2):151-156.

Spector J, William GF. Chemical, thermal, and biological ocular exposures. *Emerg Med Clin North Am*. 2008;26(1):125-136.

Do Not Confuse Orbital Cellulitis With Preseptal Cellulitis

Meghan Cain, MD

Periorbital infections are a common complaint for pediatric emergency department (ED) patients. The location of the infection in relation to the orbital septum, a fibrous layer that runs from the orbital bones to the eyelids, helps determine the type of infection and treatment strategy. Infections of the eyelids and soft tissue anterior to the septum are referred to as preseptal cellulitis. When the orbit, globe, or other structures posterior to the septum are involved, this constitutes orbital cellulitis (Fig. 64.1). Both processes tend to occur with spread of infection from adjacent structures. Preseptal cellulitis is often secondary to bug bites or small wounds but may also develop from a chalazion, hordeolum, or conjunctivitis. Orbital cellulitis typically spreads from sinusitis.

It can be difficult to clinically differentiate between preseptal and orbital cellulitis, especially in young children. Both are associated with fever, pain, and significant eyelid erythema and swelling. The key signs indicative of orbital cellulitis include decreased extraocular movements, proptosis, vision

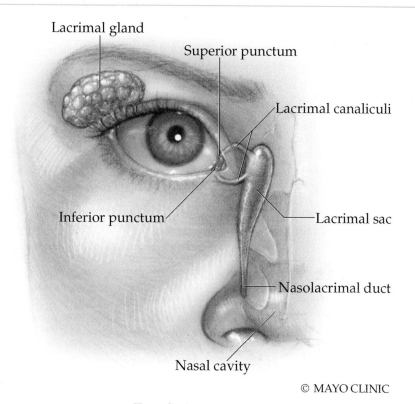

Lacrimal gland

Superior punctum

Lacrimal canaliculi

Inferior punctum

Lacrimal sac

Nasolacrimal duct

Nasal cavity

© MAYO CLINIC

Tear drainage system

Figure 64.1 Nasolacrimal system. (Used with permission of Mayo Foundation for Medical Education and Research, all rights reserved.)

changes, and papilledema. Preseptal cellulitis usually has minimal injection of the eye when compared to orbital cellulitis. If the soft tissue swelling is severe enough, this can make complete examination of the eye very limited, especially in preschool and younger aged child. In the ill-appearing child or those where a complete examination cannot be performed, it should be assumed that the infection is orbital until proven otherwise.

Insect bites and other local allergic reactions may be mistaken for cellulitis. Typically, this child will present without fever, may be itchy, and a punctate bite mark can be located with close inspection. Periorbital cellulitis would be unlikely to be bilateral, as opposed to allergic swelling which is often bilateral and associated with chemosis. A local vesicular rash with or without scleral hemorrhages suggest a viral source such as *varicella zoster* or *herpes simplex*. Common bacterial pathogens in cellulitis include strep species, *Staphylococcus aureus*, *Haemophilus influenzae*, and anaerobes. *Pseudomonas* and fungal infections should be considered in immunocompromised patients.

Preseptal Cellulitis Treatment

In a well-appearing child, preseptal cellulitis is treated with oral antibiotics and close follow-up. Antibiotic choice is typically amoxicillin–clavulanic acid or a third-generation cephalosporin for 10–14 days. Dual coverage for MRSA with either clindamycin or trimethoprim-sulfamethoxazole depends on local resistance patterns. These patients should have close follow-up in 24-48 hours, with admission for IV treatment in the absence of improvement.

Orbital Cellulitis Treatment

If orbital cellulitis is suspected a CT scan with contrast is the best imaging modality for confirmation; however, this may be normal in the first 24-48 hours. MRI can be helpful in patients with concern for intracranial spread; however, this can be difficult to obtain emergently if sedation is required. Orbital cellulitis can lead to meningitis if infection is inadequately treated; thus, a lumbar puncture should be considered if there are signs of intracranial spread. Other complications of orbital cellulitis include abscess, cavernous sinus thrombosis, and sepsis.

All children with orbital cellulitis require admission for IV antibiotics, typically with a third-generation cephalosporin and vancomycin. Anaerobic coverage with metronidazole should be added until intracranial spread can be excluded. Blood cultures are recommended before starting IV antibiotics. Culture of conjunctival drainage may not accurately reflect the causative organism and are not required. Ophthalmology should be consulted for any child with concern for orbital cellulitis. If there is associated sinusitis, consultation with otorhinolaryngology is also recommended. Adjuncts including nasal decongestants, nasal steroids, and topical ophthalmic antibiotics can be used to help treat associated sinusitis or conjunctivitis.

KEY POINTS

- Well-appearing children with preseptal cellulitis may be treated with oral antibiotics ensuring close out-patient follow-up.
- Orbital cellulitis requires admission for IV antibiotic therapy and ophthalmology consultation.
- CT scan of the orbits with contrast is the imaging test of choice to distinguish between preseptal and orbital cellulitis.

Suggested Readings

Givner LB. Periorbital versus orbital cellulitis. *Pediatr Infect Dis J*. 2002;21(12):1157-1158.
Goldman RD, Dolansky G, Rogovik AL. Predictors for admission of children with periorbital cellulitis presenting to the pediatric emergency department. *Pediatr Emerg Care*. 2008;24(5):279-283.
Wald ER. Periorbital and orbital infections. *Pediatr Rev*. 2004;25(9):312-320.

"Eye Spy" Abnormal Pupils: Be Aware That an Abnormal Pupillary Exam Is Often a Sign of Underlying Problems

Emily Wagner, MD and Geoffrey P. Hays, MD

The Normal Pupil

As the opening of the iris, the pupil can vary in size with response to light intensity and neurologic stimuli. Pupillary dilation is controlled by the sympathetic nervous system, ending with the dilator muscle of the iris (CN V). The constriction of the iris is caused by the parasympathetic activation of the iris sphincter muscle (CN III). A normal pupillary examination should evaluate for circular shape, symmetry between pupils, direct and consensual reaction to a light source, and symmetric red reflex. Abnormalities in these or associated corneal clouding, proptosis, scleral injection, or pain with extraocular movements can indicate disease.

Small Pupil (Miosis)

For bilateral miosis, ask about medication/toxin exposure! Toxidromes causing miosis include the cholinergic toxidrome, the narcotic toxidrome, and the sedative/hypnotic toxidrome. *Unilateral miosis may be Horner syndrome* caused by a disruption somewhere along the sympathetic nerve chain (absence of dilation stimulus). *Look for* ptosis, miosis, and anhidrosis! Evaluation should focus on imaging to find the lesion as etiology ranges from birth trauma, neuroblastoma, pulmonary malignancy, carotid artery dissection, and stroke.

Large Pupil (Mydriasis)

Again, consider meds and toxins for bilateral mydriasis. Mydriatic toxidromes include the anticholinergic and sympathetic toxidromes. Examples include antihistamines, cocaine, methamphetamine, or opiate withdrawal syndrome. Unilateral mydriasis can be from elevated intraocular pressure. Do not miss this diagnosis! Differential diagnosis includes glaucoma (rare in children!), medication exposure, and trauma with retrobulbar hemorrhage or tear in the pupillary constrictor ring. *If unilateral progresses to bilateral*, beware impending brain herniation from increased intracranial pressure! Consider trauma, brain tumor, and causes of cerebral edema including hyperammonemia.

Misshapen Pupil

In the setting of trauma, a teardrop pupil may indicate a globe rupture with possible orbital floor fracture. Extraocular movements may be restricted due to muscle entrapment. Fluorescein staining may show a positive Seidel sign (fluid leaking from the rupture site). Emergency treatment includes emergent ophthalmologic consultation, antiemetics (to avoid vomiting-induced worsening of globe rupture), and placement of eye shield. Give intravenous antibiotics, and ensure tetanus vaccine is current. Avoid direct ophthalmologic therapy and do **not** check intraocular pressures if an open globe is suspected. *A keyhole pupil or coloboma* may give you a clue to an underlying genetic condition such as CHARGE syndrome or Kabuki syndrome. The coloboma may be unilateral or bilateral and has likely been present since birth. A new finding in an infant should prompt outpatient genetic consultation.

Discolored Pupil

The normal response to shining a light at the pupil is a red pupillary reflex. Leukocoria (white pupillary reflex) requires emergent ophthalmology consultation for evaluation of retinoblastoma or other serious neoplasm. This is to be distinguished from corneal clouding, which is visible without shining a light and is seen with cataracts, glaucoma, or systemic disease with ocular manifestations (eg, Sturge-Weber syndrome and galactosemia).

Abnormally Reactive Pupil

Sluggish or nonreactive pupils should be correlated to mental status. Again, DO NOT MISS increased intracranial pressure from trauma, tumors, or infection. Head imaging to identify the lesions and neurosurgical consultation should be performed without delay. Consider toxin ingestion such as antidepressants, antipsychotics, and herbal OTC medications. May indicate the presence of a syndrome. Specific examples include hyperammonemia resulting from a metabolic disorder and congenital central hypoventilation syndrome.

KEY POINTS

- Abnormal pupils can be clues to serious pathology! Ask a family member if the patient has a history of abnormal pupil shape prior to the presentation to the ED.
- Small pupil: think Horner syndrome (emergent conditions include stroke, encephalitis/meningitis, internal carotid dissection) and toxidromes.
- Large pupil: evaluate for elevated intraocular or intracranial pressure or toxidromes.

- Misshapen pupil: teardrop pupil indicates globe rupture in the setting of trauma. A coloboma is congenital and should make you consider other genetic anomalies.
- Discolored pupil: leukocoria is a retinoblastoma until proven otherwise.
- Abnormally reactive pupil: do not miss increased ICP.

Suggested Readings

James R. Red reflex examination in neonates, infants, and children. *Pediatrics.* 2008;122(6):1401-1404.
Khan Z. Horner syndrome. *StatPearls: NCBI Bookshelf.* 2019.
Raoof N. Disorders of the Pediatric pupil. *Int Ophthalmol Clin.* 2018 Fall;58(4):11-22. Review.
Tintinalli, J. *Emergency Medicine: A Comprehensive Study Guide.* New York, NY: McGraw-Hill Education; 2016.

Nasolacrimal Duct Disorders: More Than Just Tears

Meghan Cain, MD

The nasolacrimal system is a complex pump system that pulls tears into the nose, stimulated by eye blinking. Tears are drawn from the eye, into the lacrimal sac via the canaliculi when the eye is closed. Upon eye opening, tears are pumped down the nasolacrimal duct into the nose. Normal tear production is not complete until 6 weeks of age; therefore, it is common for newborns to cry without visible tearing during the first weeks of life.

Nasolacrimal duct obstruction (NLDO), also known as dacryostenosis, is the most common cause of excess tear production in infants. This most often results from a failure to cannulate the distal portion of the duct at the valve of Hasner. Most patients present in the first few months of life with increased tearing, matted lashes, and mucopurulent eye drainage, often from the lateral canthus. The infant may also have a history of recurrent conjunctivitis. The lower eyelid becomes irritated due to increased tearing, but there is not associated nasal discharge or conjunctival injection. The lack of nasal discharge is helpful for differentiation from congenital glaucoma, which would demonstrate photophobia, buphthalmos, and corneal clouding.

NLDO can be confirmed with bedside testing. Using a finger or swab to create pressure over the lacrimal sac with massage in an upward motion will express mucopurulent material, consistent with obstruction. Additionally, fluorescein staining can be used to confirm the diagnosis. If the dye is still present in the eye 5 minutes after instillation, the infant has NLDO.

Over 90% of cases will clear spontaneously within the first 6 months, and most of those that persist will resolve by a year. Warm compresses and downward duct massage should be used for conservative treatment. Topical ophthalmic antibiotics can be used if there is concern for a secondary associated conjunctivitis. If the patient is 6-10 months of age, or has recurrent dacryocystitis, the patient can be referred to ophthalmology for consideration of duct probing. There is also an increased risk of amblyopia in infants with NLDO, and ophthalmology referral is warranted with any concerns.

Dacryocystitis is infection of the nasolacrimal sac presenting with swelling of the nasal aspect of the lower eyelid and periorbital area. This most commonly presents in infants with NLDO. Symptoms include erythema and swelling of the skin over the nasolacrimal sac along with tenderness and purulent drainage.

Patients with dacryocystitis should be treated with both oral and topical antibiotics. Gram-positive organisms are the most common source. Oral cefpodoxime (10 mg/kg/d po in two divided doses) or amoxicillin-clavulanate (25-45 mg/kg/d po in two divided doses) should be first line. Intravenous cefuroxime (50-100 mg/kg/d iv in three divided doses) is used in the ill-appearing child. A swab of the discharge should be sent for culture to target antibiotic coverage. Warm compresses and topical ophthalmic antibiotics are used as adjuncts to help clear the infection. Patients should be seen for follow-up within 2-3 days for reevaluation. Rarely, this can progress to severe infection such as preseptal cellulitis, orbital cellulitis, or meningitis.

Dacryocystocele (aka dacryocele, amniotocele) is secondary to blockage of the nasolacrimal sac at both the proximal and distal ends. These infants present shortly after birth with a blue, firm cyst below the medial canthal tendon. If this cystic structure protrudes into the nose, there may also be associated respiratory distress. The obstruction may be relieved by digital massage; however, these patients should have urgent referral to ophthalmology due to the risk of dacryocystitis and nasal obstruction.

KEY POINTS

- Patients with NLDO should be managed conservatively unless there are signs of infection.
- After 6-10 months of age, infants with NLDO should be referred to ophthalmology for probing.
- Dacryocystitis should be treated with systemic antibiotics; topical therapy alone is not sufficient.
- Patients with dacryocystocele require urgent ophthalmologic referral.

Suggested Readings

Bagheri N, Wajda B, Calvo C, et al. *The Wills Eye Manual: Office and Emergency Room Diagnosis and Treatment of Eye Disease*. 7th ed. Philadelphia, PA: Wolters Kluwer; 2017.
Lederman C, Lederman M. Ophthalmologic emergencies. In: Gershel JC, Crain EF, eds. *Clinical Manual of Emergency Pediatrics*. 6th ed. Cambridge, United Kingdom: Cambridge University Press; 2018.
Örge FH, Boente CS. The Lacrimal System. *Pediatr Clin*. 2014;61:529-539.
Schnall BM. Pediatric nasolacrimal duct obstruction. *Curr Opin Ophthalmol*. 2013;24:421-424.

Conjunctivitis: A Sight for Sore Eyes

Yvette Wang, MD and Elise Zimmerman, MD, MS

The conjunctiva is a thin, clear membrane lining the inner surface of the eyelids and outer surface of the globe up to the limbus. Conjunctivitis, commonly known as "pink eye," is inflammation of the conjunctiva and presents with conjunctival hyperemia or injection. Patients may also have eye discharge, eyelid swelling, and feelings of eye grittiness or burning. There are many causes of conjunctivitis. Viruses are the most common cause of infectious conjunctivitis, though bacterial conjunctivitis occurs more frequently in children than adults. Conjunctivitis is typically benign.

Infectious

Bacterial conjunctivitis typically causes acute unilateral conjunctivitis that quickly spreads to the opposite eye. There is often associated purulent eye discharge, with matting of the eyelashes. The major pathogens are nontypeable *H influenzae*, *S pneumoniae*, *M catarrhalis*, and *S aureus*. Bacterial conjunctivitis typically has a self-limited course, lasting 7-10 days. Topical antibiotic agents including fluoroquinolones, trimethoprim/polymyxin B, and erythromycin can reduce the duration of symptoms and transmission of disease. Patients with contact lenses should remove their contact lenses and be referred urgently to an ophthalmologist as these patients are at higher risk of developing corneal ulcers.

Neonatal conjunctivitis occurs less frequently with the use of prophylactic erythromycin ointment. Consider gonorrhea and chlamydia as causes of conjunctivitis with purulent discharge in the first 2 weeks of life. Classically, gonorrhea conjunctivitis occurs days 2-5 after delivery, while chlamydia conjunctivitis presents on days 5-14 after birth. Infants with gonorrhea conjunctivitis should undergo hourly saline eye lavage, be treated with parenteral antibiotics, and be admitted to the hospital. Oral erythromycin should also be started to cover chlamydial infection until eye cultures are negative in order to prevent chlamydia pneumonitis. Nasolacrimal duct obstruction can be confused with conjunctivitis, as both can present with eye discharge. However, the conjunctiva is typically clear with nasolacrimal duct obstruction.

Adenovirus is the most common cause of viral conjunctivitis. Watery or mucoid discharge, preauricular lymphadenopathy, and concurrent pharyngitis, including upper respiratory symptoms, suggest this etiology. Supportive treatment, such as the use of cool compresses and removal of eye discharge with a clean cloth to decrease transmission of infection, is recommended. Antibiotic therapy is not indicated.

Herpes simplex virus (HSV) can cause conjunctivitis in both neonates and children. This diagnosis should be considered in neonates with perinatal risk factors for HSV infection (e.g., active HSV lesions at the time of vaginal delivery). The presence of vesicles on the face should also raise concerns for this diagnosis. On fluorescein staining, herpes keratitis has a classic dendritic pattern. Conjunctival cultures should be obtained. Neonates should be started on intravenous acyclovir and topical antiviral therapy and should be admitted to evaluate for disseminated HSV infection. Topical corticosteroids should be avoided.

Noninfectious

Allergic conjunctivitis is an inflammatory response of the conjunctivae to environmental allergens, such as pollen. Seasonality and eye itching, along with bilateral eye redness, suggest an allergic etiology. Chemosis (edema of the conjunctiva) may also be present. These symptoms are treated with artificial tears and topical antihistamines.

Systemic illnesses such as Kawasaki disease, Stevens-Johnson syndrome, and Parinaud oculoglandular syndrome can also cause conjunctivitis. Kawasaki disease typically causes bilateral conjunctivitis with limbic sparing, in addition to fever, lymphadenopathy, rash, mucositis, and extremity changes. Patients with Stevens-Johnson syndrome have severe conjunctivitis with purulent discharge. The conjunctivitis is typically preceded by fever and an influenzalike illness, followed by cutaneous and mucosal lesions. Parinaud oculoglandular syndrome presents with unilateral conjunctivitis with ipsilateral tender lymphadenopathy and is most frequently an atypical presentation of catscratch disease.

In general, conjunctivitis is benign and self-limiting. However, for patients with severe pain or changes in visual acuity, or those wearing contact lenses, consider more concerning etiologies such as gonococcal, pseudomonal, and HSV infections. Also consider other etiologies for eye redness, especially in patients with preceding trauma. These higher-risk conditions may require ophthalmology evaluation.

KEY POINTS

- Conjunctivitis is most commonly viral. Antibiotics can decrease the duration of symptoms of bacterial conjunctivitis but are not indicated in the treatment of viral conjunctivitis.
- In neonates with conjunctivitis, consider gonorrhea, chlamydia, and HSV. Patients with these causes need parenteral treatment and admission for ongoing management.
- Those with contact lenses should remove and discard their contact lenses.

Suggested Readings

Azari AA, Barney NP. Conjunctivitis: a systematic review of diagnosis and treatment. *JAMA*. 2013;310(16):1721-1729.
Prentiss KA, Dorfman DA. Pediatric ophthalmology in the emergency department. *Emerg Med Clin N Am*. 2008;26:181-198.
Richards A, Guzman-Cottrill JA. Conjunctivitis. *Pediatr Rev*. 2010;31(5):196-206.

AIRWAY

Not Considering an Infant's Airway as a "Difficult Airway" from the Beginning

Jenna Lillemoe, MD and Ari Cohen, MD, FAAP

It would be helpful if infants could be managed as "little adults" when procedures are performed. Regrettably, this is not the case for infants (aged 0-1) who require intubation as they have many features that together constitute a "difficult" airway. There are a few simple steps that providers can take in preparation and technique to optimize success in securing the neonatal airway.

Anatomic Challenges

The infant's airway poses several clinical challenges. In addition to having smaller anatomic landmarks, infants have multiple anatomic features that impede visualization of the vocal cords making intubation more difficult.

Young infants have relatively short necks and large occiputs, which positions the airway anteriorly and can cause difficulty in visualizing the glottis. A small towel roll placed beneath the neck and shoulders, avoiding hyperextension, can help to improve the position of the anatomic landmarks by aligning the external auditory meatus along a horizontal line with the sternal notch.

The tongue and epiglottis in infants are larger relative to the oral cavity. These structures can collapse or protrude into the airway, further obscuring a provider's view. Infants also have a short and relatively narrow trachea that is easily compressed. Therefore, the common practice of applying cricoid pressure should be used with caution, as this maneuver can further obstruct an already narrow upper airway.

Procedure Preparation

Appropriate supplies can make all the difference for successful intubation of an infant. This includes a proper laryngoscope, endotracheal (ET) tubes, and suction supplies. Although less commonly used for older patients, straight laryngoscope blades are essential for infant intubations. Straight blades more effectively lift an infant's tongue and epiglottis, allowing for better visualization of the vocal cords. The use of some video laryngoscopes can be challenging due to the size of the infant mouth, often making direct laryngoscopy necessary. Uncuffed ET tubes are typically preferred to reduce damage to the airway and resistance of airflow, although cuffed tubes can also be used.

Having the appropriate size materials can greatly increase your chances for success; therefore, it is advisable to have a few options of laryngoscopes and ET tubes at the bedside prior to attempting intubation (Table 68.1). Depth of tube insertion should also be carefully estimated to prevent right mainstem bronchus intubation, a very common complication in small infants.

Rapid sequence intubation medications should be considered for all infant intubations, as small infants can still be feisty, making an already difficult procedure even more challenging. Medications for both sedation and paralysis should be considered, especially if the infant is awake and vigorous. The

Table 68.1 ■ Neonatal Airway Tools			
	Newborn	Small Infant	Infant
Weight (in kg)	3-5	6-7	8-9
Laryngoscope blade	0-1 straight	1 straight	1 straight
Tracheal tube	3.0-3.5 uncuffed	3.5 uncuffed	3.5 uncuffed
Tracheal tube length (cm at lip)	9.5-10	10.5-11	10.5-11

use of sedation medications is of standard practice in these cases but use of paralytics in all infants is controversial.

Despite a "difficult" airway, infants can usually be easy to bag-mask ventilate with proper head positioning. It is critical, however, to use careful technique to also avoid excessive pressure on the face as this may lead to bradycardia as well as potentially obstruct the airway. Good bag-mask ventilation techniques may be the most important airway skill to have and refine. If additional support is needed for an intubation, proper bag-mask ventilation technique can be used until additional help arrives.

KEY POINTS

- Infants have "difficult" airway anatomy. Simple strategies can help align the airway for better visualization.
- Take time to prepare with size appropriate supplies.
- Perfect proper bag-mask ventilation techniques.

Suggested Readings

Kleinman ME, de Caen AR, et al. Pediatric basic and advanced life support: 2010 international consensus on cardiopulmonary resuscitation and emergency cardiovascular care science with treatment recommendations. *Pediatrics.* 2010;126(5):e1261-e1318.

Litman RS, Fiadjoe JE, et al. The pediatric airway. In: Cote CJ, Lerman J, Anderson B, eds. *A Practice of Anesthesia for Infants and Children.* 5th ed. Philadelphia, PA: Saunders-Elsevier; 2013.

Not Knowing the Differences Between the Pediatric and Adult Airways Can Lead to Failure to Intubate the Pediatric Airway

James C. O'Neill, MD, FACEP and Shad Baab, MD

To successfully intubate a pediatric patient, one should be aware of the differences between the pediatric and adult airways. Knowing these differences enables the practitioner to acquire the positioning that will ensure success. Pediatric airways are similar to adult airways starting at age 10. Knowledge of pediatric airway differences is even more important if the patient is below the age of two. There are obvious differences between the adult and pediatric airways. The pediatric patient's mouth, oropharynx, and airway are smaller, but it is important to note that the tongue and tonsils are larger in comparison. The epiglottis in the pediatric airway is larger, differently shaped, and floppier then the adult equivalent. Because of these differences, the Miller or other straight blades are used to intubate children. We recommend using a Broselow tape to help with equipment selection. The narrow straight blade is used to push the tongue to the left during the procedure and is used to pick up the epiglottis. Significant care must be taken to be gentle and avoid hitting the tonsils since they are large and are likely to bleed with trauma.

The pediatric airway is more anterior than the adult airway. Practitioners used to intubating adults will often see the esophageal opening where they are expecting the airway. Be prepared to look more anterior than in the adult patient. Additionally, in younger children, the pediatric airway looks remarkably like the esophageal opening due to being not fully developed. It is easy to confuse the two. The pediatric airway is more cephalad than the adult airway.

Another important difference that is often overlooked is the difference in size of the pediatric occiput. The adult patient often requires a pillow under the head to place him or her in "sniffing position" to align airway axes. Pediatric patients often require a folded blanket under the shoulders to align the airway for intubation. This can be dramatic with younger children with relatively larger occiputs.

Additionally, the narrowest portion of the pediatric airway is the cricoid ring, directly below the vocal cords. This is especially frustrating when, after visualizing the vocal cords, attempts to pass a tube are stopped just beyond the vocal cords. It is essential to have tube sizes that are an extra half or whole size smaller ready during intubation attempts. This is essential with patients who might have swelling at or below the vocal cords with disease processes such as croup or bacterial tracheitis. Cuffed tubes are preferred as long as they are available. If there is not a cuffed tube available, one often has to listen for an "air leak" from the tube. The air leak ensures that the cricoid ring is not so tight around the tube that scarring and subglottic stenosis could occur over time.

Finally, there is a very short distance between being past the vocal cords and into the right main stem. Often there is only one centimeter of distance once past the vocal cords before a tube is in the right main stem. It is especially important to be in the correct location as soon as possible since a child's basal oxygen consumption is faster than an adult's. Children rapidly drop oxygen saturations when there is a right main stem intubation. Since breath sounds are often difficult to perceive in a noisy emergency department bay, we recommend using the Broselow tape to choose initial tube depth. This should be confirmed with the usual techniques, including chest radiograph.

KEY POINTS

- Knowing the differences between the pediatric and adult airways will help you perform the intubation of the airway successfully.
- Equipment sizes and tube depth are best selected with a tool such as the Broselow Tape. Chronically ill children who require airway management are often not the expected size for their age.
- In young children, a blanket under the shoulders is especially helpful for positioning if the patient has a large occiput.

Suggested Readings

Phipps LM, Thomas NJ, Gilmore RK, et al. Prospective assessment of guidelines for determining appropriate depth of endotracheal tube placement in children. *Pediatr Crit Care Med.* 2005;6(5):519-522.

Shah AN, Frush K, Luo X, Wears RL. Effect of an intervention standardization system on pediatric dosing and equipment size determination: a crossover trial involving simulated resuscitation events. *Arch Pediatr Adolesc Med.* 2003;157(3):229-236.

Walls RM, Murphy MF. *Manual of Emergency Medicine Management.* 4th ed. Philadelphia, PA: Lippincott Williams & Wilkins; 2012.

70

Get Rid of Your Discomfort With Percutaneous Transtracheal Ventilation

David Skibbie, MD, MA, FACEP, FAAEM

Introduction

It might be argued that percutaneous transtracheal ventilation is an imprecise term, as it is more accurately a method of rescue oxygenation. Generally, this procedure is considered in young children in "can't intubate, can't oxygenate" (CICO) scenarios. Although oxygenation through a small-bore catheter is purported to be minimally effective, jet ventilation and oxygenation via a small bore conduit is routinely employed in laryngeal surgery, since endotracheal intubation would make such procedures impossible. Emergency transtracheal oxygenation can be a highly effective method of rescue, given proper equipment and preparation.

Patient Selection

Cricothyrotomy allows for placement of a large bore airway device but is typically limited to adults and children 8 years of age or greater. For children <8 years, placement of a small bore cannula is the only anatomically viable method for rescue oxygenation in CICO scenarios. Certain pathologies (including croup and subglottic stenosis) obliterate the subglottic space and thus are not amenable to placement of a cannula in the cricothyroid space. In such situations, the cannula must be placed transtracheally.

Cannula Selection

Intravenous cannulas, 12-16 gauge, are commonly used for this procedure, although they tend to kink. Wire-reinforced catheters are available and effectively combat this issue, so are strongly recommended over IV catheters.

Cannula Placement

The cricothyroid membrane is the safest location to place a transtracheal catheter, since the thyroid and cricoid cartilages form a solid cartilaginous cage posteriorly.

The Cricothyroid Cannula Procedure

1. Locate the cricothyroid space by palpating the superior edge of the thyroid cartilage, identified by a V-notch in the midline. Slide your finger down the thyroid cartilage until you palpate the cricoid cartilage, identified as a prominence just below the thyroid cartilage. The cricothyroid membrane is the area between the two.
2. Attach a syringe containing 1-2 cc of sterile saline to the cannula. Puncture the cricothyroid membrane transversely while simultaneously aspirating. Intraluminal placement is identified with free flow of air into the syringe; the catheter-stylet assembly must be advanced 2-3 mm beyond this point to place the cannula fully into the airway. If the posterior wall is contacted, withdraw a few millimeters and reconfirm intraluminal placement.
3. Rotate the syringe-cannula assembly to point inferiorly, slide the cannula into the airway, and remove the needle.

The Transtracheal Cannula Procedure

1. Locate the superior aspect of the trachea, just below the cricoid cartilage. The tracheal rings are palpable in this area. Puncture is made between the first and second tracheal rings.
2. Attach a syringe containing 1-2 cc of sterile saline to the cannula. Puncture the trachea at 45 degrees inferiorly while simultaneously aspirating. Since the trachea is more deformable than the cricothyroid complex, the posterior wall is often punctured; slight withdrawal allows the trachea to rebound. Intraluminal placement is confirmed with free flow of air into the syringe.
3. Slide the cannula into the airway and remove the needle.

Methods for Oxygenation

Jet Ventilator

A jet ventilator is the most controllable device for transtracheal oxygenation, as it allows selection of a precise maximum pressure. Pressure is increased until diaphragmatic movement is noted. An initial pressure is selected (5-10 cm H_2O is reasonable), and oxygen flow is triggered. Long expiratory times are generally recommended with this device; however, since airway pressure is limited by the device, barotrauma is unlikely. Hypoxia and atelectasis are the pertinent issues when cannula oxygenation is employed. These are best combatted with longer inhalation intervals.

Other Devices

There are several commercial devices designed for the purpose of transtracheal oxygenation. In general, these are oxygen conduits that include a luer-lock connector, a connection device for an oxygen flowmeter, and fenestrations which are closed manually to provide oxygen flow to the patient.

Finally, and perhaps most simply, a bag-valve device can be connected to the cannula using a 3.0 ETT adaptor. Unfortunately, BVM methods are difficult to control, may not provide adequate airway pressures, and may dislodge the cannula.

KEY POINTS

- Preparation provides the greatest likelihood of success.
- IV cannulas tend to kink; use a wire-reinforced cannula.
- The pressure obtained from a jet ventilator can be controlled precisely so is the preferred oxygenation device.
- Bag-valve methods are difficult to control, may not provide enough pressure, and may dislodge the catheter.

Suggested Readings

Chapter 6. Hebert RB, Bose S, Mace, SE, ed. Cricothyrotomy and percutaneous translaryngeal ventilation. In: *Roberts and Hedges' Clinical Procedures in Emergency Medicine and Acute Care*. 7th ed. Philadelphia, PA: Elsevier Saunders; 2014:130-133.
Chapter 19. Bair AE, Caro DA, ed. Surgical airway techniques. In: *The Walls Manual of Emergency Airway Management*. 5th ed. Philadelphia, PA: Wolters Kluwer; 2018:224-230.

71

Treating All Noisy Breathing as the Same

Emily C. MacNeill, MD and Nicholena Richardson, MD

"There's no such thing as an easy pediatric intubation" is an important motto to live by. This statement is especially applicable to a child whose breathing you can hear when you enter a room. Thankfully, the need to definitive control of airway is infrequent. Management of these patients will be reviewed after a discussion of normal anatomy, physiology, and the pathology that can occur.

Normal Anatomy and Physiology

The young pediatric patient is more susceptible to the following issues: airway obstruction (larger occiput, larger tongue, large and floppy epiglottis, and flexible trachea), respiratory failure (decreased slow-twitch skeletal muscle, lower glycogen stores in respiratory muscles, flatter diaphragms, and smaller airways with increased resistance), and faster desaturation during apnea (lower functional residual capacity, higher metabolic rates, and fewer alveoli). These factors make pediatric airway management a high stakes game.

Pathology

Children under 2 years of age are among the pediatric patients at the highest risk for respiratory distress. Acute problems are either infectious or noninfectious. Though vaccination has led to a decrease in some infectious causes of airway obstruction, infection continues to be the most common causes of acute upper airway obstruction in the children. There are many chronic etiologies of pediatric airway obstruction (Table 71.1). Most of these issues resolve as the child grows, and the laryngotracheal structures become more cartilaginous. Superimposed infections can lead to decompensation, and it is crucial to understand how these pathologies would make intubation exceedingly difficult.

Management

When faced with a pediatric airway obstruction, history and physical exam are key. Chronic symptoms may warrant investigation, but perhaps not emergent action. Acute problems, however, usually require acute intervention. You must utilize your physical exam skills to isolate the location of the airway obstruction. Inspiratory stridor suggests that the obstruction is above the vocal cords, while expiratory stridor indicates an obstruction below the vocal cords.

Pain, fever, and fear lead to worsening airway obstruction in the small child, thus remaining calm, keeping children with their caregiver, and administering antipyretics and analgesics are all crucial steps. Do not forget that steroids and racemic epinephrine are often helpful to avoid further action.

Airway management does not necessarily equal intubation. Alternatives include high-flow nasal canula (HFNC) and noninvasive positive pressure ventilation (NIPPV). HFNC can generate a PEEP effect of up to 4-6 cm H_2O using flow rates of 1.5-2 L/kg/min in infants, which has been shown to effectively decrease the work of breathing. NIPPV decreases work of breathing, reverses hypoventilation, and maintains upper airway patency, but it requires a cooperative and alert patient. If the onset of respiratory distress is acute and severe, you are concerned for a foreign body, or other methods are failing, intubation may be necessary. Proper preparation and ensuring all available adjuncts (pediatric bougies, multiple sized tubes, supraglottic airways, and equipment for jet ventilation) are ready at the bedside is imperative.

Table 71.1 ■ Common Congenital Airway Anomalies

	Time Course	Presentation	Further Investigations	Normal Course	Treatment
Laryngomalacia	1st wk	Inspiratory stridor Worse in supine position (feeding and sleeping)	None	Resolves spontaneously by age 2	Surgery only if necessary
Vocal cord paralysis	Congenital (birth) or acquired	Bilateral birth Unilateral—weak cry, feeding difficulties, stridor and recurrent aspiration	Brain imaging for bilateral Thoracic imaging for unilateral	Spontaneous recovery in 70%	CO_2 laser (usually after 1 y)
Tracheomalacia		Expiratory stridor		Most resolve 6-12 mo	
Subglottic stenosis		Recurrent episodes of croup-like illness		Persistent symptoms	Bougie dilatation, cricoid split, tracheal resections
Hemangioma	Asymptomatic at birth, presents 3 wks to 3 mo	Biphasic stridor		Worsens until 2-5 y when it spontaneously involutes	Propranolol, systemic or lesional steroids, laser/open excision

KEY POINTS

- Utilize the physical exam to isolate the location of the airway issue; inspiratory stridor is above the cords and expiratory stridor is below.
- The most important piece of information to gather is whether this is acute or chronic in onset.
- You may have to intervene, but do not jump to intubation! Never anticipate a pediatric intubation to be easy.

Suggested Readings

Mandal A, et al. Upper airway obstruction in children. *Indian J Pediatr.* 2015;82(8):737-744. www.ncbi.nlm.nih.gov/pubmed/26104110

Santillanes G, Gausche-Hill M. Pediatric airway management. *Emerg Med Clin North Am.* 2008;26(4):961-975. www.ncbi.nlm.nih.gov/pubmed/19059095

Schibler A, Franklin D. Respiratory support for children in the emergency department. *J Paediatr Child Health.* 2016;52(2):192-196. www.ncbi.nlm.nih.gov/pubmed/27062623

72

Don't Rush to Intubate an Infant After PGE1 Administration

Erica Scott, MD and Kathleen Kinney Bryant, MD, FACEP

Sneaky Congenital Heart Defects Can Be Deadly

Fetal circulation is maintained by several circulatory ducts, most importantly the ductus arteriosus (DA). In utero, endogenous prostaglandins are produced to maintain the patency of the DA. The DA begins to close within 24–72 hours after birth. This closure is caused by decreased production of endogenous prostaglandins and increased arterial oxygen saturation (PaO_2). Fetal echocardiography and postnatal congenital heart defect (CHD) screening by pulse oximetry are helpful in the early identification of infants with ductal-dependent CHD. Despite these screening tests, infants with CHD may be missed and present to the emergency department (ED) in extremis. For infants who are cyanotic, murmurs are good indicators that a ductal-dependent lesion may be present. In noncyanotic infants, a better indicator is abnormal pulses, specifically diminished femoral pulses.

Prostaglandins

Alprostadil (PGE1) is a naturally occurring prostaglandin that can be used to prevent or reverse ductus closure in neonatal resuscitation. PGE1 must be administered as an infusion. The majority of PGE1 (60%-80%) is metabolized on first pass through the lungs. The initial dose of PGE1 is 0.05-0.1 µg/kg/min, then titrated until PaO_2 increase is noted. The PaO_2 usually increases within 10–15 minutes after PGE1 is started, but in some cases the ductus may not reopen for several hours. Transposition of the great vessels with a restrictive atrial septum and obstructed total anomalous pulmonary venous drainage are two examples where there is a delayed response to PGE1. Once a clinical response is noted, the lowest effective dose of PGE1 should be used to maintain the patency of the ductus and allow stabilization of the infant until definitive intervention. PGE1 has many adverse effects, most significant being apnea (especially in infants <2 kg), fever, seizures, flushing, bradycardia, hypotension, and diarrhea.

To Intubate or Not?

There are no specific guidelines for intubating infants with ductal-dependent CHD. Intubation for respiratory support based on initial presentation may precede PGE1 administration. Apnea secondary to PGE1 infusion is another common consideration for intubation. Recent studies have shown that infants not intubated prior to the start of PGE1 or due to apnea after PGE1 can be safely transported without mechanical ventilation. Additional studies have addressed the risk of prophylactic intubations prior to transport in stable infants requiring PGE1 infusions.

Endotracheal intubation carries its own risks. In infants, one of the more serious complications can be preload reduction with resulting hypotension requiring further medications for circulatory support. Further risks include mechanical complications such as esophageal intubation, endotracheal occlusion, displacement requiring emergent reintubation, and equipment failure. Prophylactic intubation may not be necessary simply because of PGE1 initiation if the child is not having respiratory distress. Apnea is more likely to occur in nonventilated infants when the PGE1 infusion rate is >0.015 µg/kg/min, so low-dose PGE1 (<0.015 µg/kg/min) is not a reason to electively intubate an infant prior to transport. As mentioned above, elective intubation prior to transport has been demonstrated to be a significant predictor of major transport complications. Other potential airway management options include noninvasive ventilation including intermittent bagged valve mask for brief apnea, CPAP, high-flow nasal cannula, and noninvasive positive pressure ventilation. In infants being treated with PGE1 not requiring emergent intubation, the risks for prophylactic intubation must be carefully weighed against the potential benefits.

KEY POINTS

- Early PGE1 is lifesaving in infants with suspected ductal-dependent CHD.
- There are many adverse effects of PGE1, including apnea. Apnea should not prompt stopping or lowering a PGE1 infusion.
- Prophylactic intubation after PGE1 can increase potential complications.
- Alternative respiratory support options include BVM ventilation for short apneic episodes or noninvasive ventilation.

Suggested Readings

Carmo K, Barr P, West M, et al. Transporting newborn infants with suspected duct dependent congenital heart disease on low-dose prostaglandin E1 without routine mechanical ventilation. *Arch Dis Child Fetal Neonatal Ed.* 2007;92:F117-F119.

Hundalani SG, Kulkarni M, Fernandes CJ, et al. Prostaglandin E1 for maintain ductal patency in neonates with ductus-dependent cardiac lesions. *Cochrane Database Syst Rev.* 2014;12.

Meckler GD, Lowe C. To intubate or Not intubate? Transporting Infants on Prostaglandin E1. *Pediatrics.* 2009;123:e25-e30.

Penny DJ, Shekerdenmian LS. Management of the neonate with symptomatic congenital heart disease. *Arch Dis Fetal Neonatal Ed.* 2001;84:F141-F145.

Singh Y, Mikrou P. Use of prostaglandins in duct-dependent congenital heart conditions. *Arch Dis Child Educ Pract Ed.* 2018;103:137-140.

Thinking Lack of Wheezing Is a Good Finding With Severe Asthma

Julia E. Martin, MD, FACEP

Not all asthmatics wheeze and not all wheezing is asthma. Wheezing can be bronchiolitis, status asthmaticus, anaphylaxis, foreign body aspiration, pneumonia, heart failure, and airway obstruction. A good history and physical examination will help narrow your differential.

Asthma is a combination of airway inflammation and bronchoconstriction, resulting in airflow obstruction. While wheezing is the hallmark of asthma, the most common presentation is cough. To wheeze, you need two things: obstruction and airflow. In severe asthmatics, there is little-to-no airflow—so there is little-to-no wheezing. Exacerbations have two phases: the early bronchospastic phase, which responds well to bronchodilators, and the later inflammatory phase, which is treated with steroids. Delay in treatment leads to decreased responsiveness to bronchodilators and increased likelihood of hospitalization.

Diagnostic testing for exacerbations is nearly worthless. Chest x-ray (CXR) and blood gases rarely change management. Exacerbation remains mainly a clinical diagnosis, and management should be based on therapy response.

Treatment

First-line management for all acute asthma exacerbation are inhaled beta-agonists and systemic steroids. Beta-agonists, such as albuterol, treat bronchospasm and should be used aggressively in moderate-to-severe exacerbations. It should be given early and repeated frequently in severe cases. In severe cases, continuous albuterol nebulizations are more effective than intermittent treatments. Inhaled anticholinergic agents, such as ipratropium, are also helpful in moderate-to-severe exacerbations and act synergistically when given with beta-agonists.

Exacerbations need systemic steroids. Compliance issues are common with oral prednisone and prednisolone, making dexamethasone a potentially more attractive choice. Steroids should be given early in the treatment course for maximum efficacy. Steroids may be given orally or IV since time to onset is similar for both routes.

Magnesium causes smooth muscle relaxation, thus helping reduce bronchoconstriction. It has been found useful in management of acute moderate-to-severe exacerbations.

Epinephrine also causes bronchodilation. In extreme cases, injectable IM epinephrine may be given. Inhaled racemic epinephrine—while well studied in croup—has not been well studied in asthma exacerbations. Case reports have found inhaled racemic epinephrine to be similar to albuterol but with increased side effects.

Respiratory support for severe cases can include noninvasive ventilation (NIV) and high-flow nasal cannula (HFNC). While NIV has been shown to be useful in severe exacerbations, it is not as well tolerated compared to HFNC and often requires anxiolysis. HFNC studies are limited, but case reports of successful outcomes do exist. Intubated patients in status asthmatics have significant risk for complications, and thus, all efforts should be made to avoid intubation whenever possible. Close monitoring with pulse oximetry and end-tidal CO_2 tends to be helpful adjuncts to predicting respiratory failure.

Watch Out

1) The intubation process in severe asthmatics is extremely hazardous; **plan for potential decompensation**. Anticipate subsequent hypotension, and give IV fluids prior to intubation to "prime the pump." It is also good to have vasopressors readily available as well. Patients in respiratory failure have exhausted their respiratory reserves and will likely decompensate quickly during intubation. Securing a definitive airway should be done by the most experience person available. Placement of the largest CUFFED endotracheal tube appropriate for the patient is important for oxygenation, ventilation, and suctioning.

2) After confirming tube placement, **assure appropriate ventilator settings**. Their lungs are generally hyperinflated due to air trapping, predisposing them to increased barotrauma. Expiratory phase time is prolonged due to airway obstruction, and ventilator settings should reflect this. Adjusting the inspiratory/expiratory (I:E) ratio time of 1:3 or 1:4 is extremely important to minimize further air trapping. Use smaller title volumes (5-6 mL/kg) to minimize air trapping. These setting will likely lead to permissive hypercarbia but will allow improved oxygenation.

3) Deterioration of an intubated asthmatic patient warrants a prompt evaluation for inappropriate ventilator settings, equipment failure, tube obstruction, displaced ET tube, and pneumothorax.

KEY POINTS

- Asthma exacerbation is a clinical diagnosis, and management is based on physical findings and response to therapy rather than diagnostic testing.
- First-line therapy includes inhaled beta-agonists and systemic steroids. The earlier the better.
- Take all efforts to avoid intubation if at all possible. Mechanically ventilated status asthmaticus patients have significant risks for decompensation. Pay close attention to ventilator settings.

Suggested Readings

Powell CV. Acute severe asthma. *J Paediatr Child Health*. 2016;52(2):187-191.
Rehder KJ. Adjunct therapies for refractory status asthmaticus in children. *Respir Care*. 2017;62(6):849-865.

74

Giving Albuterol to All Kids With Bronchiolitis

Rachel Cafferty, MD and Julia Fuzak Freeman, MD, FAAP

The adage "less is more" is quite fitting when discussing bronchiolitis management. Current guidelines emphasize supportive care over medical interventions for uncomplicated bronchiolitis, with a "rest is best" philosophy. Understanding the features of bronchiolitis, apnea risk factors, and management principles is key to avoiding overtreatment.

Bronchiolitis Basics

Bronchiolitis is a clinical syndrome of viral etiology affecting infants and children <2 years of age. It is most common, and often most severe, in infants aged 2-6 months. Classic presentation involves an upper respiratory infection prodrome (rhinorrhea and cough) followed by lower respiratory involvement manifested by tachypnea and/or retractions. Symptoms may last up to 2 weeks but often peak in severity between days 3 and 5 of illness. Inflammation, edema, and epithelial necrosis of the small airways (bronchioles) produces the characteristic diffuse wheezing and crackles on auscultation. A "changing examination" (fluctuations between clear, well-aerated lungs and then intermittent wheezes or crackles) is a hallmark of the disease. While respiratory syncytial virus (RSV) is the most common pathogen, other respiratory viruses (adenovirus, human metapneumovirus, coronavirus, parainfluenza, and influenza) can cause the same and equally severe clinical picture.

Apnea Risk Factors

Apnea is a life-threatening complication of bronchiolitis in young infants. Independent risk factors for apnea in bronchiolitis include prematurity (particularly <34 weeks gestation) or low birth weight (<2.3 kg), young age (<8 weeks), neuromuscular disease, and caregiver report of a witnessed apneic event. Infants with extremes of respiratory rate (<30 breaths/min or >70 breaths/min) and hypoxemia (SpO_2 < 90%) are also at risk of apnea. While patients with airway anomalies, chronic heart or lung conditions, or immunodeficiencies need to be assessed carefully, previously healthy term infants >2 months of age without significant respiratory distress or hypoxemia have an overall lower risk of apnea.

Management Strategies

Bronchiolitis is a clinical diagnosis that is based on history and physical examination findings. In previously healthy patients who are >2 months of age and at low-risk for apnea, management focuses on supportive care (suctioning and maintaining hydration) and supplemental oxygen for hypoxemia. Patients with significant respiratory distress or apnea may require additional respiratory support, such as high-flow nasal cannula or noninvasive positive pressure ventilation. Nebulized bronchodilators, hypertonic saline, and systemic glucocorticoids have been used with variable results. Current evidence shows no clinical benefit and some deleterious effects from these therapies, which are no longer recommended in the routine treatment of bronchiolitis. Despite a present wheeze, bronchodilators are largely ineffective and not indicated for patients with uncomplicated bronchiolitis. Viral testing is also not routinely indicated, as the identification of a specific respiratory pathogen will not affect treatment, outcome, risk-stratification, or resource utilization. In febrile infants with bronchiolitis (particularly with prolonged fever or hyperpyrexia), providers should consider secondary causes of fever such as acute otitis media, urinary tract infection (UTI), or more rarely pneumonia, on a case-by-case basis. Literature suggests that the incidence of concurrent UTI with bronchiolitis may be less than previously estimated. Chest radiography is also not routinely indicated and has been linked to increased inappropriate antibiotic usage despite relatively low rates of superimposed bacterial pneumonia in patients with bronchiolitis.

It is notable that low-risk infants with bronchiolitis recover without significant medical intervention, reaffirming the principle of "less is more" in treatment of this disease.

KEY POINTS

- Bronchiolitis is characterized by a fluctuating pulmonary examination and serial examinations can aid in making the diagnosis.
- Independent risk factors for apnea in bronchiolitis include prematurity, young age, low birth weight, neuromuscular disease, tachypnea or bradypnea, hypoxemia ($SpO_2 < 90\%$), or out-of-hospital apneic event(s).
- RSV positivity does not predict disease severity or does it increase a patient's risk for apnea.
- Bronchiolitis management centers on a "less is more" philosophy, with a focus on supportive care measures such as hydration and suctioning. Supplemental oxygen, high-flow nasal cannula, or noninvasive positive pressure ventilation may be beneficial for patients with hypoxia, respiratory distress, or apnea.
- Diagnostic testing and medications are generally not indicated and are discouraged.

Suggested Readings

Ralston SL, Lieberthal AS, Meissner HC, et al. American Academy of Pediatrics Clinical Practice Guideline: the diagnosis, management, and prevention of bronchiolitis. *Pediatrics*. 2014;134(5):e1474-e1502.

Schroeder AR, Mansbach JM, Stevenson M, et al. Apnea in children hospitalized with bronchiolitis. *Pediatrics*. 2013;132(5):e1194-e1201.

Tyler A, Krack P, Bakel LA, et al. Interventions to reduce over-utilized tests and treatments in bronchiolitis. *Pediatrics*. 2018;141(6).

75

Treating Patients With Cystic Fibrosis and Pneumonia With Typical Treatments for Community-Acquired Pneumonia

Maneesha Agarwal, MD, FAAP, FACEP

Cystic fibrosis (CF) is one of the most common genetically inherited diseases in Caucasian populations, although other races can be affected as well. This autosomal recessive disease is caused by mutation of the cystic fibrosis transmembrane conductance regulator (CFTR) that impacts the function of a chloride channel that is expressed in nearly every cell of the body. When this chloride channel malfunctions, patients develop thick secretions and poor ciliary clearance, resulting in thick, viscid mucus. This pathophysiology affects multiple organs, including the lungs, pancreas, hepatobiliary tract, intestines, and reproductive tract. Most patients are diagnosed in the neonatal period by newborn screening and confirmatory sweat test.

While CF is a multi-organ disease, the lungs are most commonly affected. Thick viscous mucus in their lungs plays host to bacterial colonization, resulting in chronic airway infection and inflammation. By early childhood, patients develop bronchiectasis and progressive lung dysfunction.

At times, CF patients have worsening of their chronic infection, termed a pulmonary or CF exacerbation. This typically manifests as worsening cough, increased sputum production, fever, weight loss, worsening radiographic findings, worsening pulmonary function tests, elevated inflammatory markers, and leukocytosis as compared to baseline.

While patients may be infected by typical community-acquired pneumonia pathogens, such as *Streptococcus pneumoniae* or *Haemophilus influenzae*, CF patients are prone to infection by other organisms. The most predominant microorganism is *Pseudomonas aeruginosa*, although other pathogens such as methicillin-resistant *Staphylococcus aureus* (MRSA), *Stenotrophomonas maltophilia*, *Achromobacter* species, *Burkholderia cepacia*, atypical *Mycobacterium*, and *Aspergillus fumigatus* should be considered. Many of the implicated organisms may exhibit antibiotic resistance. *Pseudomonas* is particularly challenging to treat given its ability to develop a biofilm where antibiotics may not effectively penetrate.

Patients with CF are typically treated with double coverage, high-dose, broad-spectrum antibiotics for at least 14 days. Antibiotics commonly used include broad-spectrum penicillins, cephalosporins with antipseudomonal activity, aminoglycosides, fluoroquinolones, and macrolides. Inhaled antibiotics may also be considered. It is **highly recommended** to discuss optimal antibiotic coverage with the patient's pulmonology team as they are usually aware of the patient's known pathogens and associated antibiotic susceptibilities. Patients are typically admitted for tailoring of antibiotics, aggressive pulmonary toilet, optimization of nutrition, addressing comorbidities (eg, diabetes), and close monitoring while arranging transition to outpatient care.

Considerations Beyond the Lung

While pulmonary disease accounts for ~80% of all CF deaths, be mindful that CF is a multi-organ disease. Other complications and manifestations to consider when caring for a CF patient in the emergency department include the following:

- Hemoptysis—this is a life-threatening emergency due to erosion into a bronchial vessel. In addition to standard resuscitation therapies (eg, airway support, transfusion), management requires the emergent involvement of subspecialists including pulmonology, interventional radiology, and cardiothoracic surgery for possible bronchoscopy, arterial embolization, or lobectomy. If the patient has a sensation of "tickling" in one lung, that is the likely source of bleeding; the patient should be positioned so the affected lung is dependent, hopefully tamponading the source of bleeding and containing the blood to a single lung field.
- Pancreatic insufficiency and autodigestion—this may manifest as insulin-dependent diabetes, pancreatitis, or deficiencies of the fat-soluble vitamins (eg, vitamin K deficiency leading to hemorrhage). Associated complications, such as hyperosmolar, nonketotic coma, are also possible.
- Sinusitis—this is common and may be associated with nasal polyps, manifest as pansinusitis, and require surgical intervention.
- Distal intestinal obstruction syndrome (DIOS)—thick inspissated stool may result in fecal blockage at the ileocolic junction, potentially resulting in intestinal rupture. It may also serve as the lead point for volvulus or intussusception. DIOS warrants aggressive cleanout, including possible admission and gastrografin enemas. Constipation may also occur. CF patients are also prone to rectal prolapse.
- Hepatobiliary disease—this includes cirrhosis, portal hypertension, cholelithiasis, and esophageal varices.
- Nephrolithiasis and nephrotoxicity from chronic medication use (eg, aminoglycosides).

KEY POINTS

- CF patients with a respiratory infection warrant double antibiotic coverage with activity against *Pseudomonas*. Attempt to involve the patient's primary pulmonologist to optimize care.
- While stabilizing the patient with massive hemoptysis, involve your consultants.
- Remember that CF is a multi-organ disease. Lower your threshold to investigate symptoms further; for example, abdominal pain might represent DIOS, volvulus, nephrolithiasis, etc.

Suggested Readings

Elborn JS. Cystic fibrosis. *Lancet* 2016;388:2519-2531.
Goetz D, Ren C. Review of cystic fibrosis. *Pediatr Ann* 2019;48:e154-161.
Rowe SM, Miller S, Sorscher EJ. Cystic fibrosis. *N Engl J Med.* 2005;352:1992-2001.

76

Not Recognizing Risk Factors for PE in Children

Sephora N. Morrison, MBBS, MSCI, MBA, CPE and James Chamberlain, MD

Pulmonary embolism (PE) is rare in children. Studies reveal an incidence of 8.6-57 in 100 000 hospitalized children and 0.14-0.9 in 100 000 of the general population of nonhospitalized children, with peaks in infancy and adolescence. The diagnosis must be considered as more children with chronic illnesses, who may be susceptible to PE, are surviving through improvements in health care practices. Children without chronic illnesses also remain at risk for PE in certain cases.

PE evolves from venous thrombi, which can form in the setting of Virchow triad of stasis, endothelial injury, and/or hypercoagulability. PE risk is increased when these elements coexist or overlap. Approximately 50% of PEs occur from a thrombus or thrombi travelling to the lungs from another site, commonly the lower extremities. Thromboemboli can also travel from upper extremities or other sites.

Clinical History

Diligent history taking may lead to the discovery of essential clues from current, past medical history, and/or medications prompting consideration of PE. Conditions that affect the endothelium lead to hypercoagulable states and/or stasis must be explored during system review, current and past medical history (Table 76.1).

Signs and Symptoms

PE diagnosis may be delayed up to 7 days after initial presentation. Often PE is not considered until there is cardiorespiratory deterioration in a critically ill child. Symptoms that should prompt consideration

Table 76.1 ■ Virchow Triad Category Conditions	
Virchow Triad Category	Condition
Endothelial injury	Inflammatory illnesses: rheumatologic, cardiac, renal, and liver
	Systemic and local infections
	Central venous catheters, including ventriculoatrial shunts
	Disruptions to laminar flow: corrective heart surgery, total parental nutrition
Hypercoagulable states	Inherited conditions: factor V Leiden mutation, protein S, C and antithrombin deficiency
	Acquired conditions: nephrotic syndrome, malignancy
	Medications: cancer regimens, hormonal therapy, including oral contraception
Stasis	Immobilization: extended sitting, long flights, pregnancy, recent surgeries, trauma, fractures, prolonged bed rest

Table 76.2 ■ Performance Characteristics of Tests for PE Detection	
Test	Performance Characteristics
D-Dimer	Sensitivity 79%, specificity 69%, positive likelihood ratio 2.5, negative likelihood ratio 0.3
Electrocardiography	Nonspecific findings including ST-T segment changes, sinus tachycardia, right bundle branch block, right axis deviation
Chest radiography (CXR)	Findings are often abnormal in 88% of cases and include cardiac enlargement, pleural effusion, atelectasis, parenchymal opacity
Ultrasonography	Useful in identifying thrombus source, 97% sensitivity and 94% specificity for proximal thrombus
Echocardiography	Most useful if clot visualized within central pulmonary arteries or heart
Pulmonary angiography	Unknown sensitivity and specificity in pediatrics. Invasive, expensive, time-consuming, high radiation with significant risks
Ventilation-perfusion scan	High probability scan has 85% chance of PE, low probability scan has 20% chance of PE
Multidetector computed tomography	With 2 or more risk factors: sensitivity 75%-89% and specificity 94%-99%
Magnetic resonance image	MRA most useful in combination with other techniques. High-spatial resolution 3D MRA: sensitivity 75%-100% and specificity 95%-100%. Time-resolved MRA: sensitivity 92% and specificity 94%

of PE include shortness of breath accompanied by chest pain, which are easier to elicit from older children. Concerning signs include tachypnea, tachycardia, hypoxia, pallor, unilateral extremity pain or swelling, right heart failure, cough, hemoptysis, syncope, and obesity.

Clinical Scores and Pediatrics

Several clinical decision rules help determine the likelihood of PE in adults. These include the Wells and PERC (Pulmonary Embolism Rule out Criteria) scores, which use clinical history and signs to guide testing. The performance characteristics of these scores are suboptimal to identify PE risk in pediatric patients, with sensitivity and specificity of 86% and 58%-60% for Wells and 100% and 24% for PERC, respectively. Current attempts to develop pediatric-specific scores require validation through further study.

Testing

No test conclusively rules out PE (Table 76.2). The most reliable and readily available test for PE is helical computed tomography. The D-dimer lab test, often used in adults, may be useful in adolescents but is unreliable in the setting of chronic illness and obesity. Other testing, including electrocardiography, pulmonary angiography, ventilation-perfusion scanning, magnetic resonance imaging, echocardiography, and ultrasonography, may be helpful in some cases but are either unreliable or logistically difficult to perform in the pediatric ED patient.

KEY POINTS

- PE, though generally rare in children, is more commonly seen in those with chronic medical illnesses.
- Vigilance for common pediatric PE risk factors (trauma, immobility, recent surgery, indwelling catheters, oral contraceptive use, and inflammatory conditions) can augment detection.
- Engaging our inner detective will help us break free from the box of common diagnosis due to low suspicion and misleading symptoms.

Suggested Readings

Agha BS, et al. Pulmonary embolism in the pediatric emergency department. *Pediatrics*. 2013;132(4):663–667.

Albisetti M, Chan A. Venous thrombosis and thromboembolism in children: risk factors, clinical manifestations, and diagnosis. In: Armsby C, ed. *UpToDate*. 2017. https://www.uptodate.com/contents/venous-thrombosis-and-thromboembolism-in-children-risk-factors-clinical-manifestations-and-diagnosis. Retrieved from March 27, 2019.

Hennelly KE, et al. Detection of pulmonary embolism in high-risk children. *J Pediatr*. 2016;178:214–218.e3.

Patocka C, Nemeth J. Pulmonary embolism in pediatrics. *J Emerg Med*. 2012;42(1):105–116.

Zaidi AU, Hutchins KK, Rajpurkar M. Pulmonary embolism in children. *Front Pediatr*. 2017;5:170.

Overlooking the Concurrent Injuries in Children With Rib Fractures

Anna Handorf, MD and Ari Cohen, MD, FAAP

Rib fractures are uncommon in children due to the plasticity of the pediatric skeleton. One study showed that only 2% of all children evaluated for trauma had rib fractures. As such, rib fractures in young children are a marker of more severe trauma with high risk for concurrent injuries.

The most common causes of pediatric rib fractures are accidental and nonaccidental trauma (NAT). Less common causes include birth trauma, metabolic bone disease, skeletal dysplasia, infection, and toxicity. Accidental trauma is typically due to high velocity and high impact forces, causing injury to intrathoracic structures without concurrent rib fractures. Conversely, NAT is typically due to compression, which is high force but low velocity. This mechanism does not typically cause intrathoracic injury, yet can result in rib fractures. Rib fractures are a marker for abuse and that increases the risk for concurrent injuries and mortality.

Pediatric rib fractures indicate multisystem trauma and should prompt evaluation for concurrent injuries, particularly intracranial and intra-abdominal.

Nonaccidental Trauma Concerns

The prevalence of incidental rib fractures among children <2 years old is reported to be <0.1%. Additionally, rib fractures have a positive predictive value of 95% for NAT in this age group. Excluding children with confirmed accidental trauma or metabolic bone disease, this statistic increases to 100%. As such, a full NAT workup is indicated if rib fractures are present in any child without a trauma history or bone disease.

In one study, 63% of children younger than 3 years of age with rib fractures were due to abuse. Rib fractures that are posterior, multiple, bilateral, or in multiple stages of healing are suggestive of NAT. Importantly, new rib fractures may be difficult to detect on standard chest films, as callous formation occurs over 10-14 days. Oblique views of the ribs can increase detection. If NAT is suspected, assessment for associated injuries (Table 77.1) is essential.

NAT Evaluation Essentials

A normal physical examination does not eliminate the concern for occult injuries, particularly intra-abdominal. If NAT is suspected, the initial workup should include laboratory studies and imaging. Important labs are a complete blood count, electrolytes, coagulation studies, aspartate aminotransferase/alanine aminotransferase/lipase to screen for intra-abdominal injury, a urinalysis to assess for hematuria, and toxicology screens for altered mental status.

Table 77.1 ■ Physical Examination Findings Concerning for NAT		
	<6 Months	6-12 Months	1+ Years
Head	Injuries to the ears, side of face, neck, and top of shoulders		
Oral	Frenulum tears or unexplained injuries		
Trunk/extremities	Groin/genital injury; injury to inner aspects of extremities		
Burns	Patterned, immersion, injury to perineum/lower extremities		
Bruising	Any bruise	Patterned, trunk or head, or any unexplained	
Fractures	Fractures in different stages of healing		
	Scapular, spinous process, sternal fractures		
	Fractures excluding skull or clavicle fracture	Fractures excluding simple linear skull fracture	Long bone fractures (excluding supracondylar humerus); no trauma history
Intracranial	Any subdural hemorrhage		Unexplained subdural hemorrhage
Visceral	Any visceral injury		Unexplained visceral injury

A head CT scan should be obtained to assess for occult bleeding or fractures. A skeletal survey is indicated to assess for additional fractures in patients under 24 months old and to be considered up to 60 months old. Ophthalmologic evaluation is indicated for children <5 years old within 72 hours to assess for retinal hemorrhages.

Early consultation by social work, a child protective services team, and the state child protection agency is imperative.

KEY POINTS

- Pediatric rib fractures are unusual given plasticity of the pediatric skeleton.
- Rib fractures in children <5 years are rarely accidental and can indicate concurrent injuries.
- NAT requires a multidisciplinary approach to ensure thorough workup and safe disposition.

Suggested Readings

Barsness K, Cha E, Bensard D, et al. The positive predictive value of rib fractures as an indicator of nonaccidental trauma in children. *J Trauma*. 2003;54(6):1107-1110.

Darling S, Done S, Friedman S, et al. Frequency of intrathoracic injuries in children younger than 3 years with rib fractures. *Pediatr Radiol*. 2014;44:1230-1236.

Kessel B, Dagan J, Swaid F, et al. Rib fractures: comparison of associated injuries between pediatric and adult population. *Am J Surg*. 2014;208:831-834.

Paine C, Fakeye O, Christian C, et al. Prevalence of abuse among young children with rib fractures a systemic review. *Pediatr Emerg Care*. 2019;35(2):96-103.

Ruest S, Kanaan G, Moore J, et al. The prevalence of rib fractures incidentally identified by chest radiograph among infants and toddlers. *J Pediatr*. 2019;204:208-213.

78

Do Not Miss Undiagnosed Congenital Heart Disease: In Babies With Heart Disease, Color Matters!

Sean Larsen, MD and Jenny Mendelson, MD

Children with congenital heart disease (CHD) can present in a variety of ways to the emergency department (ED). Their diagnosis may be known or unknown. They may be cyanotic or normally saturated. They may be unrepaired or have had surgical interventions for palliation and/or correction of their defect. This chapter will focus on the recognition and management of infants with critical congenital heart defects (CCHDs) such as transposition of the great arteries, hypoplastic left heart syndrome, pulmonary atresia with intact ventricular septum, tetralogy of Fallot, total anomalous pulmonary venous return, tricuspid atresia, and truncus arteriosus. CCHD lesions usually require surgical repair or intervention within the first year of life to prevent significant morbidity or mortality. Luckily, improved quality of fetal echocardiography and universal newborn pulse oximetry have dramatically increased early diagnosis.

Nevertheless, some children manage to slip through the cracks and may present to the ED with undiagnosed CCHD. Generally, newborns (<1 month) with obstructive lesions will present with either cyanosis (right-sided) or severe shock and gray appearance (left-sided). After this, CCHD patients tend to present with congestive heart failure. Lesions that under circulate the lungs present with cyanosis, while those that over circulate the lungs will be acyanotic, but exhibiting signs such as tachypnea, difficulty with feeding, and failure to thrive.

No matter the color, infants <1 month with suspected CCHD should be considered ductal dependent until proven otherwise. Start prostaglandin (PGE1) infusion early, with a dose of 0.05-0.1 µg/kg/min. Common side effects of PGE1 infusion include tachycardia, hypotension, and apnea. If the child has not already been intubated for respiratory failure, be prepared for intubation if needed. Though ketamine is frequently used for intubation in kids, it is not a great choice in CCHD due to the increase in systemic vascular resistance and catecholamine depletion. Instead, consider solely fentanyl for induction.

It may be difficult to distinguish between respiratory and cardiac etiology in an infant with respiratory distress and hypoxia. In these cases, the hyperoxia test should be administered. Though classically serial arterial blood gases (ABGs) were measured before and after 10 minutes of 100% O_2, pulse oximetry results can be used instead. If partial pressure of O_2 on ABG is <100 mm Hg, or if pulse oximetry reading remains low, this is suggestive of a cyanotic CHD. If >150 mm Hg on ABG or pulse ox significantly improves, this is suggestive of a primary respiratory problem. A pulse ox differential >3% between the right upper extremity (preductal) and either lower extremity (postductal) suggests a ductal-dependent lesion.

When children with known CHD present to the ED, ask the parents what lesion they have, what surgeries have been performed, and especially what the child's normal O_2 saturations are. In children with known mixing defects, more oxygen may cause harm. Oxygen will reduce pulmonary vascular resistance and may disrupt the balance between pulmonary and systemic blood flow resulting in pulmonary overcirculation and systemic hypoperfusion. Be cautious when fluid resuscitating a known or suspected CHD. These children may still need 40-60 mL/kg or more in sepsis or severe hypovolemia but consider using 5-10 mL/kg boluses and frequently reassessing for signs of volume overload including pulmonary crackles and hepatomegaly.

Early consultation with pediatric cardiology is a must to help guide treatment and disposition decisions. Use of color classifications, the hyperoxia test, electrocardiogram, and chest x-ray may help point to a diagnosis. While bedside ultrasound may be performed, it is not a substitute for formal echocardiography, which should be performed in the ED emergently.

KEY POINTS

- The critical congenital heart lesions typically present to the ED in one of four ways: right-sided obstructive ductal-dependent lesions are BLUE, left-sided obstructive ductal dependent lesions are GRAY, and shunting or mixing lesions can be PINK if predominantly left-to-right or BLUE if right-to-left.
- In infants <1 month and concern for CCHD, start PGE1 at 0.05 µg/kg/min, monitor for side effects, and be prepared to intubate.
- Use multiple 5-10 mL/kg boluses when resuscitating CCHD patients. Frequently reassess watching for signs of fluid overload (crackles and hepatomegaly).
- More oxygen is not always better! In many mixing defects, sats of 75%-85% are acceptable and pushing higher can cause harm. Ask parents what is normal for their child.

Suggested Readings

Judge P, Meckler G. Congenital heart disease in pediatric patients: recognizing the undiagnosed and managing complications in the emergency department. *Pediatr Emerg Med Pract.* 2016:13(5):1-26.

Plana MN, Zamora J, Suresh G, Fernandez-Pineda L, Thangaratinam S, Ewer AK. Pulse oximetry screening for critical congenital heart defects. *Cochrane Database Syst Rev.* 2018;3:CD011912.

Strobel AM, Lu le N. The critically ill infant with congenital heart disease. *Emerg Med Clin North Am.* 2015;33(3):501-518.

Poor Feeding, Cough, and Fussiness? Common Complaints Deserve a Comprehensive Workup for Pericarditis in the Postoperative Congenital Heart Disease Patient

Tyler Kingdon, MD and Julia Schweizer, MD, FAAP

Though there are many possible postoperative complications that can present subacutely (ie, postop infection) or months to years later (ie, shunt occlusion), this chapter will focus solely on postoperative pericarditis. Complaints such as cough, fussiness, and poor feeding can often be discharged from the emergency department (ED) as an upper respiratory infection with minimal workup. However, any pediatric patient within 6 weeks of cardiac surgery deserves a thorough evaluation focused on ruling out pericarditis and pericardial effusion.

History

In addition to addressing the chief complaint, be sure to ask a few specific to postop CHD patient to assure their safety. Obtain details regarding quantity of feeds, time to complete a feed, and symptoms during feeds. Timing, height of, and change in fevers should be noted as well as characteristics of a cough. In verbal patients, pericarditis chest pain may be described as a sharp, central chest pain that radiates to the shoulders and improves with sitting up. Parents should be asked what surgery the patient had and how long ago it occurred. The window for acute pericarditis within is 6 weeks postoperatively, thought it most often occurs within 1-2 weeks. Certain cardiac surgeries place patients at higher risk for pericarditis including atrial septal defect closures, Fontan, and Glenn procedures. That said, any surgery that enters the pericardial sac can result in pericarditis.

Physical Examination

Patients with pericarditis are commonly tachycardic and/or tachypneic. They are variably febrile and may be low hypotensive if they have developed tamponade. Listen for distant heart sounds or a friction rub. A friction rub is best detected during expiration with the patient leaning forward and is pathognomonic for pericarditis. If a patient has developed cardiac tamponade, this is identified by a triad of hypotension, jugular venous distension, and muffled or distant heart sounds. Pulsus paradoxus occurs when systolic blood pressure decreases by 20 mm Hg on inspiration and is a common finding in tamponade.

Evaluation

Initial evaluation should start with an electrocardiogram (ECG). The patient should be placed on continuous cardiorespiratory monitoring while in the ED as they are at high risk for arrhythmias. Initial ECG changes include ST elevation throughout all leads except aVR and V1, with upright T waves and PR segment deviation opposite P-wave polarity. Electrical alternans may be present if there is a significant effusion. Laboratory studies including a complete blood count and electrolytes should be obtained. Erythrocyte sedimentation rate and C-reactive protein are elevated in ~80% of cases. Lactate dehydrogenase, alanine transaminase, creatine kinase, and troponin levels are cardiac specific and can be elevated in 30%-50% of cases. Imaging should include a chest x-ray to evaluate the cardiac border and potentially a bedside ultrasound to characterize a pericardial effusion. In stable patients, a complete echocardiogram should be obtained as quickly as possible to quantify cardiac function.

Diagnosis

Postoperative pericarditis is diagnosed *with at least two of the following findings*: pericardial friction rub, new ST elevations or PR depressions on ECG, new or worsening pericardial effusion, or typical pericardial chest pain. Diagnosis can be supported by lab findings and pericardial inflammation seen on echocardiogram or advanced imaging.

Treatment/Resuscitation

Initial evaluation always includes the airway, breathing, and circulations (ABCs) as these patients can present acutely ill with circulatory and/or respiratory compromise. A patient with cardiac tamponade warrants a pericardiocentesis immediately. Removal of as little as 15-20 mL of fluid, depending on the patient's size, can quickly improve hemodynamics. Remember that some pediatric heart disease patients have baseline saturations below 90% (particularly those with single ventricle anatomy), so titrate supplemental oxygen to their baseline. Fluid administration should be used sparingly as hypotension or tachycardia in these patients is often fluid resistant and the underlying pericarditis or effusion needs to be treated. Lastly, the mainstay of treatment of postoperative pericarditis is high-dose nonsteroidal anti-inflammatories, supportive care, and admission to the ICU or cardiology team depending on patient presentation.

KEY POINTS

- A workup for pericarditis is almost always warranted in patients who present within 6 weeks of a pericardiotomy, even with nonspecific symptoms.
- Diagnosis of pericarditis will involve ECG or echocardiographic changes such as ST elevation or new pericardial effusion.

Suggested Readings

Adler H, Charron P, Imazio M, et al. 2015 ESC Guidelines for the diagnosis and management of pericardial diseases: the task force for the Diagnosis and Management of Pericardial Diseases of the European Society of Cardiology (ESC)Endorsed by: the European Association for Cardio-Thoracic Surgery (EACTS). *Eur Heart J.* 2015;36(42):2921-2964.

Baskar S. Pediatric Pericarditis, *American College of Cardiology.* 2016 June 8. https://www.acc.org/latest-in-cardiology/articles/2016/06/08/11/43/pediatric-pericarditis

Heching HJ, Bacha EA, Liberman L. Post-pericardiotomy syndrome in pediatric patients following surgical closure of secundum atrial septal defects: incidence and risk factors. *Pediatr Cardiol.* 2015;36:498-502.

A Faint Chance of Danger—Do Not Assume Pediatric Syncope Is Just Orthostasis Without Ruling Out These Diagnoses

Beatrice Leverett, MD and Forrest T. Closson, MD

Syncope is defined as a transient loss of consciousness resulting from a disruption or alteration in cerebral perfusion that usually has a cardiac, neurologic, neurocardiogenic, metabolic, toxin-mediated, or psychiatric cause. In pediatric patients, the vast majority of syncope cases are benign. Approaches to the emergency department evaluation of pediatric syncope vary widely and, unfortunately, often include diagnostic tests that are expensive, invasive, and largely unnecessary. A strategic approach centered on a thorough history and physical examination is clinically high yield and reduces unnecessary testing.

Pediatric syncope is usually divided into two broad categories: cardiac and noncardiac. Several noncardiac conditions can cause syncope; in these cases, historical clues, signs, and symptoms are present and can aid in catching a serious diagnosis. In general, for pediatric patients presenting with isolated syncope, the potentially life-threatening causes are almost exclusively of cardiac origin.

Cardiac causes can be divided into structural disease (including hypertrophic cardiomyopathy, arrhythmogenic right ventricular dysplasia, anomalous coronary artery, myocarditis, valvular dysfunction, and dysrhythmias (including Brugada syndrome, long and short QT syndromes, supraventricular tachycardia, Wolff-Parkinson-White syndrome, and heart block). The evaluation for all cardiac causes of pediatric syncope consists of the same key elements: the history, the physical examination, and an electrocardiogram (ECG).

Findings that warrant concern, and thus should prompt further cardiac evaluation, include exertional syncope, a family history of cardiac disease or unexplained sudden death, an abnormal physical examination finding supporting a cardiac cause, and an abnormal ECG. In 2013, Tretter and Kavey reported that the presence of any one of these had a sensitivity of 100% and a specificity of 60% for cardiac disease in pediatric patients presenting with syncope. In 2015, Hurst and colleagues also identified exertional syncope as a highly sensitive and specific finding, along with chest pain preceding the exertional syncope, syncope preceded by palpitations, and syncope without prodrome. The presence of any two of these features had a sensitivity and specificity of 100% for cardiac disease.

Conversely, specific historical elements can suggest a benign cause and support the decision not to proceed with an exhaustive workup. The most common cause of fainting in children is neurocardiogenic, or vasovagal, syncope, in which an inappropriate increase in parasympathetic activity leads to bradycardia and transient cerebral hypoperfusion, resulting in a brief loss of consciousness. This type of syncope is associated with a characteristic prodrome, with the loss of consciousness preceded by lightheadedness, visual changes, diaphoresis, pallor, and nausea. Common triggers include hyperthermia, volume depletion, prolonged standing or abrupt positional changes, and emotional distress. A presentation that includes this prodrome and a clear trigger is clinically reassuring.

Because syncope is common in pregnancy (5% of pregnant women experience syncope and 30% experience presyncope), a urine pregnancy test should be added to the workup for menstrual-age female patients. In the absence of symptoms or examination findings pointing to another cause, such as neurologic disease or metabolic derangements, additional studies, such as laboratory values, chest radiographs, and head computed tomography, are unlikely to be clinically useful and should not be ordered routinely.

KEY POINTS

- Syncope is a common presenting symptom in the pediatric emergency department and is usually benign. Dangerous causes of isolated syncope in pediatric patients generally have a cardiac source.
- An effective initial evaluation of pediatric syncope requires only a thorough history, a physical examination, and an ECG (along with a urine pregnancy test for menstrual-aged female patients). Other tests are usually low yield and should not be ordered unless they are specifically indicated based on the history and examination.
- Red flags in the evaluation of pediatric syncope include exertional syncope, syncope preceded by chest pain or palpitations, syncope with no prodrome, a family history of cardiac disease or unexplained sudden death, persistent vital sign or examination abnormalities, and abnormal ECG findings.

Suggested Readings

Fant C, Cohen A, Vazquez MN. Syncope in pediatric patients: a practical approach to differential diagnosis and management in the emergency department [digest]. *Pediatr Emerg Med Pract.* 2017;14(4 Suppl Points & Pearls):S1-S2.

Goble MM, Benitez C, Baumgardner M, Fenske K. ED management of pediatric syncope: searching for a rationale. *Am J Emerg Med.* 2008;26(1):66-70.

Hurst D, Hirsh DA, Oster ME, et al. Syncope in the pediatric emergency department—can we predict cardiac disease based on history alone? *J Emerg Med.* 2015;49(1):1-7.

Tretter JT, Kavey RE. Distinguishing cardiac syncope from vasovagal syncope in a referral population. *J Pediatr.* 2013;163(6):1618-1623.e1.

Chest Pain: Do Not Let a Normal Examination Falsely Reassure You

Erica Marburger, MD and Whitney Minnock, MD

Chest pain in children is a common presenting complaint in the emergency department (ED). Fortunately, <5% of children will have a cardiac etiology of their pain. Generally, a thorough history and physical examination can exclude serious causes of pediatric chest pain. However, there are a few pathologic entities that can present with relatively normal physical examinations.

Cardiac

Coronary artery abnormalities are a rare cause of chest pain in the pediatric population. History of previous cardiac surgery or exertional chest pain should increase concern for coronary artery abnormalities, as the examination may be normal. Additionally, keep in mind that coronary artery aneurysms are a potential long-term complication of Kawasaki disease.

Hypertrophic cardiomyopathy (HCM) is characterized by left ventricular hypertrophy with left ventricular outflow tract obstruction. HCM can produce symptoms of fatigue, palpitations, and syncope. Since HCM is genetic, be sure to inquire about history of HCM in the family or history of sudden death in a first-degree relative under the age of 50. On examination, patients may have a harsh crescendo–decrescendo systolic heart murmur heard best at the apex, which increases with Valsalva maneuver. Over 90% of patients with HCM will have abnormal electrocardiogram (ECG) findings of prominent Q waves, left axis deviation, deep inverted T waves, and left ventricular hypertrophy.

Pericarditis is usually the result of a viral infection and inflammation of the pericardial sac accompanied with chest pain that classically improves when leaning forward. On examination, the patient may be febrile and you may hear a friction rub if leaning forward. However, the examination may be normal early in the illness. Diffuse T-wave abnormalities or dysrhythmias can be seen on ECG.

Respiratory

Asthma is the most common pulmonary cause of pediatric chest pain, often described by patients as "chest tightness." Acute asthma exacerbations are generally associated with dyspnea and wheezing; however, especially in those patients with exercise-induced asthma, asthma can cause chest pain without any active wheezing.

A spontaneous pneumothorax causes sharp, sudden chest pain accompanied by dyspnea. Risk factors for development of spontaneous pneumothorax include tall, thin body habitus, smoking, and male gender, particularly as patients reach adolescence. Additionally, risk is increased with underlying lung diseases, such as cystic fibrosis or asthma. Decreased breath sounds on the effected side are diagnostic, but if the pneumothorax is small, the patient may have normal vital signs and a normal physical examination.

Pulmonary infections, including bronchitis, pneumonia, or empyema, should be considered particularly if history of fever or cough is provided. And in patients with sickle cell disease, always consider acute chest syndrome with complaints of chest pain.

Gastrointestinal

Gastroesophageal reflux (GER) is a relatively common cause of chest pain in the pediatric population, as reflux of stomach acid into the lower esophagus manifests as burning epigastric and central chest pain. Examination will be relatively normal. History of "burning" pain associated with eating or worse when lying flat is suggestive of GER. Other possible gastrointestinal causes of chest pain include esophagitis, peptic ulcer disease, or gastritis.

Musculoskeletal

Up to 30% of pediatric chest pain seen in the ED is musculoskeletal pain. Of the causes of musculoskeletal chest pain, costochondritis is the most common in children. It is characterized by sharp, stabbing pain along the contiguous costochondral. It should always be a diagnosis of exclusion.

Psychiatric

Psychogenic chest pain is usually seen in older children as a result of anxiety, panic disorder, and hyperventilation. Psychogenic chest pain is generally accompanied with anxiety, palpitations, abdominal pain, difficulty breathing, or nausea. Hyperventilation itself can cause chest pain due to respiratory alkalosis, which has been hypothesized to lead to spasm of the diaphragm and/or coronary vasoconstriction. Finally, even in pediatrics, we should not forget that use of stimulants, such as cocaine, amphetamines, bath salts, or synthetic marijuana, can cause chest pain due to cardiac ischemia from increased demand and vasoconstriction.

KEY POINTS

- Less than 5% of pediatric chest pain is cardiac.
- Chest pain associated with syncope or exertion is concerning for a cardiac etiology.
- The most common cause of noncardiac chest pain in the pediatric population is musculoskeletal pain, specifically costochondritis.
- Take a thorough history of present illness and inquire about potential risk factors to help lead you to the correct diagnosis particularly when the physical examination is nonrevealing.

Suggested Readings

Collins SA, Griksaitis MJ, Legg JP. 15-minute consultation: a structured approach to the assessment of chest pain in a child. *Arch Dis Child Educ Pract Ed*. 2014;99:122-126.
Reddy SRV, Singh HR. Chest pain in children and adolescents. *Pediatr Rev*. 2010;31:e1-e9.

Tachycardia: Don't Assume Tachycardia Is Just "Stranger Danger"

Kristin Kahale, MD and Whitney Minnock, MD

Tachycardia is a common presentation seen in emergency department (ED). When first assessing tachycardia, age is an important factor. An infant may present as poor feeding or irritability versus an adolescent who may present for palpitations or syncope during exercise. A child may only present with a "funny feeling" and describe that they just "do not feel right." Tachycardia is not necessarily due to cardiac etiology. For example, sinus tachycardia is commonly due to benign etiologies such as fever, pain, or anxiety or due to serious pathologies such as sepsis or dehydration.

If considering cardiac or possible dysrhythmia, your initial management should begin with a 12-lead ECG. Important factors to consider for dysrhythmias are rate, QRS width, and clinical stability. The role of the emergency physician should be aimed at management of dysrhythmias, determination of need for hospitalization, and necessity of cardiology follow-up and evaluation.

Sinus Tachycardia

Sinus tachycardia is considered a rate higher than average by age group, with origin from the sinus node. A p wave will precede every QRS complex. Presence of sinus tachycardia may be due to from stress, pain, fever, and dehydration. However, its presence can be associated with conditions such as sepsis, hyperthyroidism, anemia, and accidental drug ingestions, so keep that in mind. Treatment of the underlying etiology is the ultimate treatment of sinus tachycardia. Though it can be benign, it should prompt further history and evaluation. Vitals are vital.

Supraventricular Tachycardia

Considered the most common childhood dysrhythmia, supraventricular tachycardia (SVT) is most commonly a narrow complex tachycardia. It is characterized by a narrow QRS (<80 ms), rates >220 bpm in infants and >180 bpm in adolescent or child with little rate variation, and absence of normal P waves. Infants may appear ill with vague symptoms such as poor feeding and irritability, which can be confused for infection.

The mechanism of SVT is most commonly due to an accessory pathway. A short PR interval with a delta wave is a common feature of Wolff-Parkinson-White (WPW) syndrome, but it is not always present in those with an accessory pathway. AV nodal re-entry tachycardia is a less common culprit of SVT in the pediatric population. Fortunately, initial management is the same regardless of mechanism. In stable patients, try vagal maneuvers first. If this does not work, adenosine should be given through a proximal IV. Occasionally, SVT will not convert with adenosine and the addition of an antiarrhythmic agent such as propranolol, amiodarone, or procainamide can be used in consultation with a pediatric cardiologist. Unstable SVT should be managed by synchronized cardioversion. Patients with SVT who respond to adenosine may be discharged with cardiology follow-up.

Atrial Flutter and Atrial Fibrillation

Atrial flutter and fibrillation are less common causes of tachyarrhythmias in children but are more commonly seen in children with congenital heart disease (particularly after surgery) and dilated cardiomyopathy. Presence of atrial flutter or fibrillation in addition to an accessory pathway or hypertrophic cardiomyopathy places the child at increased risk for sudden cardiac death. If unstable, consider cardioversion. Overdrive pacing 10-20 bpm faster than the atrial rate may also be considered in consultation with a pediatric cardiologist. Consider hyperthyroidism as a cause of atrial fibrillation.

Ventricular Tachycardia

Ventricular tachycardia (VT) is fortunately uncommon in children. Morphology is characterized by wide QRS complexes (>100 ms). Common mimics of VT include SVT with aberrancy and AIVR. When VT is present, one must consider serious etiologies such as electrolyte abnormalities, myocarditis, cardiac tumors, or toxicologic. Recurrent exercise-induced syncope is often caused by VT. Most will have an underlying condition such as prolonged QT interval. An unstable wide complex tachycardia must be treated with synchronized cardioversion. For shock-resistant wide complex tachycardia, antiarrhythmics such as amiodarone or lidocaine should be considered.

KEY POINTS

- Infants with tachydysrhythmias may present with vague symptoms such as irritability, poor feeding, and tachypnea. Adolescents commonly present with palpitations and syncope.
- Classify tachydysrhythmias by hemodynamic stability and QRS width.
- Initial evaluation should include a 12-lead ECG. Rhythm strip is not sufficient.
- Most common tachydysrhythmia in pediatrics is SVT.
- Sinus tachycardia is treated by management of underlying disorder.

Suggested Readings

American Heart Association. 2005 American Heart Association (AHA) guidelines for cardiopulmonary resuscitation (CPR) and emergency cardiovascular care (ECC) of pediatric and neonatal patients: pediatric basic life support. *Pediatrics*. 2006;117:e989-e1004.

Crosson J, Hanash C. Emergency diagnosis and management of pediatric arrhythmias. *J Emerg Trauma Shock*. 2010;3(3):251.

Doniger SJ, Sharieff GQ. Pediatric dysrhythmias. *Pediatr Clin North Am*. 2006;53:85.

Schafermeyer R, Tenenbein M, et al. *Strange and Schafermeyer's Pediatric Emergency Medicine*. 5th ed. New York: McGraw-Hill; 2018.

Secondary Signs of Endocarditis: Know Them by Heart

William Martin, MD and Sean Thompson, MD

Infective endocarditis (IE) is infection of the endocardium and/or the heart valves (native or endogenous), typically with bacteria or fungi. The diagnosis can be elusive but carries a high morbidity and mortality. Although many characteristics of IE are common between adult and pediatric patients, several features are unique to children.

Pediatric IE is less common than adult IE; however, the frequency appears to be increasing. Trends indicate congenital heart disease (CHD) and hospitalization of critically ill children to be significant risk factors. This shift is secondary to the near eradication of rheumatic heart disease along with increased survival rates and interventions that occurs in the CHD population, which in some studies accounts for ~50% of all pediatric IE cases. In those with a previously normal heart, the increased critical care management and survival of premature infants and critically ill children play a significant role in the development of IE. This change in risk factors should change how we determine risk for IE in children.

In those with CHD, risk is dependent on the type of CHD and in what stage of repair the patient is currently. Those with unrepaired cyanotic CHD, repaired CHD with prosthetic material/device (especially within the first 6 months), repaired CHD with residual defects at site of repair, and cardiac transplant patients are at significantly increased risk. In premature or critically ill children, placement of central venous lines (CVLs) and other invasive equipment may introduce bacteria into the blood stream and often make contact the right side of the heart causing microscopic endothelial damage and perturbed blood flow, all of which increase the risk of developing IE.

Occasionally, presentation can be fulminant and children can present acutely ill. More often, the signs and symptoms of IE are nonspecific, even more so in the pediatric population. Common symptoms include general malaise, headache, arthralgias, myalgias, rigors, and diaphoresis, but the most common presenting symptom is fever. Neonates often present with feeding difficulties, respiratory distress, and unstable vital signs, with or without temperature changes. Classic signs such as Roth spots, Janeway lesions, Osler nodes, and splinter hemorrhages are exceedingly rare in children and virtually nonexistent in infants. In the pediatric population, manifestations such as heart failure, embolic phenomena, new or changing murmur, and petechial rash occur only 25%-50% of the time. In right-sided IE, the patient may present with shortness of breath and low-grade fever and imaging may show septic emboli in the lungs. Left-sided IE is more likely to present with systemic embolic complications including liver abscess, petechiae, and mycotic aneurysms.

The diagnosis for IE continues to be made in accordance with the modified Duke criteria. In most pediatric populations, a transthoracic echocardiogram is sufficient to diagnose IE; however, in cases of prior cardiothoracic surgery, a transesophageal echocardiogram is recommended.

Staphylococcus aureus and *Streptococcus viridans* remain the leading causative organisms for IE, although other organisms such as gram-negative rods and yeast (especially in premature infants with a CVL) can also be culprits. Empiric antibiotics (typically vancomycin and gentamicin) should be started while cultures are pending. It is recommended to draw three blood culture sets from three different sites prior to starting antibiotics when possible. In summary, understanding and identifying the risk factors can help increase our suspicion and aid in the diagnosis of pediatric IE.

KEY POINTS

- Congenital heart disease and children with recent central venous access are at significantly increased risk of developing IE.
- The most common symptom of IE in the pediatric population is fever. Other classical signs such as Osler nodes, Janeway lesions, and splinter hemorrhage are exceedingly rare.
- IE should be considered in patients that are toxic appearing and/or present with unexplained prolonged fever, especially if they have significant risk factors.

Suggested Readings

Baltimore RS, Gewitz M, Baddour LM, et al.; American Heart Association Rheumatic Fever, Endocarditis, and Kawasaki Disease Committee of the Council on Cardiovascular Disease in the Young and the Council on Cardiovascular and Stroke Nursing. Infective endocarditis in childhood: 2015 update: a scientific statement from the American Heart Association. *Circulation*. 2015;132(15):1487-1515.

Day MD, Gauvreau L, Shulman S, Newburger JW. Characteristics of children hospitalized with infective endocarditis. *Circulation*. 2009;119(6):865-870.

Elder RW, Baltimore RS. The changing epidemiology of pediatric endocarditis. *Infect Dis Clin North Am*. 2015;29(3):513-524.

Lin YT, Hsieh KS, Chen YS, Huang IF, Cheng MF. Infective endocarditis in children without underlying heart disease. *J Microbiol Immunol Infect*. 2013;46(2):121-128.

Viruses Can Be Real Heart Breakers—Do Not Let the Myocarditis Patient Blend in With All the Respiratory Viral Illnesses

Josephine Stout, MD and Jenny Mendelson, MD

Heart failure in young children without congenital heart disease (CHD) is relatively rare. It can be difficult to recognize as these patients may present with atypical symptoms which can mimic viral infection, dehydration, or sepsis. In children without CHD, the most common cause of congestive heart failure is acquired cardiomyopathy, frequently caused by myocarditis. It is particularly rare in infants but increases slightly with age. In the United States, the most common cause of myocarditis is viral infection. Symptoms are typically more severe in infants than in older children, including fatigue, irritability, difficulty breathing or eating, and pale, cool, or mottled skin. Physical examination may reveal persistent tachypnea and tachycardia, delayed capillary refill, hepatomegaly, gallop rhythm on auscultation, and lung crackles from pulmonary edema. As heart failure worsens, symptoms may progress to lethargy, shock, and cardiorespiratory collapse.

When there is concern for myocarditis and heart failure, start with an electrocardiogram (ECG) and chest x-ray. ECG will frequently demonstrate nonspecific findings of sinus tachycardia, ST-T wave abnormalities, and low-voltage QRS complexes. ST changes and dysrhythmias may also be present. Remember that T wave inversion is normal until adolescence, especially in V1-V3. Rightward axis deviation is also normal in infants for the first 1-2 months of age due to relative right ventricular hypertrophy in neonates. Chest x-ray may be normal in myocarditis, but an enlarged cardiac silhouette, pulmonary congestion, pulmonary edema, or pleural effusion should raise suspicion for heart failure, especially with an abnormal ECG.

Cardiac specific lab markers such as troponin and beta-natriuretic peptide (BNP) can help to distinguish between a patient with a respiratory infection and one with cardiac dysfunction. Both are frequently elevated in children with myocarditis or heart failure. While an elevated troponin or BNP may help confirm your suspicion for heart failure and myocarditis, normal results do not rule these conditions out. Additionally, the normal range for BNP varies with age in children, so be mindful when interpreting results. If there is clinical suspicion for heart failure, an echocardiogram should be done to evaluate cardiac structure and function. Point of care cardiac ultrasound by the ED provider can be useful to rapidly assess global cardiac function but is not a substitute for a formal echocardiogram. Typical findings in myocarditis include left ventricular or biventricular dysfunction, ventricular dilation, and reduced left ventricular ejection fraction.

Management of myocarditis depends on hemodynamic status and symptoms. All patients should have intravenous access and cardiorespiratory monitoring. Supplemental oxygen is also indicated in any patient with hypoxia, evidence of poor perfusion, hypoxemia, or shock. Intubation may be indicated in patients with impending respiratory failure or hemodynamic instability and can beneficially reduce afterload and improve cardiac output. However, these patients are at high risk for periintubation cardiac arrest and should be optimized prior to attempting. Patients who appear volume overloaded but well perfused will likely benefit from early diuresis. Patients with decompensated cardiogenic shock, though volume overloaded, may not have sufficient blood pressure to tolerate diuresis initially. In such patients, hemodynamic support with inotropes (typically epinephrine first line) may be needed to restore perfusion.

Lusitropic agents, such as milrinone or dobutamine, can also be useful in children with low-output cardiac failure. They improve cardiac relaxation and diastolic filling, increase cardiac contractility and cardiac output, and decrease afterload. Bolus loading doses of these agents prior to initiation of drips should be avoided as it can increase their risk of systemic vasodilation leading to hypotension. Initiation of agents such as milrinone should be done in consultation with a cardiologist or pediatric intensivist.

KEY POINTS

- Heart failure in children can be difficult to identify and easily confused with other causes of respiratory distress and shock.
- Persistent tachycardia without a cause should raise concern for cardiac dysfunction.
- Myocarditis is the most common cause of acquired heart failure in pediatrics and is most commonly caused by viral infection.
- After a thorough history and physical examination, further workup should include ECG, chest x-ray, and select lab testing, followed by echocardiogram if abnormal.
- Lusitropic agents can cause hypotension and should be used carefully in consultation with the cardiology and intensive care teams.

Suggested Reading

Bergmann KR, Kharbanda A, Haveman L. Myocarditis and pericarditis in the pediatric patient: validated management strategies. *Pediatr Emerg Med Pract*. 2015;12(7):1-24.

Remember That Very Little of Pediatric Hypertension Is Cardiac

Marie Kotenko, MD, MPH and Whitney Minnock, MD

In adults, we typically associate hypertension with cardiovascular diseases. In pediatrics, this is rarely the case. While some cardiovascular conditions can cause hypertension in the pediatric patient, like coarctation of the aorta, more commonly pediatric patients will have hypertension from obesity, renal, neoplastic, or toxicologic causes.

Defining Pediatric Hypertension

The 2017 American Academy of Pediatrics definition of elevated blood pressure in patients between 1 and 13 years old is systolic or diastolic blood pressure (SBP, DBP) ≥90th %. For children >13 years old, SBP > 120 is considered elevated. These blood pressure percentiles are based on age, gender, and height. Be sure to measure twice with an appropriately sized cuff to avoid misdiagnosis. Further scrutiny should include taking BP measurements in all four extremities, a complete neurologic exam, and abdominal and flank exams to evaluate for masses or other disturbances.

Noncardiac Causes of Pediatric Hypertension

There are many life-threatening etiologies associated with pediatric hypertension, and classifying the more common causes by age can help recognize them. In children <6 years of age, the etiology is likely renal parenchymal disease from glomerulonephritis, renal parenchymal scarring, and chronic renal failure. Poststreptococcal glomerulonephritis (PSGN) and Henoch-Schönlein purpura (HSP) have classic presentations and may account for hypertension. Questions about recent pharyngitis, rashes such as impetigo or purpuric lesions, arthralgia, edema, and sick contacts may yield clues. Scarring of the renal parenchyma can be from urologic condition. Patient should be asked about history of stones, changes in urine color or habits, frequent unexplained fevers, or infection.

In the school-aged child, neoplastic syndromes such as pheochromocytoma may present with pediatric hypertension. Catecholamine surges can lead to sweating and rashes alongside hypertension, headaches, tachycardia, and palpitations, though symptoms can often be difficult to describe. Intracranial masses and head trauma can also lead to hypertension from increased intracranial pressure.

After 6 years of age, pediatric hypertension is more likely from primary causes. In adolescents, toxicological causes must also be considered. Substances such as cocaine and amphetamines can cause hypertensive episodes that can be life threatening. Less serious toxins like caffeine can also lead to pediatric hypertension. Careful history about risk factors for substance abuse, home atmosphere, and accessibility to these substances can help direct diagnosis. When etiology is not clearly from primary or renal causes, screening with drugs of abuse panels are reasonable to ensure toxicological etiologies are not missed. In addition to illegal drug use, other substances such as medications like corticosteroids, pseudoephedrine, or birth control can also lead to hypertension. In any menstruating adolescent, preeclampsia should also be considered and pregnancy test ordered as well.

Treatment of Hypertensive Emergency

Although rare, children can have a hypertensive emergency. Given that pediatric presentations are typically secondary to another cause, the underlying disorder may present before the typical end-organ damage does. Encephalopathy is the most common form of end-organ damage seen in true pediatric hypertensive emergency and will present with lethargy, confusion, seizures, or coma. In addition to prompt treatment of the underlying cause, antihypertensives can also be used to lower blood pressure in the acute setting. Typical agents are β-blockers like labetalol or calcium-channel blockers like nicardipine. Over the first 8 hours, target reduction of systolic blood pressure by 25%. Overall treatment should be aimed at addressing underlying etiology of hypertension.

KEY POINTS

- Always think of noncardiac causes of hypertension in children.
- Confirmation of hypertension should be made in conjunction with guidelines based on patient's age, gender, and height.
- When considering cause of pediatric hypertension, it is helpful to evaluate for the most common causes by age group.
- Therapy should target systolic blood pressure reduction by 25% in first 8 hours and identification of underlying cause should take priority after initial stabilization of the patient.

Suggested Readings

Dizon A, Stauffer B. Chapter 134. Renal emergencies in children. In: Tintinali JE, Stapczynski J, Ma O, Yealy DM, Meckler GD, Cline DM, eds. *Tintinalli's Emergency Medicine: A Comprehensive Study Guide*. 8th ed. New York, NY: McGraw-Hill; 2016:885-887.
Mattoo T, et al. Evaluation of hypertension in children and adolescents. *Up to Date*. 2018.
McCollough M, Rose E. Genitourinary and renal tract disorders. In: Walls RM, Hockberger RS, Gausche-Hill M, et al., eds. *Rosen's Emergency Medicine: Concepts and Clinical Practice*. 9th ed. Philadelphia, PA: Elsevier Saunders; 2018:2177-2179.

Getting to the Heart of the Matter: Do Not Miss These Features of Pathologic Murmurs

Natasha Smith, MD and Mimi Lu, MD

Innocent Murmurs

Innocent murmurs have low-grade turbulence with normal anatomy. Up to 80% of children will display these during childhood. Innocent murmurs intensify with increased output, as occurs with fever, hyperthyroidism, exercise, fear, anxiety, or anemia. It is important to exclude endocarditis and rheumatic fever whenever fever coexists with a murmur.

Innocent murmurs have seven features, known as the Seven S's:

Sensitive: change with respiratory variation/position (louder when supine, decrease with Valsalva)
Short: brief duration (not holosystolic)
Single: no clicks or gallops
Small: nonradiating, focal
Soft: low amplitude
Sweet: not harsh
Systolic: true to its namesake!

The child should be asymptomatic from cardiac symptoms such as hepatomegaly, feeding intolerance, frequent respiratory infections, and "cardiac wheezing" from pulmonary edema. The criteria for an innocent murmur are

1) Normal physical examination apart from the murmur
2) A negative review of systems
3) No personal or family history of high-risk features of structural heart disease (ie, sudden death, teratogen exposures or maternal diabetes, rheumatic fever, or Kawasaki disease)
4) Afebrile
5) Cardiac examination is consistent with known innocent murmur patterns without additional abnormal heart sounds

If all five criteria are not met, the patient should be referred to a pediatric cardiologist for formal echocardiography.

Pathologic Murmurs

A few murmurs that can be appreciated in the ED signify a grave condition. Be cautious of murmurs with any of the following features:

1) Cardiac symptoms, cyanosis, or syncope
2) Holosystolic, strong systolic, or harsh murmurs
3) Those with strongest intensity at the left upper sternal border (LUSB)
4) Murmurs that intensify on standing
5) The presence of a systolic click, abnormal S2, additional heart sounds, or abnormal pulses
6) Murmurs that are present in the first year, and especially the first 6 hours, of life.
7) Diastolic murmurs

Hypertrophic cardiomyopathy (HCM) is the most common cause of sudden cardiac death in adolescents and is widely underdiagnosed. Obstructive HCM is due to left ventricular outflow tract obstruction during systole from asymmetric septal hypertrophy. Listen for a grade 3-4 crescendo/decrescendo systolic murmur heard best at the middle left to upper right sternal border, with increased intensity with Valsalva due to decreased venous return. In 95% of cases, the murmur will increase in intensity when standing from squatting. Conversely, the passive straight leg raising test will often decrease the murmur due to increased venous return. Eighty-five percent of patients will have decreased murmur with handgrip, which increases systemic vascular resistance (SVR).

KEY POINTS

- Innocent murmurs must meet the following five criteria at >1 year of age: (1) otherwise normal examination; (2) asymptomatic; (3) personal/family history is negative for features of structural heart disease; (4) afebrile; (5) examination is consistent with a known innocent murmur, with no abnormal heart sounds.
- Seven S's of innocent murmurs: sensitive, short, single, small, soft, sweet, and systolic.
- Refer to cardiology if (1) symptomatic; (2) abnormal examination; (3) loud/long/harsh systolic murmur; (4) strongest intensity at the LUSB; (5) louder with standing; (6) diastolic murmur or S4; (7) other abnormal heart sounds; or (8) presents in first year of life.
- Obstructive HCM is the most common cause of sudden cardiac death in pediatrics, and the murmur causes a grade 3-4 crescendo-decrescendo systolic murmur at the middle LUSB to RUSB, with increased intensity with decreased venous return.

Suggested Readings

Allen HD, Driscoll DJ, Shaddy RE, et al. *Moss and Adam's Heart Disease in Infants, Children, and Adolescents: Including the Fetus and Young Adult*. 9th ed. Philadelphia, PA: Wolters Kluwer; 2016.

Frank JE, Jacobe KM. Evaluation and management of heart murmurs in children. *American Family Physician*. 2011;84(7):793-800.

Pickoff AS. "Cardiology." *MedStudy Pediatrics Core Book 3: Cardiology*. 8th ed. MedStudy; 2017:1-51 Print.

Raees M. "Cardiology." In: Hughes HK, Lauren KK, eds. *The Johns Hopkins Hospital: The Harriett Lane Handbook*. 21st ed. Philadelphia, PA: Elsevier; 2018:156-202. Print.

87

Do Not Crash and Burn by Missing Kawasaki Disease

Carly Loner, MD and Kathleen Stephanos, MD, FAAEM

Mucocutaneous lymph node syndrome, more commonly known as Kawasaki disease (KD), is known by its defining feature of the 5-day fever. However, this disease has a wide spectrum of presentations, which can obscure the diagnoses. Diagnostic algorithms have replaced traditional criteria to prevent misdiagnosis and expedite treatment to prevent coronary aneurysm formation. KD occurs most often in males of Asian descent, though it can affect people of all ages and ethnicities. It is an autoimmune-mediated vasculitis of small- and medium-sized vessels with a seasonal pattern (more often in winter) and epidemic nature suggesting an infectious trigger. KD can involve vessels in the lungs, GI tract, meninges, or liver but preferentially affects coronary arteries. KD is typically self-limited, resolving within 12 days; however, in more severe onset of disease, and up to 25% of untreated cases, coronary aneurysms or ectasia can develop.

KD has traditionally been a clinical diagnosis based upon presence of fever ≥5 days and having at least four of five signs of mucocutaneous inflammation: bilateral conjunctivitis, oropharyngeal mucus membrane changes (strawberry tongue, erythema of the tongue or posterior pharynx), cervical lymph-adenopathy, rash (typically morbilliform and truncal), and changes in distal extremities (erythema or edema). Symptoms do not have to be present simultaneously to make the diagnosis, so a careful history is crucial.

The 2017 American Heart Association (AHA) guidelines recommend consideration of KD in infants and children with prolonged fever and one of the following clinical scenarios: irritability, unex-plained aseptic meningitis, unexplained culture-negative shock, cervical lymphadenopathy, or retro-pharyngeal phlegmon without antibiotic response. Differential diagnoses of children with persistent fever and mucocutaneous findings may include drug hypersensitivity, viral exanthem, staphylococcal scalded skin syndrome, Stevens-Johnson syndrome, scarlet fever, and toxic shock syndrome.

There is no single diagnostic lab test for KD. Presence of certain labs can support the diagnosis but do not exclude it. Most cases will be associated with systemic inflammation, with elevated C-reactive protein (CRP), erythrocyte sedimentation rate (ESR), white blood cell count (WBC), liver enzymes (from hepatic congestion), and platelets (usually a late finding). Due to associated urethritis, urinalysis may show sterile pyuria. Urine dipstick will test negative for leukocyte esterase due to the presence of predominantly mononuclear WBCs. Other lab findings include anemia, hypoalbuminemia, hyperlip-idemia, and hyponatremia.

Adolescents and older children are likely to present with classic signs of KD but may also have meningeal or gastrointestinal symptoms resulting in delayed diagnosis of KD. Children <1 year old have the greatest risk of coronary aneurysm formation and commonly present with incomplete KD. In 2010, the AHA developed an algorithm to identify incomplete KD in patients with prolonged fever. Elevated inflammatory markers (CRP ≥ 3 mg/dL and/or ESR ≥ 40 mg/dL), warrant assessment of supplemental laboratory criteria (albumin ≤3 g/dL, anemia for age, WBC ≥ 15 000 cells/mm³, urine WBCs ≥ 10 cells/high-power field) and echocardiogram. If more than three of the supplementary labs are met or echocardiogram is positive, treatment is recommended. If a child does not meet criteria, he or she should be monitored and retested for 2 additional days of fever or desquamating rash. Patients with a suspected diagnosis of KD require admission for intravenous immunoglobulin (IVIG). IVIG given within 10 days of symptom onset can significantly decrease the development of coronary artery aneurysms. Children should receive an initial large infusion of 2 g/kg over 8-12 hours as well as aspirin (30 mg/kg/d in 4 doses).

Repeat dosing may be required if the patient remains symptomatic, primarily with fever.

KEY POINTS

- There are established criteria for diagnosis of typical and incomplete KD.
- Suspect this diagnosis in any child with prolonged, unexplained fever.
- Infants are at highest risk of coronary aneurysm development and are also likely to present with subtle findings or incomplete KD, so early consideration is key.
- Early IVIG administration reduces formation of coronary aneurysms thereby preventing long-term cardiac complications.

Suggested Readings

Dietz SM, Stijn DV, Burgner D, et al. Dissecting Kawasaki disease: a state of the art review. *Eur J Pediatr.* 2017:176(8):995-1009.

Pilania RK, Dharmagat B, Singh S. Controversies in diagnosis and management of Kawasaki disease. *World J Clin Pediatric.* 2018;7(1):27-35.

Vervoot D, Donne M, Gysel DV. Pitfalls of diagnosis and management of Kawasaki disease: an update for the pediatric dermatologist. *Pediatr Dermatol.* 2018;35(6):743-747.

Pediatric Electrocardiogram Differences: Know Which Findings Are Normal in Children and Which Ones Spell Trouble

Andrea P. Anderson, MD and Sabreen Akhter, DO, DTM

It is important to recognize findings that are concerning in adults but are considered normal in kids. Pediatric norms for rate, intervals, axis, and morphology vary with age. Do not feel the need to memorize it all, as normative tables can be used for reference.

Axis

Relative right ventricular hypertrophy (RVH) is normal in newborns and resolves by age 6 months. The electrocardiogram (ECG) pattern is similar to RVH in adults: QRS axis deviation greater than +90 degree, R wave dominance in V1, and T wave inversions in V1-V3. Left axis deviation is abnormal in newborns.

Q Waves

Narrow Q waves (<3 ms) of up to 6-8 mm are normal until age 3 years in inferior and left precordial leads (II, III, aVF, V5, and V6). Q waves may indicate pathology if they are abnormally deep, wide, or appear in right precordial leads such as V1.

QRS Waves

The QRS duration lengthens during childhood, from 50-70 ms in neonates to 70-100 ms in teens. Right ventricular dominance in infants is gradually replaced by left so that the pediatric ECG is similar to an adult ECG by age 3-4 years. R wave amplitude in the right precordial leads decreases with age, while the left amplitude increases; the opposite is true for S waves.

ST Segment

ST depression or elevation of up to 1 mm in limb leads and 2 mm in left precordial leads may be normal. In adolescents, concave ST elevation can indicate benign early repolarization in leads with an upright T wave. Similarly, ST depression can indicate benign "J point depression" if concave and upward sloping. By contrast, a depressed ST segment that is downward sloping or horizontal is abnormal.

QTc Interval

Infants <6 months have a QTc < 490 ms. After 6 months, there is considerable variation, but the mean QTc throughout childhood is 410-450 ms.

T Waves

T waves in the precordial leads are upright at birth, then invert in V1-V3 after the first week of life. They remain inverted until about age 8 years but may persist into early adulthood. Inverted T waves convert to upright T waves in a predictable order: first V3, then V2 and finally V1. Upright T waves in V1 and V4R in children 3 days to 6 years can indicate RVH. T waves in V5 and V6 are usually upright.

Additional findings that may be normal in children include heart rate >100 beats per minute (bpm), marked sinus arrhythmia, RSR' pattern in V1, short PR (<120 ms), and slightly peaked P waves (<3 mm height is normal in infants under 6 months).

Supraventricular Tachycardia

Supraventricular tachycardia (SVT) accounts for 90% of dysrhythmias in children. Suspect SVT in children with a heart rate above 180 bpm or infants with a heart rate above 220 bpm *without variability*. SVT is marked by rapid, usually narrow (<80 ms), regular QRS waves and absent P waves. In infants, SVT can present with signs of heart failure such as low weight, poor feeding, and irritability. Verbal children may describe palpations, chest pain, dizziness, or fatigue. Note that >95% of wide complex tachycardia in pediatrics are not ventricular tachycardia, but instead variants of SVT.

A rapid push of adenosine to transiently block AV nodal conduction is the first-line treatment for stable SVT. Vagal maneuvers such as a bag of ice on an infant's face can be attempted while preparing adenosine. Second-line therapies include calcium channel blockers such as verapamil to slow AV node conduction, procainamide to slow conduction through the atria, or amiodarone to prolong the AV nodal refractory period.

Wolf-Parkinson-White (WPW) syndrome is subtype of SVT marked by an accessory conduction pathway. When in sinus rhythm, ECG reveals a short PR interval and characteristic "delta wave" or slurred upslope at the start of a widened QRS. In WPW, adenosine or other AV nodal blockade can precipitate a lethal reentry tachycardia especially if the QRS is wide; in this rare case, procainamide or amiodarone can be used. Of course, if a patient has unstable SVT, immediate synchronized cardioversion is the first move.

Hypertrophic Cardiomyopathy

Hypertrophic cardiomyopathy (HCM) classically presents as the healthy teen who collapses while playing basketball, requiring bystander CPR and defibrillation, sometimes with a history of syncope and a family history of early sudden death. ECG findings include increased precordial voltages, ST segment changes, deep, narrow, "daggerlike" Q waves in lateral and inferior leads, and signs of left atrial hypertrophy. HCM is a high mortality diagnosis, resulting in ventricular arrhythmias which can cause sudden death.

KEY POINTS

- Inverted T waves in precordial leads V1-V3 are normal in children; they flip to upright in a predictable order from left to right, typically by early adolescence.
- RVH with right axis deviation is normal in newborns and resolves by 6 months.
- Supraventricular tachycardia should be suspected with heart rate >180 bpm in children or >220 bpm in infants and ECG shows a narrow, regular QRS with absent p waves.

Suggested Readings

Burns E. Paediatric ECG Interpretation. Life in the Fast Lane. https://litfl.com/paediatric-ecg-interpretation-ecg-library/. Last updated March 16, 2019.

Davignon A, Rautaharju P, Boisselle E, et al. Normal ECG standard for infants and children. *Pediatric Cardiology.* 1980;1:123-131.

Evans WN, Acherman RJ, Mayman GA, et al. Simplified pediatric electrocardiogram interpretation. *Clin Pediatr.* 2010;49(4):363-372.

Goodacre S, McLeod K. Paediatric electrocardiography. *BMJ.* 2002;324:1382.

Do Not Be Shocked! Know the Meaning of the First Three Letters of a Pacemaker's Code

Ryley McPeters, MD and Stephen Mac, MD, FAAP

Introduction

Pacemakers are typically placed in pediatric patients for the treatment of bradycardia, AV block, or life-threatening tachyarrhythmias. Implantable cardioverter-defibrillators (ICD) can also be used to treat life-threatening tachyarrhythmias. Pacemakers include a generator (hardware and battery) and leads extending into the myocardium. A pulse created by the generator travels down the leads depolarizing the myocardium. Leads can be placed in the right atrium, right ventricle, or left ventricle. Pacemakers are described by a unique 5-letter code. The first three letters are the most important, remembered using the mnemonic PaSeR. The first letter (Pa) describes the chamber being **Pa**ced, while the second letter (Se) identifies which chamber is **Se**nsed. These can be O (no chamber), A (atrium), V (ventricle), or D (dual A + V). The third letter (R) describes the **R**esponse to sensing which can be O (none), T (triggered), I (inhibited), or D (dual I + T). So, a pacemaker labeled VVI would have a ventricle that is paced and sensed and a pulse generator which inhibits pacing output in response

Evaluation

A focused history should start with the type of pacemaker, indication for placement, and date of implantation and any revisions. History concerning for pacemaker-related complications include palpitations, weakness, dyspnea, hiccups (diaphragmatic stimulation), syncope, dizziness, and pain/erythema around the pacemaker site. Physical examination should focus on vitals and cardiopulmonary examination including an assessment for trauma or infection of the implantation site. An electrocardiogram (ECG) should be performed with and without a magnet placed on the generator and should be compared to previous ECGs. Labs should evaluate for thyroid or electrolyte abnormalities or acidosis. AP and lateral chest x-ray may reveal lead dislodgement, fracture, perforation, or migration. An overpenetrated x-ray can also provide manufacturer and identification information if the patient is unable to do so or does not have their device information card. Pediatric cardiology should be consulted early. The device representative can be an excellent resource also and can interrogate the device if there are concerns for malfunction.

Early Complications

Early complications occur within the first 6 weeks post-operatively. Typically, these complications are related to the surgical procedure itself, venous access, or lead positioning or displacement. Post-operative infection is most often seen in immunocompromised patients or patients on steroids or blood thinners. Infections can be progressive from a single stitch to the surgical pocket or the entire pacing system and can lead to bacteremia or endocarditis.

Late Complications

Late complications are rare and are typically related to battery malfunction or device failure. Device failure is divided into three categories: failure to capture, failure to pace, and failure to sense. Failure to capture occurs when an impulse is sent down the lead but myocardial depolarization does not occur. In this case, pacemaker spikes can often be seen on the ECG with no induced cardiac response. Failure to pace occurs when the pacemaker does not provide a stimulus for the myocardium to fire. When this happens, the patient's heart rate is typically below the set lower limit of the device, and there are no pacemaker spikes nor pacemaker-induced QRS complexes seen on the ECG. Failure to sense occurs when the pacemaker does not recognize depolarization traveling up the lead wire. This can be described as oversensing or undersensing. Oversensing is marked by improper interpretation of the electrical activity by the pacemaker, whereas undersensing occurs when the pacemaker is unable to correctly interpret the native cardiac activity.

Management

Emergency department management of patients with pacemaker failure is based on symptoms and hemodynamic status. If the device fails, place pacer pads in anticipation of transcutaneous pacing. Atropine or epinephrine may be helpful in patients with profound bradycardia or shock. With pacemaker-mediated tachycardia or dysrhythmias, place a magnet over the device to terminate these rhythms. The magnet changes the pacemaker to a fixed, asynchronous mode, and the patient's heart rate will be determined by the device's preset rate. When a magnet is applied to an ICD, stop shock delivery without affecting the pacing function. Early consultation with a pediatric cardiologist is always recommended.

KEY POINTS

- The first three letters of a pacemaker's code describes the chamber being paced, the chamber being sensed, and the mode of response.
- A focused history should include whether the patient is pacemaker dependent, the type of pacemaker implanted, the date of implant, and the program settings.
- A magnet placed on the pacemaker will return the pacemaker to its preset rate.
- Early pediatric cardiology consultation is recommended for pacemaker malfunction.

Suggested Reading

Allison M, Mallemat H. Emergency care of patients with pacemakers and defibrillators. *Emerg Med Clin North Am.* 2015;33(3):653-667.

Hall, E, Fairbrother, H. Pacemaker and AICD management in the Emergency Department. EMDocs.net. June 2015.

Martindale J, deSouza IS. Managing pacemaker-related complications and malfunctions in the emergency department. *Emerg Med Pract.* 2014;16(9):1-21.

Shaw K, Bachur R. Evaluation of the patient with a cardiac device. *Fleisher and Ludwig's Textbook of Pediatric Emergency Medicine.* 7th ed. ; 2016:654-655 Chapter 94.

Singh H, Batra A, Balaji B. Cardiac pacing and defibrillation in children and young adults. *Indian Pacing Electrophysiol J.* 2013;13(1):4-13.

ABDOMEN

Be Aware of the Varied Presentation of Pediatric Appendicitis

Vishal Naik, MD and Anupam B. Kharbanda, MD, MSc

For many, the appendix is a structure that typically bears little significance in day-to-day function. For others, the appendix becomes an object of great significance as it begins a journey from inflammation to perforation. With a variety of vague presentations possible in the pediatric patient, it falls on the ED clinician to establish the diagnosis of appendicitis via the least invasive method possible.

History and Examination

Diagnosed in more than 75 000 children annually in the United States, appendicitis results from obstruction of the appendiceal lumen from a fecalith or other inflammatory process. Pediatric patients old enough to verbalize will typically complain of generalized abdominal pain localizing to the right lower quadrant as the inflamed appendix irritates the peritoneum. Younger patients, however, present with more vague symptoms such as fussiness, irritability, or refusal to walk. The clinician must have a high index of suspicion for appendicitis as time to diagnosis is strongly linked to morbidity. For the younger child, the differential should include torsion (testicular and ovarian), urinary tract infection (UTI), constipation, nephrolithiasis, and gastroenteritis, among others. For postpubertal children, history should include last menstrual period and prior sexual history to account for an expanded differential including ectopic pregnancy, sexually transmitted disease, pelvic inflammatory disease (PID), and endometriosis.

Examination findings generally attempt to illicit peritoneal signs in the child and vary by age and disease progression. In children of all ages, the clinician should observe the child ambulate or jump. Classic findings such as pain at McBurney's point or Rovsing's sign may be present. Caution must be taken as recent studies reveal that a significant minority of children will present atypically, lacking classic appendicitis examination findings. Psoas and/or obturator signs suggest a retrocecal appendix but are infrequently present. For the postpubertal child, the clinician should also perform a thorough genitourinary examination. Children who appear toxic or refuse to move should raise suspicion for a more progressed disease state such as perforation or abscess formation.

Diagnostics

Physical examination and basic laboratory testing (ie, CBC) of a child with suspected appendicitis are utilized to guide diagnosis and management. Clinical scores such as the Alvarado, Pediatric Appendicitis Score (PAS), or Pediatric Appendicitis Risk Calculator (pARC) employ a mixture of leukocyte/neutrophil count, history, and physical examination findings to risk stratify patients for potential appendicitis. In general, equivocal scores indicate imaging/further workup, while low-risk patients can be discharged with close follow-up.

A component of many clinical decision pathways, the CBC with differential is a key factor in risk stratifying children for appendicitis. A lower WBC indicates a lack of inflammation and, subsequently, a higher negative predictive value for acute appendicitis. A mild elevation in WBC is most characteristic of acute appendicitis with higher levels signifying abscess, perforation, or pneumonia. Other laboratory tests, such as the urinalysis and urine pregnancy test, help rule out other conditions like nephrolithiasis, UTI, and ovarian pathology.

If the decision is made to image, ultrasound should first be considered. Ultrasound, in the hands of a pediatric-trained sonographer, is equivalent to CT in the diagnosis of acute appendicitis. If ultrasound results are indeterminate, current research recommends admission for serial sonography or transfer to a center with pediatric radiology. CT scan is indicated when complex appendicitis is suspected (ie, perforation or abscess formation).

Management

During the diagnostic evaluation for acute appendicitis, efforts should be made to hydrate and ensure adequate pain and nausea control. Opioid use does not mask peritonitis and will likely lead to improved sonography. Ideally, surgical consult is made early. Following diagnosis, empiric antibiotics should be started. If acute appendicitis has been diagnosed at night, the patient can safely be admitted for surgery to be performed during the daytime in the presence of a full surgical team.

KEY POINTS

- Have a high index of suspicion for acute appendicitis, especially in younger children who may present with vague symptoms.
- Clinical decision support systems or scores (Alvarado, PAS, pARC) should be utilized to guide evaluation.
- The CT scan should be reserved for children where complex appendicitis is suspected.
- Children diagnosed with acute appendicitis should be started on empiric antibiotics.

Suggested Readings

Hansen LW, Dolgin SE. Trends in the diagnosis and management of pediatric appendicitis. *Pediatr Rev.* 2016;37(2):52-58.

Lipsett SC, Bachur RG. Current approach to the diagnosis and emergency department management of appendicitis in children. *Pediatr Emerg Care.* 2017;33(3):198-203.

Snyder MJ, Guthrie M, Cagle S. Acute appendicitis: efficient diagnosis and management. *Am Fam Physician.* 2018;98(1):25-33.

Pyloric Stenosis: Diagnosis the Stenosis Before It Becomes "Classic"

Corinne Shubin, MD and Jessica Wall, MD, MPH, MSCE, FAAP

Background

Infantile hypertrophic pyloric stenosis is the most common gastrointestinal disease of infants and is characterized by an abnormal thickening of the pylorus, resulting in gastric outlet obstruction. The etiology of pyloric stenosis remains unknown; however, risk factors include formula feeding, young maternal age, exposure to erythromycin, and being a firstborn male.

Clinical Presentation

Infants with pyloric stenosis typically present between 2 and 5 weeks of life with projectile vomiting. Emesis is typically nonbilious and progressively projectile, and infants with pyloric stenosis generally show continued interest in feeding after vomiting. Other common presenting symptoms include failure to thrive or poor weight gain, constipation, irritability, jaundice, or dehydration. Signs on physical examination include visible peristalsis or a palpable "olivelike" mass in the right upper quadrant. However, over the last several decades with increased use of ultrasound resulting in earlier diagnosis of pyloric stenosis, <20% of patients have a palpable olivelike mass on examination at the time of presentation.

Diagnosis

Historically, the upper gastrointestinal contrast radiology was utilized to diagnose pyloric stenosis by demonstrating abnormal contrast transmission through the gastric outlet. Currently, ultrasound is the gold standard for diagnosis and can be performed by point-of-care in the emergency department or radiology. A pyloric muscle of >2 mm thick or >12 mm long is diagnostic of pyloric stenosis. Laboratory evaluation can demonstrate a hypochloremic, hypokalemic metabolic alkalosis; however, as patients are presenting earlier, many do not show these electrolyte derangements. Approximately two-thirds of infants with pyloric stenosis have an elevated bicarbonate level, but the majority of patients have normal potassium and chloride levels.

This is likely due to an early diagnosis of pyloric stenosis with ultrasound. Ultrasound is a safe, noninvasive and easy means of diagnosis in the emergency department. Ultrasound screening for infants with a concerning history for pyloric stenosis will likely confirm a diagnosis before the infants develop growth, metabolic or electrolyte disturbances.

Management

The definitive management of pyloric stenosis is laparoscopic pyloromyotomy; however, this does not need to be done emergently, and patients should be medically optimized prior to surgical intervention. It is important correct any hemodynamic instability, dehydration, or electrolyte disturbances. Infants with pyloric stenosis should have intravenous access placed, balanced crystalloid fluid boluses given as needed for dehydration, be started on glucose containing maintenance intravenous fluids, and be admitted or transferred for definitive management.

KEY POINTS

- Infants may not have the "classic" olivelike mass palpable in the right upper quadrant or electrolyte derangements.
- Ultrasound of the pylorus is key to diagnosing pyloric stenosis. Consider ultrasound in patients with a concerning history to avoid growth, metabolic and electrolyte disturbance.
- Definitive management is surgical, but the patient must be stabilized medically prior to surgical treatment.

Suggested Reading

Glatstein M, Carbell G, Boddu SK, Beradini A, Scolnik D. The changing clinical presentation of hypertrophic pyloric stenosis: the experiences of a large, tertiary care pediatric hospital. *Clin Pediatr (Phila)*. 2011;50(3):192-195.

Taylor ND, Cass DT, Holland AJ. Infantile hypertrophic pyloric stenosis: has anything changed? *J Paediatr Child Health*. 2013;49(1):33-37.

Roberto G, Said E. Infantile hypertrophic pyloric stenosis: an epidemiological review. *Neonatal Netw*. 2018;37(4):197-204.

The Inception of an Intussusception: Look for the Bowel Within a Bowel Even if Symptoms Are Not "Classic"

Carl Mirus IV, MD and Kathleen Stephanos, MD, FAAEM

Intussusception is a form of bowel obstruction caused by the involution of proximal bowel into the adjacent distal bowel. It is a common etiology of pediatric abdominal pain, which can occur in any bowel region but is frequently at the ileocecal junction. Intussusception is often idiopathic and easily managed; however, delays in diagnosis can result in obstruction and ischemia leading to necrosis, perforation, peritonitis, and even death.

History and Physical Examination

Intussusception is the most common cause of intestinal obstruction in children 3 months to 5 years old, occurring twice as often in males. A history of conditions associated with bowel wall inflammation or thickening (ie, cystic fibrosis or inflammatory bowel disease) should raise suspicion as this can act as a lead point (the site triggering involution of the bowel). The commonly taught triad of symptoms (colicky pain, abdominal mass, and red currant stools) exists in <50% of children. Rather, intussusception often presents with one or more of four distinct features: intermittent abdominal pain, vomiting, pallor, and lethargy. Abdominal pain, typically intermittent and cramping, may also manifest as episodic crying, fetal positioning, or lethargy and is the most common presenting symptom. Vomiting is the second most common symptom, potentially leading to dehydration and electrolyte abnormalities. Diarrhea occurs in about 25% of patients and is often small in volume and duration. Bilious vomiting and currant jelly stools are infrequent and late findings suggestive of developing bowel ischemia.

Abdominal examination may reveal a "sausage-shaped" mass on the right, although frequently the examination is benign. Distension and significant tenderness often occur as a late finding. Differential diagnosis should include other causes of bowel obstruction (eg, volvulus, pyloric stenosis, Hirschsprung disease), infections, and appendicitis.

Diagnosis

Ultrasound is the diagnostic first-line modality. An intussusception has a hypoechoic ring with central echogenicity ("target or bull's-eye" sign). Intraperitoneal free fluid, pneumatosis, or fluid within the intussusception predicts a higher risk case that may be less amendable to enema reduction. Absence of blood flow on Doppler is concerning for bowel ischemia and warrants immediate surgical evaluation. Abdominal radiographs are less sensitive than ultrasound but may show a soft tissue density projecting into the gas of the large bowel, an obscured liver margin, or no air in the cecum. X-ray may identify bowel obstruction or pneumoperitoneum if shot in an upright or lateral decubitus view. Computerized tomography may show intussusception but is unnecessary unless attempting to characterize a mass or if the diagnosis is unclear.

Management

Initial focus should be on fluid resuscitation and electrolyte repletion. Once identified, fluoroscopically guided liquid/air enema for reduction is standard treatment. The patient should be transferred to a facility with both a radiology service equipped to perform the reduction and a pediatric surgery service due the risks of perforation or failed reduction. A commonly espoused protocol for reduction follows the rule of "3's": there should be no more than 3 attempts, each lasting no more than 3 minutes, with resolution for at least 3 days. If these conditions are not met, surgical intervention may be required.

Enema reduction should not be attempted if there are peritoneal signs on examination or evidence of perforation or mass on imaging. Pediatric surgery should be involved early but may only be needed if reduction is unsuccessful. Admission and monitoring for recurrence (occurs in up to 10%) is reasonable though asymptomatic patients with good hydration and reliable caregivers that have access to transportation and medical care may be discharged. Reoccurrences should be treated anew, with repeat nonoperative means if possible.

KEY POINTS

- Intussusception is the most common cause of intestinal obstruction in children 3 months to 5 years old.
- Common presentation is colicky abdominal pain, vomiting, and lethargy. A "sausage-shaped" mass can sometimes be felt. Current red stools are an infrequent and late finding.
- Ultrasound is the first-line modality for diagnosis of intussusception and can provide information regarding treatment prognostics.
- Reduction with air or fluid enema by a radiologist is the mainstay of treatment, however should not be performed if there are concerns of perforation.

Suggested Readings

Beasley S. The 'ins' and 'outs' of intussusception: where best practice reduces the need for surgery. *J Paediatr Child Health*. 2017;53(11):1118-1122.
Gilmore AW, Reed M, Tenenbein M. Management of childhood intussusception after reduction by enema. *Am J Emerg Med*. 2010;29:1136-1140.
Whitehouse JS, Gourlay DM, Winthrop AL, Cassidy LD, Arca MJ. Is it safe to discharge intussusception patients after successful hydrostatic reduction? *J Pediatr Surg*. 2010;45(6):1182-1186.

GI bleed: Do Not Be fooled by bleeding imposters

Kelly Patel, MD and Sandal Saleem, MD, FAAP

Gastrointestinal (GI) bleeding is a common presenting complaint to Pediatric Emergency Departments (PED). A large nationwide study showed that only 11.6% of pediatric patients with the complaint of GI bleeding were admitted to the hospital for further workup. The majority of GI bleed complaints are non–life threatening and can be worked up as an outpatient. Our job is to determine both the location and severity of acute GI bleeding in order to optimize the diagnostic and therapeutic management. For patients showing signs of hemorrhagic shock secondary to GI bleeding, do what you do best! Focus on ABCs. Transfusion goals start with bolus of Packed Red Blood Cell (PRBC) and balanced resuscitation with blood, Fresh Frozen Plasma (FFP), and platelets.

In neonates presenting with feeding intolerance, inconsolability, abdominal distension, bilious or bloody vomiting, peritonitis, hematochezia, or melena, we need to recognize signs of shock, poor perfusion, and life-threatening bleeding. The three "must not miss" diagnoses of upper and lower GI bleeding are vitamin K deficiency, necrotizing enterocolitis, and malrotation with volvulus. Stabilize the patient and then on investigate the source of bleeding. Necrotizing enterocolitis is diagnosed with abdominal x-ray showing pneumatosis intestinalis, pneumoperitoneum, ileus, and/or hepatobiliary gas. Malrotation with volvulus is diagnosed with upper GI series with oral contrast. Vitamin K deficiency in neonate at birth can also be a cause of GI bleeding, which can be remediated with plasma, factor repletion, and vitamin K. Consider this diagnosis in neonates after a home birth or with parents who refused the vitamin K at birth.

In infants and toddlers, the must not miss diagnoses of GI bleeding are intussusception, vascular malformation, and Meckel diverticulum. Intussusception should be on your differential for children from 6 to 36 months of age and symptoms of abdominal pain. The classic teaching is sudden onset intermittent, severe, crampy progressive abdominal pain, drawing legs up to abdomen in intervals, vomiting, sausage-shaped abdominal mass, and currant jelly colored bloody stool. Though 20% of patients can present with altered mental status and severe sepsis alone. After stabilization, abdominal ultrasound showing a classic "target" sign is the definitive diagnosis but can be missed during initial scanning, so rescan based on your index of suspicion. Treatment for non–ill appearing patients is air enema typically performed by radiologist. Treatment of the patient with signs of end organ damage, ischemia, and severe sepsis or shock definitive treatment is surgical. In Meckel diverticulum bleeding, the classic teaching is that it will present as painless rectal bleeding with benign abdominal examination with the rule of 2s: by 2 years of age becoming symptomatic, affecting 2% of the population, often 2 in in length, 2 types of gastric mucosa, and found within 2 ft of the ileocecal valve. Diagnosis is made with Meckel scan or T-99 for stable patients with eventual surgical options. CT angiography is used for brisk bleeding in the sick patient requiring multiple transfusions.

In older children and adolescents presenting with GI bleeding must not miss diagnoses include inflammatory bowel disease (IBD), cryptic liver disease, and intestinal ulceration. Patients with extra–intestinal symptoms of oral ulcers, clubbing, erythema nodosum, jaundice, hepatomegaly, fatigue, anemia, poor weight gain, weight loss, and chronic abdominal pain should clue you in to possible IBD. These patients will eventually require a GI workup with endoscopy. Complications from IBD include strictures, fistulas, Small Bowel Obstruction (SBO), and refractory colitis, which would all potentially require surgical intervention.

Common masqueraders of GI bleeding are usually benign and can fool parents and clinicians. These bleeding imposters can be differentiated by considering history, examination, and a few simple tests. In the neonatal period, swallowed maternal blood can be a GI bleeding imposter. The Apt test is highly specific for fetal blood and can be used to specify if blood is fetal in origin. Two other common benign GI bleed diagnoses are milk protein allergy and anal fissure. Diet and medications can impact the color of stool. Children with diets containing beet root, cranberry jam, or artificial food coloring can have reddish, brick colored stool. Iron supplements and Pepto-Bismol can be mistaken for melena while cefdinir and rifampin cause reddish stool. In these situations, a simple fecal occult will be negative and reassuring.

KEY POINTS

- Do not forget to get your ABCs and advanced resuscitation techniques in the truly ill child with a GI bleed.
- Rule out the must not miss diagnosis of pediatric GI bleeding through history and physical examination and order imaging studies as necessary.
- Consider foods and medications that may cause stool discoloration.

Suggested Readings

McMillan DD, Wu J. Approach to the bleeding newborn. *Paediatr Child Health*. 1998;3(6):399-401.
Pant C, Olyaee M, et al. Emergency department visits for gastrointestinal bleeding in children: results from the Nationwide Emergency Department Sample 2006–2011. *Curr Med Res Opin*. 2015;31(2):347-351.
Squires RH Jr. Approach to the child with upper or lower gastrointestinal bleeding. In: Rudolph CD, ed. *Rudolph's Pediatrics*. New York, NY: McGraw-Hill; 2003:1371-1375.
Saliakellis E, Borrelli O, Thapar N. Paediatric GI emergencies. *Best Pract Res Clin Gastroenerol*. 2013;27:799-817.

The Hard Truth of Constipation—Do Not Miss the Potentially Serious Causes

Jennifer E. Guyther, MD and Carmen Avendano, MD

As much as 30% of the pediatric population experience constipation. Patients present with fewer than three bowel movements per week, acute abdominal pain, stool retention, and crying. For reference, normal stooling patterns are as follows. Newborns transition from meconium to a green/brown stool and then a yellow/brown milk stool by 4 or 5 days of life. After 3 weeks of life, babies may go up to 2 weeks without passing stool. Older children stool between several times per day to once every several days. The North American Society of Pediatric Gastroenterology, Hepatology and Nutrition defines constipation as a delay or difficulty in defecation > 2 weeks that causes significant distress to the patient. Key historical questions include frequency and consistency of stools, pain or bleeding with defecation, abdominal pain, vomiting, toilet training history, soiling, appetite change, diet, and medications.

Worrisome signs include onset during the neonatal period, failure to pass meconium, weight loss or poor weight gain, delayed motor milestones, and ribbonlike stool. The differential diagnosis includes Hirschsprung disease, hypothyroidism, milk protein allergy, celiac disease, imperforate/stenotic anus, intestinal obstruction, cystic fibrosis, spinal cord dysfunction, and botulism. Special attention should be paid to the abdominal, perineal, and neurologic examination. Concerning findings include abdominal distention, sacral dimpling, midline pigment abnormalities or hair tufts, an abnormal anus, or an empty rectal vault despite palpable stool on abdominal examination. A digital rectal examination is only needed if the history or examination is abnormal.

Current evidence does not support routine abdominal radiographs or blood work for evaluation of fecal impaction. Multiple scoring systems for assessing stool burden have been proposed, but they do not have high inter-reader reliability.

Table 94.1 ■ Oral Medications Used to Treat Constipation		
Medication	Mechanism	Dose
Polyethylene glycol	Opposes absorption of water by the large bowel; not absorbed or metabolized	Typical maintenance dose is 0 4 g/kg/d (max, 100 g/d)
Lactulose	Draws fluid into large bowels, increasing peristalsis (safe at all ages)	1-2 g/kg/d
Milk of magnesia	Promotes osmotic retention of fluid (can lead to toxicity in infants)	2-5 y: 0.4-1.2 g/d 6-11 y: 1.2-2.4 g/d 12-18 y: 2.4-4.8 g/d
Mineral oil	Makes the stool slippery; slows colonic absorption of water	1-3 mL/kg/d (max 90 mL)
Bisacodyl	Acts on intestinal mucosa, altering water and electrolyte secretion	3-10 y: 5 mg/d >10 y: 5-10 mg/d
Senna	Acts on intestinal mucosa, altering water and electrolyte secretion	2-6 y: 2.5-5 mg/d 6-12 y: 2.5-12 mg/d >12 y: 15-20 mg/d
Sodium picosulfate	Acts on intestinal mucosa, altering water and electrolyte secretion	1 mo to 4 y: 2.5-10 mg/d 4-18 y: 2.5-20 mg/d

An elimination diet may be beneficial for milk protein allergy but often not for 2-4 weeks. Most children with cow's milk allergy also react to goat and sheep's milk and some to soy milk so hydrolyzed formulas such as Nutramigen and Alimentum may be preferable in these cases. Adding fiber or water to the diet does not relieve constipation unless they are deficient. Medication options to treat constipation are listed in Table 94.1.

KEY POINTS

- Constipation is a delay or difficulty in defecation >2 weeks that causes significant distress to the patient.
- Rectal examination, blood work, and radiographs are needed only if the patient's history or the physical examination raises concern.
- Always consider secondary causes of constipation such as Hirschsprung disease and botulism and look for clues in the history and physical examination findings.
- For fecal disimpaction, use polyethylene glycol (PEG) at 1-1.5 g/kg/d for 3-6 days.
- Once disimpaction has been achieved, maintenance therapy is with PEG, 0.4 g/kg/d. Lactulose is also a first-line treatment and is considered safe for all ages.

Suggested Readings

Gfroerer S, Rolle U. Pediatric intestinal motility disorders. *World J Gastroenterol* 2015;21:9683-9687.

Khan L. Constipation management in pediatric primary care. *Pediatr Ann* 2018;47:e180-e184.

Madani S, Tsang L, Kamat D. Constipation in children: a practical review. *Pediatr Ann* 2016;45:e189-e196.

Tabbers MM, DiLorenzo C, Berger MY, et al. Evaluation and treatment of functional constipation in infants and children: evidence-based recommendations from ESPGHAN and NASPGHAN. *J Pediatr Gastroenterol Nutr* 2014;58:258-274.

95

Pediatric Diarrhea—Hydration Is the Most Important Factor in Treatment

Neethu M. Menon, MD

Gastroenteritis is a common cause of pediatric emergency department (ED) visits in the United States. In developed countries, diarrhea is most commonly caused by either viral infectious agents or self-limiting bacterial pathogens. In areas with poor sanitation, cholera, invasive bacterial infections, and parasitic infestations also need to be considered.

Hydration Status and Rehydration

The primary concern for children with diarrheal illnesses is hydration status. Early dehydration is often asymptomatic. As it progresses, increased thirst, irritability or restlessness, tachypnea, decreased skin turgor, and sunken fontanelle in infants develop. Sunken eyes typically indicate further worsening. Labs such as urine specific gravity, serum electrolytes, and bicarbonate level usually are not needed but can help guide management in severe dehydration. Initial clinical assessment is the key to appropriate and timely rehydration.

It is important to start hydration as soon as possible; oral for mild to moderate dehydration and intravenous (IV) for severe cases. Thereafter, delayed reassessment or fluid orders in a busy setting may result in a fluid deficit. Consequently, consider placing an order for continuous fluids at the same time that the bolus is ordered. These fluids should include regular maintenance volumes as well as the extra amount needed to replace ongoing losses. It is equally important to watch for signs of fluid overload, especially in children with known or suspected cardiac illnesses. Nonetheless, a majority of the children will require a relatively large amount of fluids to overcome the deficits produced by the diarrhea. Though providers may be tempted to start with IV fluids, oral rehydration therapy (ORT) is the mainstay of therapy for mild to moderate dehydration. If IV hydration is initiated, ORT should be encouraged simultaneously. Infants may require 2-4 oz of ORT per episode of diarrhea, and children 4-8 oz. Remember that diarrhea leads to loss of water as well as electrolytes so it is important to provide electrolyte-containing fluids appropriate for age. Dairy products can sometimes worsen the diarrhea with temporary changes in the intestinal brush border resulting in lactase deficiency. Consequently, formula-fed infants may require temporary soy-based formula. Coconut water, fresh fruit juices, and soda should be avoided since they are sweetened with sugar, which can lead to osmotic diarrhea and hypernatremia secondary to sucrose intolerance. There are a number of commercially available oral rehydration solutions, and care providers should use a solution that has salt concentrations similar to WHO recommendations. For IV rehydration, lactated Ringer (LR) solution supplies adequate sodium and chloride, small amounts of potassium as well lactate for correction of acidosis. In the presence of hypovolemic shock, normal saline (NS) can be used too.

Therapeutics

Antimicrobial drugs are not routinely used for acute diarrheal illnesses because most illnesses are self-limiting viruses requiring only supportive care. Immunocompromised and septic patients may have underlying bacterial etiologies that require prompt therapy. Additionally, bloody diarrhea should prompt testing to identify the infectious source first, as the patient may be at risk for hemolytic uremic syndrome with antimicrobial treatment.

Antidiarrheal drugs like loperamide have no practical benefits for children with acute or persistent diarrhea. Risks outweigh benefits in children younger than 3 years of age who can experience adverse effects like lethargy, paralytic ileus, and abdominal distension. European guidelines promote the use of probiotics in children with acute gastroenteritis, but there is an absence of strong evidence. In developing countries, zinc supplementation is also incorporated with ORT.

Similar to any other acute illness, it is imperative to educate the child's family on return precautions, including to watch for signs of dehydration (including urine output and mental status), serious infection, and white or bloody stool.

KEY POINTS

- Evaluate for objective clinical features of dehydration to rapidly establish the appropriate rehydration measures.
- ORT is the primary intervention in mild to moderate dehydration but should be used as an adjunct in severe diarrhea too.
- LR IV fluid is a preferred over NS for severe diarrhea hydration.
- Empiric antimicrobial treatment should be limited to specific clinical scenarios.
- Antidiarrheal treatment should be avoided as the risks outweigh the benefits.

Suggested Readings

Cheron G, Jais JP, Cojocaru B, et al. The European Paediatric Life Support course improves assessment and care of dehydrated children in the emergency department. *Eur J Pediatr*. 2011;170:1151-1157.

Freedman SB, Pasichnyk D, Black KJ, et al. Gastroenteritis therapies in developed countries: systematic review and meta-analysis. *PLoS One*. 2015;10(6).

Li ST, Grossman DC, Cummings P. Loperamide therapy for acute diarrhea in children: systematic review and Meta-analysis. *PLoS Med*. 2007;4(3):495-505.

World Health Organization website. https://www.who.int/en/news-room/fact-sheets/detail/diarrhoeal-disease

Dehydration and Electrolyte Problems: Do Not Start IV Fluids in Children Without a Trial of PO Fluids and Antiemetics

Jonathan Higgins, MD, FAAP and Ryan Kearney, MD, MPH

Assessing Dehydration

Dehydration develops from excess fluid loss, insufficient fluid intake, or both. Common sources of fluid loss include vomiting, diarrhea, or evaporative fluid losses such as prolonged fevers, tachypnea, and heat. Dehydration severity is based on percentage decrease in body weight, though the preillness weight is rarely available in practice. Clinically, severe dehydration typically manifests as shock with changes in mental status, tachycardia, delayed capillary refill, and/or oliguria. A normal age-appropriate blood pressure is less reassuring as hypotension is a late and serious finding of shock in children. Moderately dehydrated patients often have tacky mucous membranes, decreased skin turgor, and some degree of irritability, with or without tachycardia. Patients with mild dehydration typically lack abnormal examination findings but have supporting history. The Clinical Dehydration Scale is fairly reliable to assess dehydration in children 1-36 months with gastroenteritis, albeit with limited evidence.

Managing Mild and Moderate Dehydration

Children with mild or moderate dehydration should initially receive a trial of oral rehydration therapy (ORT), with an antiemetic medication such as ondansetron if vomiting is present (0.15 mg/kg orally up to 8 mg maximum). This approach reduces interventions, ED resource use, and hospitalization while reinforcing therapy that can be continued at home.

ORT fluids balance glucose and sodium concentrations to replace electrolytes and limit the hyperosmotic intestinal fluid shifts that can worsen discomfort. Multiple commercial ORT options exist in the United States, such as Pedialyte or Enfalyte. Avoid liquids with unbalanced sugar and/or electrolyte content such as sodas, colas, sports drinks, undiluted fruit juices, and animal broths. Start ORT with small, frequent amounts and gradually increase the volume as tolerated.

Children with moderate dehydration who fail a trial of ORT may require intravenous (IV) or nasogastric fluids. Begin with a 20 mL/kg bolus of isotonic IV fluids over 30 minutes. In suspected or known heart failure patients, use 10 mL/kg boluses and frequently reassess. For nasogastric repletion, give 20 mL/kg of an appropriate ORT up to 600 mL over 60 minutes. An infrequently used but effective method of rehydration is hyaluronidase-facilitated hypodermoclysis (subcutaneous fluid administration). Using a small angiocatheter (eg, 24 gauge) in the subcutaneous tissue of the interscapular region or midanterior thigh, a subcutaneous infusion of recombinant hyaluronidase (150 units) allows a 20 mL/kg isotonic fluid to be painlessly infused SQ over an hour. Clinical signs of rehydration include normalization of vital signs, capillary refill, and willingness of the child to take fluids orally as their alertness and energy improve. Patients who fail ORT or have electrolyte/glucose abnormalities may require admission.

If starting an IV, check serum glucose and electrolytes. Hypernatremia usually reflects total body water depletion, whereas hyponatremia can result from free water reabsorption secondary to an increased antidiuretic hormone secretion. Nonanion gap metabolic acidosis can occur from bicarbonate losses in diarrhea. Serum ketones are frequently present in children with poor oral intake, but concomitant hyperglycemia should prompt a workup for diabetic ketoacidosis. Treatment of hypoglycemia often starts with oral glucose but with hemodynamic instability, altered mental status, or toxic appearance, a 2-5 mL/kg bolus of 10% dextrose should be given IV. Slow dextrose infusion rates (2-3 mL/min) may prevent insulin release and rebound hypoglycemia.

Special Circumstances and Pitfalls to Avoid

Ask how caregivers are mixing formula or ORT. If mixed incorrectly, patients are at higher risk for electrolyte derangements. Patients on enteral feeds may be unable to increase their intake enough in times of increased losses. Patients on diuretics may maintain an iatrogenic diuresis despite hypovolemia and can have more pronounced electrolyte changes. Those with known or suspected diabetes insipidus can rapidly develop hypernatremia. Even with mild symptoms, patients with certain metabolic diseases may require early dextrose-containing IV fluids as they can build up toxic metabolites (eg, lactate) rapidly. Prompt IV hydration in patients with concern for Shiga-toxin-producing bacterial enterocolitis has been shown to reduce the development and severity of hemolytic uremic syndrome.

KEY POINTS

- History and examination alone can establish severity of acute dehydration for most children.
- Children with mild-moderate dehydration should receive a trial of ORT and ondansetron before initiating IV fluids or checking laboratory studies.
- Severe dehydration requires prompt initiation of IV fluid resuscitation.
- Consider earlier intervention for children with certain chronic illnesses.

Suggested Readings

Falszewska A, Szajewska H, Dziechciarz P. Diagnostic accuracy of three clinical dehydration scales: a systematic review. *Arch Dis Child*. 2018;103(4):383-388.

Niescierenko M, Bachur R. Advances in pediatric dehydration therapy. *Curr Opin Pediatr*. 2013;25(3):304-309.

Powers KS. Dehydration: isonatremic, hyponatremic, and hypernatremic recognition and management. *Pediatr Rev*. 2015;36(7):274-283.

Spandorfer PR, Alessandrini EA, Joffe MD, et al. Oral versus intravenous rehydration of moderately dehydrated children: a randomized, controlled trial. *Pediatrics*. 2005;115(2):295-301.

Why Is My Baby's Poop White?: Do Not Forget to Check the Direct Bilirubin Level for Jaundiced Infants

Dhritiman Gurkha, MD and Whitney Minnock, MD

Jaundice in the neonatal period is a common emergency department (ED) presentation. It is caused by deposition of unconjugated bilirubin pigment in the skin and mucous membranes leading to yellowish discoloration appreciated clinically. It is important to determine if the hyperbilirubinemia is either unconjugated or conjugated as this can dramatically change the management and disposition of a patient. In this chapter, we will focus on the less common but potentially life-threatening conjugated hyperbilirubinemia (CH), specifically Biliary Atresia (BA).

Background and Definitions

The definition of CH is controversial, but a safe practical definition is any direct bilirubin value higher than the lab reference (usually above 2 mg/dL or >20% of total bilirubin). More sensitive than specific for liver disease, it is a clinical surrogate for cholestasis. This would normally be excreted into bile and eventually eliminated through intestine. In the first month of life, cholestatic jaundice is most commonly a clinical manifestation of biliary atresia. Nearly 25%-40% of BA present clinically in the first month of life as cholestatic jaundice.

The cause of BA is not known, but it has significant negative outcomes if the diagnosis is delayed. It most commonly involves an inflammatory process that leads to destruction of intra- and extra-hepatic bile tracts that causes complete biliary obstruction. This eventually leads to liver damage and cirrhosis within the age of 2-3 years. This is why it is prudent for the emergency provider to consider this diagnosis.

Clinical Assessment

It is important to ask about pale stool (lack of stercobilinogen), dark urine (presence of biliverdin), and jaundice (tissue bilirubin) as part of the history. These will be typical findings in the history of an infant with BA. Examination may be unremarkable but can reveal failure to thrive, jaundice, and hepatospleno-megaly. When there are dysmorphic features like hypertelorism with deep-seated eyes and a pointed chin, consider Alagille syndrome as the diagnosis. This is a rare genetic disorder affecting multiple systems including vision, cardiac, vascular, and skeletal anomalies requiring appropriate subspecialty care.

Investigations

Obtain serum conjugated bilirubin in addition to the total bilirubin to establish the direct hyperbiliru-binemia. The cholestatic pathology may be further supported by elevated liver enzymes, gamma-glu-tamyl transferase, and alkaline phosphatase. An abdominal ultrasound with Doppler is a vital imaging modality that may reveal an enlarged liver with an absent or atretic gallbladder. Furthermore, watch for the "triangular cord sign," a hyperechoic area due to a fibrous hepatic duct.

Management

An ED provider's role in BA management is timely identification. Once BA is diagnosed, the management is mainly surgical. Aside from the bloodwork and imaging mentioned above, one may consider chest radiograph if there is clinical concern for Alagille syndrome to look for any rib or vertebral body anomalies. BA requires urgent pediatric surgery evaluation. Timely diagnosis helps improve the outcome of the Kasai hepatic portoenterostomy (HPE) aimed at reestablishing bile flow. About 70% of patients will reestablish bile flow, if the HPE is performed within the first 60 days of life. This drops to <25% of patients with bile flow, if it is done after 90 days of life.

KEY POINTS

- Consider BA in any neonate or young infant with prolonged jaundice beyond 1 week of age, especially with acholic stools.
- Remember to order conjugated serum bilirubin in addition to total serum bilirubin.
- Ultrasound imaging of the abdomen with Doppler for initial radiologic evaluation.
- Timely pediatric surgery consultation/referral for evaluation of HPE.

Suggested Readings

A-Kader HH, Balistreri WF. Neonatal cholestasis. *Nelsons Textbook of Pediatrics.* 21th ed. ; 2020:2092-2101.e1.

Fawaz R, Baumann U, Ekong U, et al. Guideline for the evaluation of cholestatic jaundice in infants: joint recommendations of the North American Society for pediatric gastroenterology, hepatology, and nutrition (NASPGHAN) and the European Society for Pediatric Gastroenterology, Hepatology, and Nutrition (ESPGHAN). *J Pediatr Gastroenterol Nutr.* 2017;64:154-168.

Goodhue C, Fenlon M, Wang KS. Newborn screening for biliary atresia in the United States. *Pediatr Surg Int.* 2017;33:1315-1318.

Jones KL. *Smith's Recognizable Patterns of Human Malformation.* 6th ed. Philadelphia, PA: Elsevier Saunders; 2006:670-671.

Russell EA, Chumpitazi BP, Chumpitazi CE. Gastrointestinal emergencies. *Fleisher and Ludwig's Textbook of Pediatric Emergency Medicine.* 7th ed. Lippincott Williams and Wilkins; 2016:771-772.

Lets Be Blunt—Do Not Underestimate the Importance of Serial Abdominal Examinations in Pediatric Blunt Abdominal Trauma

Eva Tovar Hirashima, MD, MPH

Managing children with blunt abdominal trauma (BAT) can be challenging given the wide variation in anatomic and physiologic differences, our overreliance on computed tomography (CT), and the fact that most children with BAT are initially evaluated in general emergency departments without the guidance of a pediatric trauma surgeon. BAT is the leading cause of missed diagnosis leading to death, despite being less frequent than head or thoracic injuries.

Children may sustain multiple traumatic injuries given closer proximity of organs and a smaller body area over which the force of injury can be dissipated. Their organs are also less protected with less fat, weaker musculature, and proportionally larger viscera extending beyond the pelvic brim and below the costal margin. Furthermore, the ribs offer less protection due to increased pliability. This is why the spleen and liver are the most commonly injured abdominal organs. To complicate matters, the elastic and resilient tissues of children may not demonstrate external signs of trauma. Persistent tachycardia should alert the emergency physician (EP) to the presence of compensated shock as blood pressure is maintained until 30%-40% blood loss. Hypotension is a late and ominous finding and definitive of decompensated shock.

Hemodynamically Unstable Pediatric Abdominal Injury

Stabilization and initial management of children should proceed in a systematic fashion according to the Advanced Trauma Life Support guidelines. Children with signs concerning for BAT and hemodynamic instability unresponsive to fluid resuscitation and blood transfusion should proceed to emergency laparotomy (EL).

Hemodynamically Stable Pediatric Abdominal Injury

The Pediatric Emergency Care Applied Research Network (PECARN) BAT decision tool uses seven readily available clinical variables that help identify children at very low risk for intra-abdominal injury (IAI). Absence of all variables can obviate the need for CT, though presence of one or more variables should not be interpreted as an indication for CT imaging. In descending order of importance these are: evidence of abdominal wall trauma or seatbelt signs (SBS), Glasgow coma score <14, abdominal tenderness, evidence of thoracic wall trauma, complaints of abdominal pain, decreased breath sounds, and vomiting.

Keep in mind that hollow viscus and pancreatic injuries are often initially clinically silent with a delayed presentation. Fortunately, they may be associated with continued abdominal pain or injury patterns such as the SBS and handlebar marks. If present, observation with serial abdominal examinations can avoid a missed diagnosis.

There is no single laboratory study that can reliably predict IAI in children. However, when used in conjunction with clinical judgment, elevated transaminases (AST > 200 units/L, ALT > 125 units/L), gross or microscopic hematuria, or a hematocrit <30% should prompt further investigation. In cases of nonaccidental trauma, always the exception, an AST or ALT >80 units/L correlate with IAI, even in cases with minimal physical examination findings.

Focused Assessment with Sonography for Trauma (FAST) has a low sensitivity for IAI in children and is not a substitute for abdominal CT. Additionally, the majority of BAT in children is managed nonoperatively so a positive FAST is not necessarily an indication for EL. Although institutional variability exists, indications for CT imaging include SBS, abdominal wall bruising, abdominal tenderness, peritonitis, elevated transaminases, gross hematuria, downtrending hematocrit, or a positive FAST examination.

Trepidation regarding the next diagnostic step may be present in patients who "fail" the PECARN decision tool. However, in patients without clear-cut indications for a CT, combining serial examinations, negative screening FAST examinations, and unremarkable laboratory studies over an observation period of 12-24 hours may help exclude abdominal injuries forgoing unnecessary exposure to ionizing radiation.

KEY POINTS

- Children are more susceptible to blunt injuries and are more likely to have no external signs of trauma despite the presence of IAI.
- The PECARN decision tool can help avoid CT in those children with very low risk for IAI.
- The FAST examination is unable to rule out IAI and should not be used as the sole screening tool.
- In patients who "fail" PECARN, combining serial abdominal examinations, negative FAST examinations, and unremarkable laboratory studies may accurately rule out IAI.
- Always consider NAT in infants with inconsistent or implausible history, in these cases elevated transaminases are a useful indicator of IAI.

Suggested Readings

Adelgais KM, Kuppermann N, Kooistra J, et al. Accuracy of the abdominal examination for identifying children with blunt intra-abdominal injuries. *J Pediatr.* 2014;165:1230-1235.

Holmes JF, Lillis K, Monroe D, et al. Identifying children at very low risk of clinically important blunt abdominal injuries. *Ann Emerg Med.* 2013;62(2):107-101.

Miele V, Piccolo CL, Galluzzo M, et al. Contrast-enhanced ultrasound (CEUS) in blunt abdominal trauma. *Br J Radiol.* 2016;89:20150823.

Oh Heavens.... HUS and *Escherichia coli* 0157:H7—Do Not Rush to Give Antibiotics to Children With Bloody Diarrhea

Matthew B. Underwood, MD, FACEP

Hemolytic Uremic Syndrome Overview

Hemolytic uremic syndrome (HUS) is a consumptive coagulopathy leading to the classic triad of microangiopathic hemolytic anemia (MAHA), thrombocytopenia, and acute kidney injury (AKI). Shiga toxin-producing enterohemorrhagic *Escherichia coli* (STEC) HUS accounts for about 85%-90% of cases, and *Streptococcus pneumoniae* HUS accounts for about 5%. Terminology often refers to diarrhea positive (D+, or typical HUS) and diarrhea negative (D−, or atypical HUS) forms. The diagnosis of HUS is made with anemia (often <8 g/dL) with schistocytes and helmet cells on peripheral smear, thrombocytopenia (<140,000/mm^3), and AKI ranging from proteinuria, hematuria, elevated blood urea nitrogen (BUN), and creatinine levels to oliguria and failure requiring dialysis.

Escherichia coli 0157:H7

STEC HUS is mostly a disease of children under 5 years. Shed in the feces of cattle, sheep, and other ungulates, outbreaks of STEC are linked to ground beef, exposure to animals, and contaminated water.

After an incubation period of 3-4 days, an enterocolitis develops with nausea, fever, crampy abdominal pain, and diarrhea that becomes bloody in more than 70% of cases. HUS develops in 10%-15% of patients with STEC, usually 7-10 days after symptom onset.

Management

Children with bloody diarrhea require stool culture or PCR and Shiga toxin testing for STEC. Once diagnosed, treatment is largely supportive as there is no antidote against the toxin. Risk factors for poor prognosis include leukocyte count >25 000 cells/mL, hemoconcentration (likely reflecting dehydration), and duration of dialysis. Controversy exists regarding the use of antibiotics in suspected STEC infection. Most studies found no difference or showed potential for harm with antibiotics for D+ HUS outcomes. Current recommendations are to avoid the use of antibiotics in *E. coli* O157:H7 infections. Pediatric patients with bloody diarrhea should not be treated empirically but rather should be based on culture results.

Antimotility agents should not be used as they have shown to increase complications. Early, judicious IV fluids have been shown to reduce renal and other complications, though physicians should monitor for fluid overload if renal failure worsens. The American Academy of Pediatrics recommends immediate treatment with short-acting antihypertensive medications if there is severe hypertension (BP increase of 30 mm Hg or more above the 95th percentile).

Red blood cell transfusions should be considered at hemoglobin levels <7 g/dL or hematocrit <18%. Platelet transfusions should be avoided except for patients with significant bleeding. Dialysis is common, especially with symptomatic uremia, severe fluid overload, azotemia with BUN > 80 mg/dL, or significant electrolyte abnormalities.

Other Causes and Caveats

The second most common infectious cause of HUS is associated with *S. pneumoniae* infection. These patients, usually 1-2 years of age, typically present either as a severe pneumonia often complicated with an empyema, effusion, or meningitis. Compared to D+ HUS, they often have more severe initial disease with longer duration of oliguria and thrombocytopenia with increased transfusion and dialysis requirements. Treatment includes vancomycin and a broad-spectrum cephalosporin, because of disease severity and prevalence of resistant pneumococcus. Plasma exchange should be considered early although current evidence consists of only case reports. Additionally, the complement inhibitor eculizumab, a recombinant monoclonal antibody, is being used for familial and acquired forms of HUS. There are a few small reports of eculizumab being used for severe forms of STEC HUS with neurological manifestations, but current evidence does not support common use.

KEY POINTS

- Avoid antimotility agents and choose antibiotic treatment based on stool culture/PCR results.
- Treat patients with bloody diarrhea and early HUS with early IV volume expansion.
- Pay attention to blood pressure and initiate treatment for severe hypertension.
- Initiate broad antibiotic coverage when HUS is secondary to *S. pneumoniae*.
- Institute plasma exchange for atypical, nonpneumococcal HUS.

Suggested Readings

Ardissino G, Tel F, Possenti I, et al. Early volume expansion and outcomes of hemolytic uremic syndrome. *Pediatrics*. 2016;137(1):e20152153.

Fadi F, Zuber J, et al. Haemolytic uraemic syndrome. *Lancet*. 2017;390(10095):681-696.

Flynn JT, Kaelber DC, Baker-Smith CM, et al. Clinical practice guideline for screening and management of high blood pressure in children and adolescents. *Pediatrics*. 2017;140(3):e20171904.

Grisaru S. Management of hemolytic uremic syndrome in children. *Int J Nephrol Renovasc Dis*. 2014;7:231-239.

Sjal M, Leonard RK. *Escherichia coli* infections. *Pediatr Rev*. 2015;36:167.

100

Twist of Fate: Do Not Ignore Bilious Emesis in a Baby

Carrie M. Myers, MD and Ashley M. Strobel, MD, FACEP, FAAP

It is important to remember that malrotation is the anatomic condition, and midgut volvulus is the acute complication of that condition. When malrotation occurs *in utero*, the duodenojejunal flexure does not form properly. The cecum often lies in the right upper quadrant secured to the abdominal wall via fibrous bands of tissue ("Ladd bands"). Rather than a thick and wide mesenteric root, the intestines are secured by a narrow base. The narrow base predisposes to two potential complications: the bowel is more likely to wrap around on itself (midgut volvulus) and the duodenum is at risk of obstruction by overlying Ladd bands. Midgut volvulus occurs when the bowel twists upon itself at the superior mesenteric artery (SMA) and/or vein. This results in duodenal and mesenteric vessel obstruction leading to ischemia and bowel necrosis if not reversed within 6 hours. Therefore, early recognition is everything.

The emergency department (ED) differential of emesis in infants is broad, ranging from benign overfeeding to life-threatening surgical abdominal catastrophes. Identifying historical red flags can differentiate between the serious and the benign and prevent a delayed diagnosis. Ask open-ended questions about the emesis. Have parents describe the character and color. Ask whether the baby is still hungry after emesis, whether emesis occurs right after feeds, and how much is being fed and in what interval. Typical feeds for neonates are 2-3 oz every 2-3 hours or 20-30 minutes by breast every 2-3 hours. Any infant with bilious emesis has malrotation with volvulus until proven otherwise. However, prior to complete obstruction or during intermittent spontaneous reduction of volvulus, the emesis may be yellow. Smartphone photos from parents may be helpful. Reviewing the infant's growth chart to ensure appropriate weight gain (20-30 g/day) is vital, as growth failure can indicate serious pathology such as malrotation.

About 80% of malrotation cases present within the first month of life and 90% are diagnosed within the first year. Over 50% of intestinal malrotations with midgut volvulus within the first month of life exhibit bilious, dark green vomiting. These patients may also display classic symptoms of bowel obstruction including abdominal distention (though rare), peritonitis, and hematochezia. Hematochezia is an ominous sign that bowel ischemia and/or necrosis is already occurring. Older children may have more vague symptoms such as diarrhea and malabsorption.

Once midgut volvulus is suspected, imaging studies should be obtained emergently. Abdominal radiographs may show the classic "double-bubble" sign of duodenal obstruction, though up to 20% can be normal. The gold standard for diagnosis of malrotation is an upper gastrointestinal (UGI) series, with a sensitivity of close to 96%. Radiologist availability to perform an UGI varies depending on each medical center's resources. Contrast for an UGI may be administered orally or via nasogastric tube. Findings in an UGI series may include a duodeno-jejunal junction flexure that does not lie to the left of midline at L2 left-sided spinous pedicle and/or at the level of the duodenal bulb. A "bird-beak" appearance, or "cork-screw" sign, is often seen on the lateral. Ultrasound has a sensitivity of 80%-90% in the hands of an experienced sonographer. Reversal of the SMA and superior mesenteric vein (SMV) are called the "whirlpool sign," in which the twisted bowel takes on a swirling appearance. Computed tomography is very sensitive, but other modalities provide adequate sensitivity with less radiation exposure.

Initial ED management includes intravenous fluid resuscitation, electrolyte repletion, and gastric decompression with an age-appropriate sized nasogastric tube. Prompt consultation or transfer to a pediatric surgeon is imperative for a concerning presentation. This is a condition that must be dealt with promptly and surgically.

KEY POINTS

- Bilious emesis is never normal and should be worked up as a surgical emergency until proven otherwise.
- Feeding history and growth chart evaluation for proper weight gain can give clues to underlying malrotation.
- The diagnostic test with greatest sensitivity for diagnosis of malrotation is an upper GI series, so avoid false reassurance with a normal plain abdominal x-ray.

Suggested Readings

Applegate KE, Anderson JM, Klatte EU. Intestinal malrotation in children: a problem-solving approach to the upper gastrointestinal series. *Radiographics.* 2006;26:1485-1500.

Langer JC. Intestinal Rotation Abnormalities and Midgut Volvulus. *Surg Clinics of N Am.* 2017;97:147-159.

Tullie LGC, Stanton MP. Bilious vomiting in the newborn. *Surg (United Kingdom).* 2016;34(12):603-608. doi:10.1016/j.mpsur.2016.10.003.

Walters MM, Robertson RL. Chapter 4 Gastrointestinal imaging. *Pediatric Radiology.* Philadelphia, PA: *The Requisites.* 4th ed. Elsevier; 2017:100-101.

Let Your Light Shine!: Do Not Confuse a Hydrocele for a Hernia

Kevin Landefeld, MD and Matthew Carlisle

A concerned parent brings their infant into the emergency department (ED) for evaluation of swelling of the right groin extending into the right scrotum. The child is well appearing and playful but does have a mass of the right inguinal region and scrotal swelling. Does this child need an urgent surgery or can they follow up with their pediatrician during the next wellness check?

Two of the more common causes of inguinal masses and scrotal swelling are inguinal hernia and hydrocele. Other considerations should include lymphadenopathy, lipoma, and undescended testes (all typically causing inguinal swelling), or varicocele, testicular torsion, malignancy, spermatocele, and epididymal cyst (all typically causing testicular/epididymal swelling or mass). An inguinal hernia is a protrusion of abdominal contents into the inguinal canal as a result of a patent processus vaginalis. Hernia contents often include bowel and can contain ovaries in females. Inguinal hernias occur in 1%-4% of newborns but are more frequent in the premature. Risk factors also include male sex (6:1 male to female ratio), family history, connective tissue diseases, genitourinary abnormalities, and any process that increases abdominal pressure. In comparison, a hydrocele is a fluid-filled connection along the descent of the testicles into the scrotum. A communicating hydrocele is a narrow patent processus vaginalis that allows the passage of fluid only. A hydrocele of the spermatic cord is an irregular closure of the processus vaginalis distally then proximally leading to a fluid collection. It is located in the inguinal canal, is nonmobile, and can easily be mistaken as an inguinal hernia.

History and physical are important elements in differentiating an inguinal mass in a child. Parents may report intermittent groin swelling or swelling that may only be present with processes increasing abdominal pressure such as standing, crying, straining, or coughing. An intermittent or fluctuating swelling indicates a continuity with the peritoneal cavity seen in inguinal hernias and communicating hydroceles. It is important to ensure the child is not having increased fussiness, decreased appetite, or vomiting as it may indicate an obstruction associated with incarcerated hernia. On physical examination, first look for asymmetry of the child's groin or genitalia. In male patients, it is important to palpate the testicle in the scrotum to rule out undescended testicles. Standing the child up or observing while crying or coughing may make the swelling more apparent. A communicating hydrocele in the scrotum will transilluminate with a light held behind it, while an inguinal hernia into the scrotum generally will not. However, a neonate may be an exception as the neonatal bowels may transilluminate as well. An inguinal hernia should be reducible with gentle pressure, while a hydrocele of the spermatic cord is a fixed and nonmobile mass. If after physical examination and history, it is unclear whether it is an inguinal hernia or a hydrocele, an ultrasound (US) can help to differentiate. On US, an inguinal hernia containing bowel gas shows as hyperechoic transverse lines with shadowing behind it. Additionally, bowel may be identified by its peristalsis motion. A simple hydrocele will be a nonmobile hypoechoic collection.

It is important to differentiate inguinal hernias from hydrocele because of the differences in morbidity and treatment approaches. A communicating hydrocele or hydrocele of the spermatic cord managed conservatively with observation until at least 1 year of age as it may spontaneously absorb. In contrast, an inguinal hernia needs urgent surgical repair due to the high rate of incarceration, especially in the first year of life. It is recommended that surgical repair be performed within 2 weeks from diagnosis of an asymptomatic inguinal hernia, as one study shows a 7% incarceration rate. For incarcerated inguinal or even difficult to manually reduce hernias, the patient may need to be admitted for surgical repair in 24 to 48 hours.

KEY POINTS

- Groin swelling might not be evident unless the patient is standing, crying, or coughing.
- Prematurity and male sex are significant risk factors for inguinal hernia in a child.
- Inguinal hernia in an infant requires urgent surgical repair due to high incidence of incarceration.
- A hydrocele of the spermatic cord is located within the inguinal canal, is nonmobile, and is usually observed till 1 year of age for spontaneous resolution.

Suggested Readings

Basta AM, Courtier J, Phelps A, et al. Scrotal swelling in the neonate. *J Ultrasound Med*. 2015;34:495–505.
Kapur P, Caty MG, Glick PL. Pediatric hernias and hydroceles. *Pediatr Clin North Am*. 1998;45(4):773–789.
Palmer LS. Hernias and hydroceles. *Pediatr Rev*. 2013;34:457.
Tintinalli JE, Stapczynski JS, Ma OJ, eds. *Tintinalli's Emergency Medicine*. 8th ed. New York, NY: McGraw Hill; 2016.

Time Is Stoma: G-Tube Dislodgement Is a Time-Sensitive Emergency

Ashley M. Strobel, MD, FACEP, FAAP

Kids are encouraged to be kids, whether or not they have chronic medical problems. More children are living and playing with gastrostomy (G) or gastrojejunostomy (GJ) tubes. Tube dislodgement is common and can be managed effectively in the emergency department (ED). Once an enteral tube falls out, replacement is a time-sensitive emergency and the child should be roomed immediately for two reasons.

Table 102.1 ■ Steps for "Dilating Up" a Stoma After Difficulty Replacing a Dislodged GT

- Get your GT with same diameter FR and length
- Use a bladder straight catheter (8, 10, 12, 14 FR) 2-3 sizes below the original GT size
- Lube the catheter and insert gently into the stoma
- Fill balloon with water
- Wait 5-10 minutes while rotating the catheter in the stoma
- Remove water from the balloon and remove the urinary catheter (consider placing a guide wire and using seldinger technique)
- Increase the FR of the urinary catheter and repeat steps 1-4 until the catheter is the same size diameter (FR) as the original GT FR or 2FR bigger
- Place the correct size GT and confirm placement.

First, the G-tube may be the child's only access to vital nutrients and medications. Complex care children require special, often unpalatable, formulas and medications. The special formulas may prevent catabolism with accumulation of toxic metabolites, or prevent periods of hypoglycemia. Some children can take solids or liquids by mouth and supplement with the enteral tube. However, each child's stage in feeding tolerance and diet progression varies, so it is important to ask parents to gauge risk for imminent hypoglycemia or accumulation of toxic metabolites. Some children are on continuous feeds while others are on bolus feeds, and knowing the feeding schedule is important to their ED care. Consider frequent point-of-care glucose evaluations and communicate this plan with nursing and family. An IV may be required to maintain euglycemia and prevent catabolism during periods without feeds.

Second, enteral tubes form a gastrocutaneous fistula as the stoma matures after surgical or endoscopic placement. The tract matures within 6-8 weeks of tube placement. Tube replacement within 4 hours of dislodgement is imperative before stoma stenosis occurs, which may incur additional surgery for replacement. While awaiting the new G-tube, a Foley or bladder catheter should be placed into the stoma to maintain patency. Nutrients, medications, and fluids can be delivered through this catheter if needed. Maintaining the tract should never be delayed for transfer, specialty consultation, or equipment gathering. Delay in stoma catheterization most commonly occurs in three common scenarios and should be avoided: if the tube is immature and surgical consultation is required per institutional protocol, if the child has a GJ tube requiring replacement by specialty consultation. However, delay should not occur due to an ED not stocking the child's tube, as a bladder catheter can temporize and prevent stoma closure.

Prior to bedside replacement, three features of the device must be known: the type of enteral tube (adjustable length or low profile, nonballoon or with balloon device, etc.), tube diameter, and tube length.

Confirmation of placement can be done one of three ways: aspiration of gastric contents, injection saline and aspiration of gastric contents mixed in that volume of saline, or instillation of 20-30 mL water-soluble contrast followed by abdominal x-ray 1-2 minutes later to confirm contrast is in the gastrointestinal tract rather than the peritoneum. While replacement confirmation should be documented, radiographic confirmation rarely reveals inadequate tube placement. To avoid length of stay increases, limit radiographic confirmation to: immature track replacement, evidence of replacement difficulty or stoma stenosis.

KEY POINTS

- Maintaining the tract and preventing hypoglycemia or accumulation of toxic metabolites should not be delayed for transfer, specialty consultation, or equipment gathering
- A simple urinary catheter in the stoma can allow critical feeding access and maintain stoma patency
- Assessment for and prevention of hypoglycemia is imperative
- All emergency physicians and triage nurses at any emergency department must recognize GT dislodgement as a time-sensitive emergency, and be prepared to assist the family

Suggested Readings

Bhambani S, et al. Replacement of dislodged gastrostomy tubes after stoma dilation in the pediatric emergency department. *West J Emerg Med.* 2017;18:770-774.

http://pemcincinnati.com/blog/g-tube/

http://www.nationwidechildrens.org/feeding-tube-changing

Juern J, Verhaalen A. Videos in clinical medicine. Gastrostomy-tube exchange. *N Engl J Med.* 2014;370:e28.

"Not Aggressively Treating Patients With Nephrotic Syndrome Presenting With Fever"

Rebecca C. Bowers, MD, FACEP and Vinayak Gupta, MD

The first recorded description of nephrotic syndrome (NS) dates back to the 15th century. We are thankful—and assume that everyone else is too—that the diagnostic methodology of nephropathology no longer involves taste, making the diagnosis of NS a bit more palatable today. NS is important for emergency clinicians to understand as there are many complications including thromboembolism, abnormal lipid metabolism, anemia, hyperparathyroidism, and infection.

In its simplest form, NS occurs when diseased kidneys allow the spillage of proteins from the blood into the urine. There are numerous underlying causes including infection, glomerular disease, toxins, idiopathic, vasculitides, and malignancy. Diagnostic criteria include urine protein/Cr ratio >2 (think 3+ protein on urine dipstick), hypoalbuminemia <2.5 g/dL, clinical edema, and hyperlipidemia with cholesterol >200 mg/dL. Edema can be in dependent areas or widespread throughout the body and is due to changes in oncotic pressure from hypoalbuminemia. Interestingly, in children, the edema commonly manifests as periorbital edema. Realistically, in the ED, you will likely develop the diagnosis by your history, noting edema on examination and finding hypoalbuminemia and proteinuria on laboratory studies. So congratulations! ... you have diagnosed nephrotic syndrome! Before patting yourself on the back, though, make sure to thoroughly evaluate for serious infection, especially in the setting of fever. The risk of infectious complications is very high in children with NS, with a recent study revealing 76% of patients developing infection.

Children with NS are predisposed to infection due to changes in cellular and humoral immunity. Common infections include upper respiratory tract infection, UTI, pneumonia, cellulitis, and spontaneous bacterial peritonitis (SBP). These infections can be hard to discern, as some patients may not be symptomatic. Specifically, with UTIs, one study notes 28% of patients with culture-positive UTI were not symptomatic. Furthermore, while *Escherichia coli* is the most common cause of UTI, non-*E. coli* species account for up to 40% of culture species, so it is important to choose appropriate antibiotic coverage as your hospital antibiogram dictates.

A rare, but important illness to consider in patients found to have NS is SBP. If a child with NS presents with fever and abdominal pain, be sure to consider this as part of your differential. Some patients may not have enough ascites to rapidly obtain a sample for definitive diagnosis in the emergency setting. It is important to treat empirically for SBP in the setting of fever and abdominal pain in NS if you cannot readily obtain fluid for testing. You should consider other intra-abdominal diseases such as appendicitis and intussusception, but do not forget about SBP. One study suggests that a low serum albumin of <1.5 g/dL on initial presentation of NS is associated with increased risk of peritonitis throughout the course of the illness.

Infections may happen at any time throughout the course of illness. Not all infections will present at the time of diagnosis. Since most causes of NS in children are autoimmune related, the treatment typically involves immunosuppressant therapy and initiating therapy to a child with a new diagnosis should involve a nephrologist. As might be expected, though, children on immunosuppressant therapy are at a higher risk of secondary infections.

We understand a wee bit more about NS today compared to the 15th century. While diagnosing and treating NS in conjunction with a nephrologist is important, it is also very important to assess and evaluate cases for possible occult bacterial infections as part of their presentations. Do not disregard symptoms or signs that suggest associated complications.

KEY POINTS

- Infection is an often overlooked cause of morbidity in children with NS and should be aggressively evaluated, often treated empirically, and not underestimated.
- Children with NS have an even higher risk of infection if they are taking steroids or other immunosuppressant medications.
- Children with NS are more susceptible to SBP and other serious bacterial infections so vigilance is required as they may initially appear well.

Suggested Readings

Alfakeekh K, Azar M, et al. Immunosuppressive burden and risk factors of infection in primary childhood nephrotic syndrome. *J Infect Public Health.* 2019;12(1):90-94.

Hingorani SR, Weiss NS, Watkins SL. Predictors of peritonitis in children with nephrotic syndrome. *Pediatr Nephrol.* 2002;17(8):678-682.

Wei CC, Yu IW, et al. Occurrence of infection among children with nephrotic syndrome during hospitalizations. *Nephrology.* 2012;17(8):681-688.

104

Renal: Nephritis: "Not Having a Strategy to Evaluate Hematuria in a Child"

Landon A. Jones, MD

Mom ... Why does my pee look like that?! While hematuria is a panic-inducing experience for parents, it only takes 1 mL of blood to discolor 1 L of urine. In general, hematuria is defined in three ways: normal (<5 red blood cells per high-power field [RBCs/HPF]), microscopic (>5 RBCs/HPF), or macroscopic (visible by the naked eye).

After reassuring the family that the child is not likely exsanguinating from the hematuria, it is time to assess whether this is truly hematuria. There are a number of mimics of hematuria such as myoglobinuria (eg, rhabdomyolysis, extreme exercise, myopathies), hemoglobinuria (eg, hemolysis), drugs, toxins, uric acid crystals, and foods. While the urine dipstick may return positive for blood, a urine microscopy is needed to truly see if it is hematuria (ie, the presence of whole red blood cells). Urine microscopy may also reveal urine sediment such as casts. If urine dipstick is positive for blood but microscopy is negative for RBCs, urine discoloration is secondary to either myoglobinuria or hemoglobinuria. If the urine dipstick is negative for blood, other causes of urine discoloration may need to be explored.

Now it is time to explore whether this is glomerular vs nonglomerular. Nonglomerular causes can include urinary tract infections, urolithiasis, hypercalciuria, urethritis, trauma, aortic fistulas, bladder masses, cancers, etc. The workup is usually dependent on the child's symptoms and signs. A glomerular cause is called a glomerulonephritis (GN). There are other glomerular diseases that less commonly result in hematuria; these are nephrotic syndromes and thrombotic microangiopathies (eg, hemolytic uremic syndrome) and will not be discussed here.

GN is defined as a triad of hematuria, hypertension, and acute kidney injury (AKI). There are few congenital causes of GN; most are acquired and immunologically mediated. Also, most causes of GN are postinfectious and—lucky for us—usually spontaneously resolve. Do not ignore hematuria, though. At a minimum, our job is to emphasize/arrange timely follow up in well-appearing children. While there are numerous causes of nephritis in children, the three most common causes of nephritis are postinfectious GN (PIGN), IgA nephropathy, and vasculitis. It may sound simple, but the MOST important factors in developing a diagnosis are a thorough history and physical examination. It takes an additional 15-30 seconds to ask about recent infections, associated symptoms, previous episodes of hematuria, family history, etc.

The most common cause of nephritis is postinfectious (PIGN). Think poststreptococcal GN, but realize that strep pharyngitis is not the only culprit—both upper respiratory infections (about 1-2 weeks prior) and skin infections (3-5 weeks prior) can cause this too. Further evaluation with a CBC, CMP, antistreptolysin O (ASO) titer, complement C3 and C4 levels, and anti-DNase B and others may be needed after a consultation with nephrology.

Another common cause of nephritis is IgA nephropathy, which often presents as recurrent gross hematuria in the setting of infection. Like PIGN, it is immune-mediated. Unlike PIGN, though, the nephritis of IgA nephropathy develops much sooner (1-2 days) after the onset of infection. Labs would be similar to PIGN above.

IgA vasculitis (aka Henoch-Schonlein Purpura) is another common cause. It is a small vessel vasculitis and symptoms depend on the location of the vasculitis: joints (arthralgias), skin (pathognomonic rash), GI (abdominal pain), and renal (nephritis)—so a thorough physical examination is very important. If there is hematuria, labs should assess for AKI and—since it is a vasculitis causing the pathognomonic rash—thrombocytopenia should not be present.

The biggest pitfalls in the setting of pediatric nephritis are: (1) ignoring/overlooking the hematuria, (2) failing to emphasize/arrange timely follow up and, (3) failing to recognize associated hypertension and AKI. A systolic blood pressure (SBP) of 140 mm Hg in an adult can be easily glazed over. In a child, though, an SBP of 140 may be severe hypertension that needs to be acutely addressed. Unless age specific BPs are referenced, this might be easily overlooked.

KEY POINTS

- While most causes of GN are postinfectious and spontaneously resolve, we still need to have a strategy to evaluate hematuria in a child.
- Do not overlook the associated signs of GN of hypertension and AKI.
- At a minimum, arrange or emphasize need for timely followup for hematuria.

Suggested Readings

Brown DD, Reidy KJ. Approach to the child with hematuria. *Pediatr Clin N Am*. 2019;66(1):15-30.
Viteri B, Reid-Adam J. Hematuria and proteinuria in children. *Pediatr Rev*. 2018;39(12):573-587.
Wenderfer SE, Gaut JP. Glomerular diseases in children. *Adv Chronic Kidney Dis*. 2017;24(6):364-371.

Overlooking Spontaneous Bacterial Peritonitis in Patients With Nephrotic Syndrome

Jeremiah Smith, MD, FAAP

In the pediatric emergency department, our job is to not only find the needle in the proverbial haystack but also not miss the rock in the middle of the road. Spontaneous bacterial peritonitis (SBP) is not common with appropriate therapies; however, it is still a known complication of nephrotic syndrome that carries a high mortality if missed.

Nephrotic Syndrome

Nephrotic syndrome is characterized by massive loss of protein in the urine due to a defect in the glomerular filtration barrier not caused by a single diagnostic entity. The four classic features of nephrotic syndrome are proteinuria, hypoalbuminemia, edema, and hyperlipidemia. The evaluation of nephrotic syndrome begins as always with a thorough history and physical examination. A typical evaluation will include CBC, chemistries with albumin and LFTs, creatinine, complement levels, and a chest x-ray. In select patients, you may obtain ANA (antinuclear antibody), viral testing (HIV, HBV, HBC), kidney biopsy, and specific histologic testing. Treatment is specific to the underlying cause and made with expert consultation.

Spontaneous Bacterial Peritonitis

Infection can be common in children with nephrotic syndrome for multiple reasons. SBP has an incidence as high as 15% for a number of reasons. Urinary loss of immunoglobulin and complement, impaired lymphocytic function, use of immunosuppressive agents, and ascites provide a natural culture media for bacterial growth, contributing to this increased rate of infection. Additionally, the loss of opsonizing factors likely increases susceptibility to encapsulated organisms such as *Streptococcus pneumonia*.

The typical presentation includes fever, rapid onset of abdominal pain, and abdominal tenderness in a child with known nephrotic syndrome. Abdominal pain and tenderness has been found in 70%-92% and 88% of all children with SBP, respectively. The abdomen may be taut, and gentle percussion can cause severe abdominal pain. Children will often find a position of maximum comfort with hips and knees flexed.

Laboratory/diagnostic testing along with imaging is used to help with the initial diagnosis. A CBC will oftentimes show an elevated WBC and neutrophil count. Inflammatory markers such as CRP and ESR may be elevated, and electrolyte abnormalities may be present. An elevated lactate may be present as well. Abdominal x-rays are used to evaluate for signs of free intraperitoneal air, air fluid levels, or ascites. Additional imaging such as ultrasound may be indicated as well.

Diagnosis is typically confirmed with paracentesis and evaluation of the ascitic fluid (AF). The AF may appear turbid or cloudy. Laboratory criteria for SBP include the following: WBC should be >500 cells/mm^3, ANC > 250 cells/mm^3, protein count >3 g/dL or >0.5 ratio of fluid to plasma protein, fluid to plasma LDH > 0.6, acidic pH < 7.31, elevated lactate, or a positive culture. There are cases of false-negative results related to lysis of neutrophils and delayed culture results leading to a potential increased mortality rate. Bedside use of leukocyte esterase reagent strips has been shown as a possible rapid and inexpensive method to diagnose SBP.

Once the diagnosis of SBP is considered, prompt diagnostic evaluation and emergent stabilization should be initiated including airway assessment and stabilization, rapid infusion of crystalloid up to 60 mL/kg for hypoperfusion, correction of electrolyte abnormalities, and dextrose as needed. Broad spectrum antibiotics should be used. It is important to note that opioid analgesia will not mask peritonitis and adequate analgesia is indicated.

KEY POINTS

- Nephrotic syndrome consists of proteinuria, hypoalbuminemia, edema, and hyperlipidemia.
- Always consider spontaneous bacterial peritonitis in any child with nephrotic syndrome and abdominal pain.
- Paracentesis and AF evaluation is used to diagnose SBP.
- Emergent stabilization and fluid resuscitation with broad spectrum antibiotics are indicated in children with suspected SBP.

Suggested Readings

Abd El-Hakim Allam A, Eltaras S, Hussin MH, et al. Diagnosis of spontaneous bacterial peritonitis in children using leukocyte esterase reagent strips and granulocyte elastase immunoassay. *Clin Exp Hepatol*. 2018;4:247-252.

Hoffman RJ, Wang VJ, Scarfone RJ. *Fleisher and Ludwig's 5-Minute Pediatric Emergency Medicine Consult*. 1st ed. Philadelphia, PA: LWW; 2012.

Niaudet P. Complications of nephrotic syndrome in children. In: Post T, ed. *UpToDate*. Waltham, MA: *UpToDate*; 2016. www.uptodate.com.

Wang C, Greenbaum LA. Nephrotic syndrome. *Pediatr Clin N Am*. 2019;66:73-85.

106

"Urine" Trouble Now—Evidence to Approach Pediatric UTI

James (Jim) Homme, MD, FACEP

Urinary tract infections (UTIs) are second only to general viral illnesses diagnosed in children presenting to the emergency department (ED) and are the leading cause of serious bacterial illness in infants. Left untreated UTIs can progress to urosepsis and potentially cause renal scarring. While early diagnosis and initiation of treatment improves outcomes, it can be challenging, especially in the preverbal child. Lack of defining signs and symptoms, challenges in obtaining urine samples, varying sensitivities and specificities of screening tests, and the delayed nature of the gold standard culture often result in an uncertain diagnosis at time of ED discharge.

UTIs are often classified as lower tract (cystitis) or upper tract (pyelonephritis). Rates of UTIs vary with age and underlying risk factors. Infants < 3 months of age are at highest risk. Other higher risk populations are any female < 12 months of age and Caucasian females < 2 years of age, uncircumcised males, any history of a UTI or known underlying urogenital abnormalities, and patients with chronic indwelling catheters. The most common pathogen detected in UTIs is *Escherichia coli* with a prevalence of >90% in healthy outpatients. Any empiric antibiotic treatment therefore should be directed at this organism. Other less common causes are *Enterococcus*, *Staphylococcus saprophyticus*, *Klebsiella*, *Enterobacter*, *Proteus mirabilis*, *Pseudomonas aeruginosa*, and *Citrobacter*.

In nonverbal infants, fever without an obvious source is the primary presentation for UTI. Some infants may have associated vomiting, irritability, or suprapubic tenderness. Fevers ≥39°C for ≥2 days with no other signs of infection also increase risk for UTI. Urine odor has not been correlated with disease. Older children will report dysuria and exhibit signs of pain with urination or hesitancy to void. Caregivers note increased frequency and urgency as well as secondary incontinence. Abdominal pain has also been associated with UTIs. Fever, vomiting complaints of back pain, or costovertebral angle tenderness on physical examination increase risk for pyelonephritis. An online calculator has been developed to aid clinicians in determining risk for UTI in children 3-23 months of age (https://uticalc.pitt.edu/).

Unlike in healthy adults where treatment may be initiated based on signs and symptoms alone, pediatric patients with symptoms concerning for UTI will only have a confirmed diagnosis ~8% of the time. Therefore, urine testing is critical. Testing approaches vary based on age and risk factors. In any high-risk patient, obtaining a sterile urine sample via catheterization or suprapubic aspiration is recommended. Clean catch midstream urine samples are also acceptable when they can be reliably produced and collected. Controversy regarding the use of samples obtained through the use of urinary bags exists. It has been shown to be a reasonable option for lower risk patients, whereby if the bag urine produces any positive finding on initial testing, it is followed by a catheterized specimen for confirmatory culture.

Screening testing for UTIs typically can be done with a urine dipstick, focusing on the leukocyte esterase and nitrite components of the test. Leukocyte esterase, produced by neutrophils detected in the urine, is highly sensitive for a UTI (~95%) but not specific. Nitrites, produced through bacterial conversion of dietary nitrates, are not sensitive but highly specific for UTI. Gram stains and urinalysis with microscopy are other more time-consuming alternative screening tests. It is generally recommended that all clean/sterile urine samples, regardless of screening results, be sent a confirmatory culture. Up to 10% of pediatric tested for UTI without pyuria will have a positive culture. Empiric antibiotic treatment based on local sensitivities should be started with any positive dipstick. The most commonly utilized antibiotics are oral first- or third-generation cephalosporins. Parenteral antibiotics are utilized in neonates and patients unable to tolerate oral therapy. Treatment in infants is always directed at more severe disease as it is impossible to differentiate between cystitis and pyelonephritis based on screening evaluation alone. Duration of treatment in older children suspected of uncompli-cated cystitis decreases with increasing age.

KEY POINTS

- *Escherichia coli* causes >90% of all urinary tract infections in childhood. Empiric antibiotic therapy should be directed at this organism.
- Up to 10% of pediatric tested for UTI without pyuria will have a positive culture.
- Urine testing with confirmatory culture is mandatory for all pediatric patients suspected of a UTI.

Suggested Readings

Shaikh N, et al. Does this child have a urinary tract infection? *JAMA*. 2007;298(24):2895-2904.
Subcommittee on Urinary Tract Infection, Steering Committee on Quality Improvement and Management. Urinary tract infection: clinical practice guideline for the diagnosis and management of the initial UTI in febrile infants and children 2 to 24 months. *Pediatrics*. 2011;128:595-610.

Funny Dermatologic Findings

Kathryn Kean, MD

The skin, the largest organ, functions as a barrier, protector, regulator of temperature and fluids, and immune system participant. Important clinical clues to systemic disease can be found on the skin exam, therefore, it is critical to recognize and differentiate the basic from not so basic skin diseases.

Diaper Dermatitis

Diaper or contact dermatitis is an inflammatory reaction of the skin triggered by direct contact with warm, wet, soiled material, or even chemicals (blue dyes in a diaper or moist wipes) for prolonged peri-ods. Harsh soaps, detergents, and severe diarrhea also predispose to this condition. The diaper rash is usually acute, well-demarcated erythema, sparing the skin folds and found on convex surfaces of the perineum, lower abdomen, buttocks, and proximal thighs. Treatment involves identifying and avoiding the offending agent, gentle cleansing, as well as topical treatments for localized patches such as thick applications of lubricants and zinc oxide barrier creams.

Seborrheic Dermatitis

Seborrhea is characterized by a confluent salmon-colored plaque with greasy yellow scale. It is usually nonpruritic and very prominent in warm, moist, intertriginous areas (ie, neck or perineum). Coinfec-tion with *Candida* or *Pityrosporum* can occur; however, there are no "satellite" lesions typically seen with these organisms. The rash becomes a dry, scaly dermatitis on the face, scalp (cradle cap), and post-auricular areas. Treatment involves antifungal washes and low potency topical steroids.

Atopic Dermatitis

Atopic dermatitis is a dry, pruritic, inflamed recurrent rash, often symmetrical in distribution, pri-marily found on both the flexural and extensor surfaces and sparing the moist regions of the body.

Associated atopic diseases such as asthma, allergic rhinitis, or other allergies are common. Food allergy is found in up to a 30% of young patients with eczema. Mainstays of treatment are skin hygiene, hydration, and topical emollients and steroids. Treatment for any signs of superinfection should be directed toward *Staphylococcus aureus*, unless the lesions resemble eczema herpeticum (punched out, crusted), then antiviral therapy is warranted. Persistent dermatitis unresponsive to conservative management should raise concern of other etiologies including fungal, psoriatic, bacterial, or lichen dermatitis.

Fungal Dermatitis

Candidal infections typically present as a sharply demarcated erythematous rash bordered with pin-point satellite papules and pustules. *Candida albicans* infection should be suspected whenever skin folds (intertriginous areas) are involved or when dermatitis does not respond to conservative treatment. Potassium hydroxide (KOH) prep examination shows budding yeast or pseudohyphae. Treatment is topical antifungals.

Dermatophyte (tinea or "ringworm") infections in the perineum are usually the result of autoinoculation from a primary patch at another location. The rashes are characterized by scaly, erythema with a raised or elevated "active" border, with central clearing. KOH preparation shows the typical hyphae and yeast ("spaghetti and meatballs"). Treatment includes topical antifungals alone, as topical steroids will worsen the dermatitis.

Bacterial Infections

Staphylococcal infections frequently complicate contact dermatitis. Lesions are characterized by erythematous-based, thin-walled pustules that often rupture and dry leaving a scaly base. Cultures can be done to confirm diagnosis but are typically unnecessary. Treatment requires (early) diagnosis and oral/topical antibiotics.

Staphylococcal scalded skin syndrome (SSSS) is typically associated with diffuse cutaneous painful blistering erythroderma sparing mucous membranes. Treatment includes admission for analgesia, IV fluids, and antistaph agents plus clindamycin.

Papulosquamous Disorders (Papules and Scales)

Psoriasis is a common disorder characterized by erythematous, well-demarcated plaques covered by a thick silvery scale typically involving the extensor surfaces of extremities and scalp. Occasionally, particularly in infants, it may present as confluent diaper dermatitis. It should be suspected when a diaper rash persists for months despite therapy for other more common etiologies. Skin biopsy will confirm the diagnosis.

Lichen planus is an inflammatory dermatitis with flat-topped, pruritic polygonal violaceous papules and plaques with a fine lacy pattern (Wickham striae) on outer surfaces. Typically seen on dorsal surfaces of extremities but may also involve the oral and genital mucosa. Treatment includes topical steroids.

Rare Rashes

Persistent dermatitis, nonresponsive to conservative management can be a sign of life-threatening like Langerhans cell histiocytosis (LCH), cutaneous lymphoma, or genetic disorders such as acrodermatitis enteropathica (AE). LCH should be suspected when the skin papules are very crusted or are associated with petechiae and systemic symptoms. Primary zinc deficiency (AE) includes the inflammatory rash around the mouth and anus, persistent diarrhea, and hair loss.

Stevens-Johnson syndrome (SJS) and toxic epidermal necrolysis (TEN) represent spectrums the spectrums of rare, potentially life-threatening disorders distinguished by severe epidermal and mucosal membrane necrosis and full-thickness sloughing of skin. Percentage of body surface area involved determines the classification. Successful treatment depends on early recognition, multidisciplinary involvement, and aggressive supportive care.

KEY POINTS

- Examine the skin in pediatrics (all of it!), so you do not miss important clinical clues to systemic disease.
- Skin fold involvement (or lack thereof) helps in differentiating between many common rashes in the genitourinary region.
- Topical treatments are mainstays as long as you know what you are treating.
- Persistent or recalcitrant dermatitis despite empiric treatment warrant referral.

Suggested Readings

Kress DW. Pediatric dermatology emergencies. *Curr Opin Pediatr*. 2011;23(4):403-406.
Shin HT. Diagnosis and management of diaper dermatitis. *Pediatr Clin North Am*. 2014;61(2):367-382.

Vaginitis in the Prepubertal Girl—A Not So Challenging Discharge Diagnosis

Mahsa Akhavan, MD

When vaginitis gets diagnosed in an infant, toddler, or preteen, the presenting complaint is one of vaginal discharge, pain with urination or concerns of a urinary tract infection. Keeping this in mind, take the time and patience to relax the patient, in order to do an external genital exam in addition to urine testing.

Vaginitis is the most common gynecologic problem in prepubertal girls. The hypoestrogenic hormonal milieu in such patients increases the susceptibility of the vaginal mucosa to infection. The etiology is usually nonspecific (25%-75%) but may be due to known pathogens. Sexual abuse should also always be considered. Symptoms the patient or caretaker may describe are dysuria, discharge, pain, bleeding or spotting, itching, or erythema of the vulvar region. On evaluation of the genital area, the skin around the vagina will look erythematous and this may extend to the anus. Pooling of discharge and/or excoriations of the genital area are additional signs. Factors associated with vaginitis include poor hygiene, retained foreign material such as toilet paper, bubble baths, obesity, tightly fitted clothing, alkaline environment, low estrogen state leading to mucosal thinning, and the lack of labial development. Caregivers of patients with vaginitis should be advised to use cotton underwear and avoid tight pants, prolonged periods of time in wet bathing suits, and bubble baths. In addition, proper peroneal hygiene should be reviewed with the suggestion of use of wet wipes instead of toilet paper. Treatment includes sitz baths, which is essentially soaking in warm water a couple of times a day for 15 minutes. With these simple actions in place, symptom resolution should occur within 2-3 weeks, usually sooner. Persistent symptoms despite conservative treatment warrant further investigation for retained foreign body or specific infections.

Specific Infections

Candida is the most common fungal infection causing vaginitis. A variety of antifungal topical or oral treatment options exist. *Streptococcus pyogenes* is the most commonly cultured bacterial etiology and is treated with topical Mupirocin or an oral penicillin. Pinworms usually present with a primary complaint of nocturnal pruritus and are diagnosed by visualization of adult pinworms or application of adhesive tape to the perianal region followed by microscopic evaluation for eggs. Treatment consists of antihelminthic agents. Detection of any sexually transmitted infection may indicate abuse although Chlamydia has been rarely shown to be transmitted during a vaginal birth and last for years until treated.

Foreign Body

When dealing with history of chronic vaginal discharge, foul odor, or spotting of blood, foreign body should be considered. The most common foreign body is toilet paper, although paper clips and hair bands are other commonly described objects. After application of a topical anesthetic, warm fluid irrigation with saline or sterile water should successfully remove the object. Consider anxiolysis or even sedation if the patient is young, difficult to examine, or very uncomfortable with the examination and removal process. Inserted button batteries have been reported and linked to grey watery discharge. If suspected, immediate removal and a thorough examination of the extent of the burn under general anesthesia are warranted.

KEY POINTS

- Vaginitis is the most common gynecologic problem in prepubertal girls.
- What sounds like a UTI is not always a UTI, and so careful genitourinary examinations should be part of the evaluation.
- Isolating an organism associated with sexual transmission should result in evaluation for sexual abuse.
- Chronic vaginal discharge or foul odor should prompt an investigation for a foreign body.
- Antibiotics are rarely needed to treat vaginitis.

Suggested Readings

Hayes L, Creighton SM. Prepubertal vaginal discharge. *Obstetr Gynaecol.* 2007;9:159-163.
Joishy M, Ashtekar C, Jain A, Gonsalves R. Do we need to treat vulvovaginitis in prepubertal girls? *BMJ.* 2005;330(7484):186-188.
Stricker T, Navratil F, Sennhauser FH. Vulvovaginitis in prepubertal girls. *Arch Dis Child.* 2003;88:324-326.
Vandeven AM, Emans SJ. Vulvovaginitis in the child and adolescent. *Pediatr Rev.* 1993;14:141-147.

GU Torsion (Male and Female)

Quinn Cummings, MD

Testicular and ovarian torsion are highly time-sensitive surgical emergencies with similar presentations, diagnostic modalities, and management. Timely diagnosis and operative management maximizes the chance of salvage, and clinicians must rapidly make the diagnosis.

History

Although sudden testicular pain with nausea and vomiting are the classic symptoms of testicular torsion, isolated lower abdominal/flank pain may be the presenting complaint in up to 20% of patients. There can be underlying minor trauma, but it usually occurs at rest, with the left testicle being affected more commonly (by contrast, the right ovary is more commonly affected). Due to the sensitive nature of the affected area, patients may not complain of testicular pain or swelling, so a testicular examination should be done on any male patient who has a complaint of lower abdominal, flank, or scrotal pain.

Ovarian torsion classically presents with sudden pelvic pain, pelvic mass, and nausea/vomiting; fever may be present in a subset of patients. Symptoms may wax and wane, suggesting intermittent torsion and detorsion. Ovarian and testicular torsion present nonspecifically in infants (irritability, vomiting, abdominal distention), making diagnosis a challenge.

Physical Examination

The physical examination varies widely between patients. In ovarian torsion, there may be abdominal or pelvic tenderness, but this can be absent in up to one-third of patients. The affected hemiscrotum may appear swollen and discolored in testicular torsion, and the testicle may be tender, edematous, and elevated with a horizontal lie. The examination finding with the highest sensitivity is absence of the cremasteric reflex, but ~30% of males with normal testes have an absent cremaster reflex, and importantly, the presence of a cremaster reflex does not rule out testicular torsion.

Investigation

If there is a high suspicion for torsion, consultation with an urologist should occur prior to imaging. Depending on the individual ED workflow, sonographic is often performed simultaneously.

Although Doppler ultrasound is the test of choice, it is only moderately sensitive, with up to 25% of confirmed testicular torsion having normal Doppler flow. This may be related to spermatic cord thickness or the degree of torsion. The other major limitation of ultrasonography is operator dependence.

Because the ovaries are intra-abdominal organs, the differential diagnosis is often broadened in female patients, as diagnoses such as appendicitis and ectopic pregnancy must be considered. As the ovary receives a dual blood supply, a normal ultrasound does not rule out the diagnosis even in the presence of symptoms, and surgical consultation may still be indicated in a concerning history and clinical examination.

Urine should be sent to evaluate for epididymo–orchitis and infection, among other etiologies if the ultrasound is not diagnostic of torsion.

Management

There is a 90%-100% rate of testicular salvage within 6 hours, making this the ideal time window for scrotal exploration and operative management. Despite historic teaching, salvage rates in patients with testicular torsion for more than 24 hours may be upward of 20%. Regardless, best available evidence and expert opinion hold that torsion of the gonads is a true surgical emergency and a time-sensitive condition. For this reason, preoperative manual bedside testicular detorsion by an emergency physician can be considered, although this often results in only partial return of blood flow; operative scrotal exploration by a urologist is still indicated. Similarly, operative management is likewise indicated in female patients and should be considered in anyone with suggestive clinical history regardless of ultrasound results. Do not delay surgical consultation in a patient with potential torsion.

KEY POINTS

- Torsion is a clinical diagnosis. Keep a high degree of suspicion and consult a surgeon early to avoid gonadal loss.
- Testicular salvage has been noted in up to 20% of cases with >24 hours of symptoms.
- Abdominal/pelvic tenderness may be absent in one-third of patients with ovarian torsion.

Suggested Readings

Bronstein M, et al. Meta-analysis of B-mode ultrasound, Doppler ultrasound, and computed tomography to diagnose pediatric ovarian torsion. *Eur J Pediatr Surg.* 2015;25(1):82-86.

Davis JE, Silverman MA. Urologic procedures. In: Roberts JR, Custalow CB, Thomsen TW, eds. *Roberts and Hedges' Clinical Procedures in Emergency Medicine and Acute Care.* 7th ed. Philadelphia, PA: Elsevier; 2019:1141-1185.

Houry D, Abbott JT. Ovarian torsion: a fifteen-year review. *Ann Emerg Med.* 2001;38(2):156.

Mellick LB. Torsion of the testicle: it is time to stopping tossing the dice. *Pediatric Emer Care.* 2012;28:80-86.

Weiss DA, Jacobstein CR. Genitourinary emergencies. In: Shaw KN, Bachur RG, eds. *Fleisher and Ludwig's Textbook of Pediatric Emergency Medicine.* 7th ed. Philadelphia, PA: Wolters Kluwer; 2016:1353.

110

Not Just Adults: Abnormal Uterine Bleeding and Teenage Menstrual Issues

Amy Pattishall, MD and Atsuko Koyama, MD, MPH

Emergency department (ED) physicians must frequently distinguish the highly variable characteristics of normal menstruation from symptoms of pathology. In developed countries, menarche usually occurs between 12 and 13 years. Due to frequent anovulatory cycles, menstrual patterns can be irregular the first 2 years after menarche; typical cycles are 21-45 days, with periods lasting 2-8 days. Abnormal uterine bleeding (AUB) and dysmenorrhea are two common menstrual concerns seen in the ED.

When evaluating menstrual complaints, a confidential sexual history is paramount, including screening for nonconsensual sexual activity and commercial sexual trafficking. An external vaginal examination should always be performed so as not to miss signs of trauma or anatomic abnormalities, such as hematocolpos. However, a virginal patient should not be traumatized with a pelvic examination. Avoid missing pelvic inflammatory disease (PID), vaginal foreign bodies, or pelvic mass by performing a bimanual examination with or without speculum in sexually active patients.

Abnormal Uterine Bleeding

AUB describes bleeding that is irregular, prolonged, or heavy. In adolescents, anovulatory cycles are the most common cause, but failing to consider the differential can result in missed diagnoses such as hematologic issues (thrombocytopenia, von Willebrand disease, and other coagulation disorders), pelvic infections, and other endocrine causes (polycystic ovary syndrome, hypothyroidism). A contraceptive history is important as adolescents using medroxyprogesterone injections, subdermal implants, or intrauterine devices (IUDs) have higher rates of AUB. Complications of pregnancy, particularly ectopic pregnancy, are potentially life threatening and should not be missed. Endometriosis should be considered in cases of AUB with pelvic pain, particularly if symptoms persist despite treatment.

Management of heavy menstrual bleeding (HMB) involves rapid assessment for hemodynamic instability or hypovolemia, for which volume resuscitation and transfusion should begin immediately. Laboratory testing should include complete blood count, pregnancy test, type and screen, and screening for sexually transmitted infections (STIs). HMB is frequently the presenting symptom of a bleeding disorder in adolescents, especially if present since menarche. Hormonal therapy can affect test results; therefore, screening before treatment is important.

Hormone treatment with combined or progestin-only pills are first-line therapy to stop AUB. IV estrogen should be restricted to patients not tolerating oral medications. Patients should be admitted if they have symptomatic or severe anemia. Discharged patients should be prescribed oral hormonal contraceptives and iron supplementation with or without antiemetics. The levonorgestrel IUD is approved for treatment of HMB and may be considered for appropriate candidates.

Dysmenorrhea

Primary dysmenorrhea, or painful menstruation not associated with any pelvic abnormality, is common in adolescents and can affect daily activities. It is associated with ovulatory cycles, therefore becomes more common with increasing age. Endometrial prostaglandin synthesis and the subsequent inflammatory response are thought to cause the symptoms typical of dysmenorrhea: uterine cramping, bloating, nausea, vomiting, diarrhea, dizziness, fatigue, backache, and headache. Symptoms may start prior to the onset of bleeding and usually resolve within 2-3 days.

Primary dysmenorrhea is a clinical diagnosis. Atypical symptoms should prompt evaluation for causes of secondary dysmenorrhea, including emergent conditions such as ectopic pregnancy and ovarian torsion and urgent conditions such as endometriosis, PID, tubo–ovarian abscess (TOA), adeno-myosis, and uterine fibroids. Pregnancy and STI testing are indicated in sexually active adolescents. Pelvic ultrasound may aid in diagnosis.

NSAIDs that inhibit cyclooxygenase (eg, ibuprofen, naproxen, mefenamic acid) started 1-2 days prior to menses onset and continued until symptoms resolve, are the first-line treatment for primary dysmenorrhea. Combined hormonal contraceptives have also been used in treating primary and some causes of secondary dysmenorrhea, such as endometriosis. Evaluation by a gynecologist is warranted if symptoms are not improving despite treatment.

KEY POINTS

- When evaluating menstrual complaints, always obtain pregnancy testing and do not forget about screening for STIs, nonaccidental trauma/abuse, sexual assault, and sex trafficking.
- Periods occurring less than every 21 days, lasting more than 7 days, requiring frequent pad/tampon changes, or causing symptoms of anemia should prompt laboratory evaluation.
- Pregnancy and its complications, ovarian torsion, PID, and TOA are not-to-miss diagnoses when evaluating possible dysmenorrhea.

Suggested Readings

American College of Obstetricians and Gynecologists. Committee Opinion No. 651. Menstruation in girls and ado-lescents: using the menstrual cycle as a vial sign. *Obstet Gynecol*. 2015;126:e143–e146.

Haamid F, Sass AE, Dietrich JE. Heavy menstrual bleeding in adolescents. *J Pediatr Adolesc Gynecol*. 2017;30:335–340.

Ryan, Sheryl A. The treatment of dysmenorrhea. *Pediatr Clin North Am*. 2017;64(2):331–342.

Wolf M, Chuang JH, Mollen CJ. Gynecology emergencies. In: Shaw K, Bachur R, eds. *Fleisher and Ludwig's Text-book of Pediatric Emergency Medicine*. 7th ed. Philadelphia, PA: Wolters Kluwer; 2016:784–803.

Straddle Injuries Management: Be Able to Distinguish Accident From Abuse

Carrie Busch, MD, MSCR

Pediatric genital trauma from straddle injury can result in significant caregiver anxiety. In addition to the physical pain and discomfort, genital injuries carry with them psychosocial implications that can complicate patient encounters. Injuries occur when urogenital soft tissues are compressed against the bones of the pelvis. Common mechanisms include falls onto a bicycle frame, playground equipment, furniture, or other objects. High-risk scenarios include a slippery surface with falls onto the rim of a bathtub or pool ledge. Inline skating accidents with rapid abduction have also been reported to result in straddle injuries.

As with all aspects of medicine, a detailed history is critical. It can be helpful to interview the child and caregiver separately. Be cautious to use open-ended questions when interviewing the child. Let them use their words to avoid suggesting an injury mechanism or using words that they may simply adopt. When a clear history is provided by the child that is consistent with the injury seen, the event was witnessed, or multiple sources of information are available, then sexual abuse is unlikely. Addi-tional investigation by law enforcement may be indicated if the child is not ambulatory, the event was unwitnessed, the history is not forthcoming, or the injuries are inconsistent with the history provided.

Blunt Injury

The majority of straddle injuries involve blunt trauma to the perineum. Injuries can include ecchymoses, abrasions, and lacerations that typically involve the labia of females and the scrotum of males. Accidental mechanisms tend to produce an asymmetric injury pattern when compared to sexual assault that is more midline. In accidental straddle injury, the urethra, hymen, vagina, and rectum are typically spared. In boys, special attention to scrotal integrity and testicular involvement is needed. Notable scrotal edema, pain, or an abnormal examination warrants a scrotal ultrasound with Doppler flow to evaluate for testicular injury.

Penetrating Trauma

While uncommon, penetrating trauma can be accidental and result in injury to the perianal, hymenal, and vaginal tissues. The mechanism reported typically involves a fall onto a pointed object. Injury has been reported while getting in the bathtub, running on a slick surface, or jumping from one bed to another. Penetrating injuries may look minimal externally but carry a high risk of associated internal injury including bowel perforations, urethral disruptions, scrotal perforations, and vaginal perforations. Penetrating injuries can mimic those seen in child sexual abuse emphasizing the need for vigilance and a good history.

Treatment

Vulvar hematomas can be large and painful resulting in distortion of the genital anatomy or urinary retention. They can typically be managed conservatively with ice and limiting activity. Hematomas that are large or rapidly expanding benefit from the placement of a Foley catheter. Rapidly expanding hematomas can cause pressure necrosis of the overlying skin or spontaneously rupture and may warrant evacuation with placement of a drain.

Genital lacerations without active bleeding can be left to heal on their own without repair. Actively bleeding injuries require identification of the source and may require a sedated examination to ensure complete visualization of the wound. Keep in mind that blood may pool in the vaginal vault and genital irrigation may be helpful to identify the source. Lacerations may respond to vaginal packing or require surgical repair.

Patients must be able to void prior to discharge. Patients may require the assistance of topical analgesia such as ice or topical lidocaine. Persistent inability to void or other indicators of urethral trauma (blood at meatus) requires further evaluation for urethral disruption.

Healing and Return Precautions

Home care for most genital trauma includes Sits baths, limiting activity, and a perineal irrigation bottle. Families can be reassured that most genital trauma will heal rapidly and without residual scarring. Families should be instructed to seek additional care for ongoing bleeding, inability to urinate, abdominal pain, or secondary injury. Follow-up is recommended 2-4 days from injury.

KEY POINTS

- A detailed history is essential to eliminate abuse.
- Penetrating injuries can be externally deceiving and have been associated with additional injuries.
- Ensuring ability to void is critical prior to disposition.
- Most genital injuries heal rapidly and without scarring.

Suggested Readings

Dowd MD, Fitzmaurice L, Knapp JF, Mooney D. The interpretation of urogenital findings in children with straddle injuries. *J Pediatr Surg*. 1994;29(1):7-10.

Spitzer RF, Kives S, Caccia N, Ornstein M, Goia C, Allen LM. Retrospective review of unintentional female genital trauma at a pediatric referral center. *Pediatr Emerg Care*. 2008;24(12):831-835.

Sugar NF, Feldman KW. Perineal impalements in children: distinguishing accident from abuse. *Pediatr Emerg Care*. 2007;23(9):605-616.

112

A Sticky Situation: Know How to Manage Labial Adhesions

Cullen Clark, MD and Kathleen Meadows, MD, FAAP

Labial adhesions (aka labial agglutination, synechia vulvae, or labial fusion) result from fusion of the mucosa of the labia minora. A fairly common finding, labial adhesions manifest predominantly in pre-pubescent females with a prevalence of 0.6%-5% in the first 5 years of life. Several mechanisms contribute to the formation of labial adhesions, most widely believed to be caused by irritation of the vaginal mucosa in the setting of a low estrogen state.

The majority of labial adhesions are asymptomatic and diagnosed by physical examination. Typically an incidental finding by caregivers or medical staff, adhesions are often found when a nurse attempts to catheterize an infant or toddler for a urine sample. When symptomatic, the patient may experience urinary incontinence (postvoid dripping), recurrent urinary tract infections, vaginitis, hematuria, vaginal pain with ambulation, and/or urinary frequency.

Inspect the vulva in the frog-leg position. Visualization of the adhesion often requires gentle traction to separate the labial majora. The examination may be uncomfortable but should not be painful for the patient. The adhesion can extend a small portion of the labia to covering the urethral meatus and vaginal introitus entirely, typically from posteriorly to anterior.

The most commonly due to vaginal irritation in prepubertal females, providers should consider other conditions such as sexual abuse, infection (candidiasis, infestation), poor hygiene (a sign of neglect), or chemical trauma.

Asymptomatic labial adhesions do not require treatment in the ED. Over 80%-90% of adhesions without signs of infection or urinary outflow obstruction can be observed as an outpatient and spontaneously resolve within a year of identification. However, those with symptoms of irritation or urinary outflow obstruction require treatment from the ED. Topical estrogens are the mainstay of treatment for labial adhesions. A small amount of estrogen 0.01% ointment applied directly and exclusively to the area of fusion has been shown to be effective in resolving adhesions in the majority of patients but recurrence rates were significant. There was no significant difference in duration of topical estrogen treatment on rate of recurrence so duration should be short to minimize side effects. The current recommendation is 2-4 weeks maximum of estrogen ointment applied twice a day or until separation of adhesions. Topical estrogens are systematically absorbed and can lead to breast budding, vaginal irritation, and scant vaginal bleeding. Side effects typically resolve upon discontinuation of medication. Recent evidence shows that topical betamethasone ointment is also an effective alternative.

In the case of recurrent, symptomatic labial adhesions, referral for manual separation may be necessary. Manual separation in the ED is NOT recommended as it can be a very painful procedure and is best performed under local or general anesthesia by a surgeon or pediatric gynecologist. It is not recommended to manually separate labial adhesions for bladder catheterization. Consider instead a bag specimen or a suprapubic tap if a sterile specimen is required. If manual or spontaneous separation occurs, give parents anticipatory guidance to continue an emollient such as petroleum jelly or low-dose steroid ointment for several days to weeks in order to reduce risk of recurrence.

The key aspect of treatment for symptomatic labial adhesions is anticipatory guidance. Labial adhesions can be a source of anxiety for parents and patients. While resolution is nearly 100% by the time of puberty, there can often be recurrence throughout the prepubertal phase. Ensure parents understand this risk and when to contact their pediatrician. Additionally, parents and patients (if applicable) should be advised on methods to prevent vaginal irritation such as wiping from front-to-back, wearing cotton underwear, avoiding bubble baths or irritating soaps/detergents, and avoiding tight-fitting, wet clothing against the labia for prolonged periods.

KEY POINTS

- Asymptomatic labial adhesions can be monitored as an outpatient without treatment.
- Nearly 100% of labial adhesions will resolve by puberty.
- Frog-leg positioning is the best means to visualize labial adhesions.
- First-line treatment for symptomatic labial adhesions is topical estrogen ointment.
- Labial adhesions should prompt questions about an underlying problem such as sexual abuse, infection, neglect, or chemical irritation.

Suggested Readings

Bacon JL, Romano ME, Quint EH. Clinical recommendation: labial adhesions. *J Pediatr Adolesc Gynecol.* 2015;28(5):405-409.

Mayoglou L, Dulabon L, Martin-Alguacil N, Pfaff D, Schober J. Success of treatment modalities for labial fusion: a retrospective evaluation of topical and surgical treatments. *J Pediatr Adolesc Gynecol.* 2009;22(4):247-250.

Nield LS. Labial adhesions. In: McInerny TK, Adam HM, Campbell DE, DeWitt TG, Foy JM, Kamat DM, eds. *American Academy of Pediatric Care.* 2nd ed. American Academy of Pediatrics; 2017.

Norris JE, Elder CV, Dunford AM, Rampal D, Cheung C, Grover SR. Spontaneous resolution of labial adhesions in pre-pubertal girls. *J Pediatr Child Health.* 2018;54(7):748-753.

Wejde E, Ekmark AN, Stenström P. Treatment with oestrogen or manual separation for labial adhesions—initial outcome and long term follow-up. *BMC Pediatr.* 2018;18(1):1-9.

Always Look Under the Diaper: Congenital Abnormalities of the Genitourinary Tract

Perry White Mitchell, MD and Matthew Carlisle, MD, MAS

Adrenal crisis and testicular cancer. These are not bread-and-butter cases seen in your emergency department (ED) every day. However, in cases of children with ambiguous genitalia, these are real, potentially life-threatening complications of which all emergency providers should be aware. In disorders of sex development, young children possess genitalia that do not fit typical male or female phenotypes. In addition to the psychological issues these children face, disorders of sex development may have life-threatening sequelae as well. In this section, we will discuss congenital adrenal hyperplasia (CAH), cryptorchidism, and hypospadias, which should be routinely considered in children presenting to the ED with ambiguous genitalia.

Physical Examination

Performing a thorough GU examination is crucial in initiating the diagnostic process of disorders of sexual development. Adequate GU examination of male children includes assessment of penile length, foreskin, testicular location/presence, urethral meatus location, scrotal anatomy, and inguinal masses. Male ambiguous genitalia may present as micropenis, hypospadias, or an empty scrotum. An ED appropriate female GU examination includes assessment of external structures such as the clitoris and labia. Speculum or bimanual examination should be deferred for most prepubertal patients. Female ambiguous genitalia may manifest as clitoral enlargement, labial fusion, or palpable labial masses, which may be testes.

Congenital Adrenal Hyperplasia

The most common etiology of ambiguous genitalia in genotypic females is CAH. Considering the associated risk of life-threatening adrenal crisis, it is imperative that this diagnosis is always considered in infants with ambiguous genitalia. CAH is caused by deficiency in one of the enzymes (most commonly 21-hydroxylase) responsible for producing steroid hormones (cortisol, aldosterone). The classic form of CAH (most severe) usually presents in infancy and is associated with adrenal insufficiency. This form of CAH is part of the genetic disease screen performed on all infants in the United States. The less common, milder form of CAH is associated with menstrual irregularity, acne, and masculine characteristics (developed during teenage/early-adult years) but not ambiguous genitalia. When evaluating a female with ambiguous genitalia, always be aware of signs and symptoms of adrenal crisis, caused by low circulating levels of cortisol and aldosterone. These signs and symptoms include hypotension, catecholamine-resistant shock, failure to thrive, vomiting, diarrhea, and severe abdominal pain. Lab derangements include hyponatremia, hyperkalemia, and hypoglycemia. Once the diagnosis is suspected, rapid treatment with intravenous fluids, hydrocortisone, and electrolyte management should be initiated. Long-term medical management of CAH is daily steroids. However, referral to a urologist is also invaluable, as surgical cosmetic correction may assist the associated psychological effects.

Cryptorchidism

Absence of testes in the scrotum should trigger concern during GU examination. Cryptorchidism is due to incomplete testicular descent into the scrotum, which is abnormal after 4 months of age. The undescended testes may be present in the abdominal cavity or the inguinal canal. Cryptorchidism can occur concomitantly with other disorders (eg, androgen insensitivity syndrome, Klinefelter syndrome, Prader-Willi syndrome, hypospadias, etc.). Without adequate treatment, cryptorchidism carries risks of testicular cancer, intra-abdominal testicular torsion, infertility, and inguinal hernia. Therefore, boys with cryptorchidism should be referred to a urologist for surgical correction, ideally between ages 4 and 12 months.

Hypospadias

Ventral displacement of the urethral opening, known as hypospadias, is one of the most common congenital abnormalities in males. Hypospadias does not usually cause immediate life-threatening issues; however, it is associated with misdirected urinary stream, inability to urinate while standing, foreskin abnormalities, and penile curvature. There is some suggestion that patients with hypospadias have an increased risk of urinary tract infection, both pre- and postrepair. Hypospadias generally occurs in isolation but associated disorders can be present. Patients with hypospadias can be difficult to catheterize so a bag specimen or suprapubic aspiration should be considered instead. Urologic consultation is recommended to redirect the urethral meatus and flow of urine.

KEY POINTS

- Always look under the diaper as ambiguous genitalia is a finding that always requires further workup and long-term management.
- Consider congenital adrenal hyperplasia in all children with ambiguous genitalia and signs/symptoms of adrenal crisis.
- Urology referral should be placed when cryptorchidism or hypospadias is detected to prevent the associated complications and to pursue surgical correction.

Suggested Readings

Hadziselimovic F, et al., eds. Examination and clinical findings in cryptorchid boys. *Cryptorchidism: Management and Implications.* Berlin, Heidelberg: Springer-Verlag; 1983:93-98.

Hindmarsh PC, Geertsma K. *Congenital Adrenal Hyperplasia: A Comprehensive Guide.* Cambridge, Massachusetts: Academic Press; 2017.

Khan DI, et al. *Ambiguous Genitalia: An Approach.* Saarbrücken, Germany: LAP LAMBERT Academic Publishing; 2013.

Always Check Under the Hood: Do Not Confuse Phimosis and Paraphimosis

Tseng-Che Tseng, MD and Rebecca Hutchings, MD

In uncircumcised males, the prepuce or foreskin naturally covers and actually adheres to the glans penis at birth. The adhesions are gradually broken down by hormonal changes, and the prepuce is usually fully retractable over the glans penis by 5 years of age. There is no need to forcibly retract the foreskin either at home or in the emergency department.

Balanitis/Balanoposthitis

Balanitis is a superficial inflammation of the glans alone, whereas balanoposthitis occurs when the inflammation involves both the glans and prepuce. Diagnosis of balanitis and balanoposthitis is made clinically based upon examination findings of erythema and swelling of foreskin. Symptoms consist of pruritus and/or pain. The main causes of inflammation are trauma, local irritation, and infection. Infectious sources are commonly derived from local colonization of *Candida albicans*, or gram-positive anaerobic and aerobic bacteria such as Group A *Streptococcus*. Infectious etiologies change as colonization changes in different age groups. For example, in sexually active adolescents, sexually transmitted organisms such as *Chlamydia trachomatis* and *Neisseria gonorrhoeae* are more commonly causative agents. Inflammation can also be caused by external irritation from soap and laundry detergents. Removal of irritant agents and improved hygiene should resolve the inflammation. If an infectious cause is suspected, balanitis and balanoposthitis should be treated with topical antifungals (ie, clotrimazole cream) and/or antibiotics (topical or oral depending on extent of symptoms). Be aware that recurrent balanoposthitis may be indicative of diabetes mellitus or an immunocompromised state; an appropriate workup should be performed when indicated.

Phimosis

Phimosis occurs when the foreskin cannot be retracted back over the glans. In pediatric patients, this is often a physiologic condition without any symptoms and generally resolves spontaneously by 5 years of age. Pathologic phimosis occurs when the foreskin is truly not retractable, which occurs due to scarring from trauma, infection, or inflammation. Signs and symptoms include inability to retract the foreskin after being able to do so at an earlier age, dysuria, pain, bleeding, and/or inability to void.

Initial management of pathologic phimosis begins with conservative treatment. Counsel parents to apply a steroid cream to the tip of the foreskin twice a day. After a few days, the child or his parents can start trying to gradually push the foreskin back as far as it will go easily without hurting. Once the foreskin can be pulled back a bit, the cream can be applied more proximally. The foreskin should then be returned to its normal position. The patient should also be referred to urology as an outpatient. If the condition persists, corrective circumcision might be recommended. Generally speaking, phimosis is not a medical emergency. Often times, it only requires reassurance to parents and counseling on not forcing the foreskin back proximally. However, it is important to assess if patient is able to urinate. If urinary outflow obstruction occurs, further intervention such as a dorsal slit procedure and circumcision might need to be performed urgently.

Paraphimosis

In contrast to phimosis, paraphimosis occurs when the proximal foreskin has been fully retracted and now cannot be replaced back over the glans. This can cause obstruction of circulation leading to strangulation of the glans, which requires emergent reduction to prevent tissue ischemia and necrosis. Diagnosis is made clinically, and the mainstay of treatment is timely manual reduction with adequate pain control. Manual reduction is achieved by pushing forcefully on the glans with the thumbs while pulling the foreskin proximally with fingers. In most instances, manual compression can reduce the swollen foreskin within the first few hours. In difficult cases, different methods have been used to aid in reducing swelling including the application of ice and the use of compression bandages. Osmotic agents such as granulated sugar or gauze covered with dextrose solution or mannitol can be applied to the glans to reduce swelling as well. If manual reduction fails, incision of constricting foreskin (dorsal slit reduction) with a nerve block will need to be performed to relieve the pressure. Of note, methods for reducing swelling should not be performed when the glans appears blue or black with firmness on palpation, an indication of penile necrosis. If signs of penile necrosis or urinary obstruction are present, emergent urology consultation is warranted. The patient will need immediate reduction, either under procedural sedation in the emergency room or in the operating room.

KEY POINTS

- Phimosis is not an emergency if the patient can urinate.
- Paraphimosis is an emergency and requires emergent reduction.
- Emergent consultation with urology for paraphimosis is required when signs of necrosis or urinary outflow obstruction are present.
- Recurrent balanoposthitis can be associated with diabetes mellitus or an immunocompromised state.

Suggested Readings

Edwards S. Balanitis and balanoposthitis: a review. *Genitourin Med.* 1996;72(3):155-159.
McGregor TB, Pike JG, Leonard MP. Pathologic and physiologic phimosis: approach to the phimotic foreskin. *Can Fam Physician.* 2007;53(3):445-448.
Simpson ET, Barraclough P. The management of the paediatric foreskin. *Aust Fam Physician.* 1998;27:381.

DERMATOLOGY

Neonatal Rashes: Know the Bad From the Not So Bad

Denisse Fernandez Goytizolo, MD and Madeline M. Joseph, MD, FACEP, FAAP

Various rashes may present in the neonatal period. Although the majority are transient and benign, they represent a significant source of parental concern. It is essential to recognize these entities from serious neonatal rashes to ensure their optimal management in the emergency department.

Rashes We Do Not Need to Worry About

Transient Neonatal Pustular Melanosis
Transient neonatal pustular melanosis (TNPM) is a transient and self-limited dermatosis. It is characterized by three sequential lesions: (1) superficial vesiculopustules of 1-2 mm of diameter that disappear in 1-2 days, (2) ruptured pustules with a collaret of fine scale, and (3) hyperpigmented macules that fade in 3 weeks to 3 months. All areas of the body may be affected, including palms and soles. TNPM requires no therapy.

Erythema Toxicum Neonatorum
Erythema toxicum neonatorum (ETN) is a self-limited rash of unknown etiology. Lesions consist of central erythematous 2-3 mm macules and papules that evolve into pustules and are surrounded by a larger area of erythema. The lesions may be a few to several hundreds and appear on the face, trunk, and proximal extremities. Palms and soles are spared. Lesions usually appear 1-2 days after birth and up to the 10th day of life. ETN fades within 5-7 days, but it may recur for several weeks. No treatment is necessary.

Milia
Milia are benign, self-limited keratinous cysts. Lesions consist in firm tiny whitish-yellow papules of 1-2 mm in diameter, most often located on the forehead, cheeks, nose, chin, gingivae, and on the midline of the palate (Epstein pearls). Milia disappear spontaneously within the first months of life.

Miliaria
Miliaria results from retention of sweat in occluded eccrine sweat ducts due to newborns being in warm, humid conditions (such as nursing or wearing of tight-fitting clothing during hot, humid weather).

- *Miliaria crystalline*: pinpoint, clear vesicles of 1-2 mm in diameter that rupture and desquamate lasting for hours to days. It appears on the head, neck, and upper trunk.
- *Miliaria rubra or neonatal prickly heat*: small erythematous papules and vesicles over the face, upper trunk, and intertriginous area of the neck.

All forms of miliaria respond to cooling of the patient by removal of excess clothing, baths, and regulation of environmental temperature. Topical agents are usually ineffective.

Neonatal Cephalic Pustulosis

The formerly called neonatal acne is a benign and self-limited condition attributed to maternal andro-gen stimulation to the neonatal adrenal glands. The lesions are papules and pustules over the face, neck, and trunk. Neonatal cephalic pustulosis (NCP) resolves without scarring in a few months. Treatment is usually unnecessary but topical azole or mild topical steroids may speed resolution.

Severe, persistent NCP accompanied by other signs of hyperandrogenism should prompt suspicion for adrenal cortical hyperplasia or other underlying endocrinopathies.

Seborrheic Dermatitis

Seborrheic dermatitis (SD) pathogenesis is unknown, but *Pityrosporum (Malassezia)* and *Candida* species have been implicated. SD presents with a nonpruritic erythematous scaling eruption on hair-bearing areas (eg, scalp [cradle cap], eyebrows) and perinasal, presternal, postauricular, and inter-triginous areas. SD may be focal or involve almost the entire body.

SD is usually self-limited and resolves within several weeks to months. A stepwise management is suggested, beginning with reassurance and watchful waiting. The scales can be removed with a soft brush after shampooing or emollient use. Tar-containing shampoos are first line followed by selenium sulfide shampoos and antifungal creams or shampoos. Mild steroid creams are another option.

Generalized SD accompanied by failure to thrive and diarrhea should prompt suspicion for immunodeficiency, and a poor response to treatment may result from pathology such as Langerhans cell histiocytosis.

Life-Threatening Neonatal Rash

Neonatal herpes simplex virus infection is usually transmitted during delivery. Manifestations occur between the 1st and 3rd week of life but can be as late as the 4th week. Neonates may present with local or disseminated disease, and skin vesicles are common with either type. Rapid diagnosis by viral cul-ture or HSV PCR is essential. The most common site of retrieval is the skin vesicle. The nasopharynx, eyes, rectum, blood, and CSF should also be tested. Treatment is with parenteral acyclovir and sup-portive care.

KEY POINTS

- The diagnosis of neonatal benign rashes can typically be made by identifying the time of appearance, characteristics of the lesions, and body distribution patterns.
- Vesicular rash in neonates should prompt suspicion for and treatment of neonatal HSV.

Suggested Readings

O'Connor NR, McLaughlin MR, Ham P. Newborn skin: Part I. Common rashes. *Am Fam Physician*. 2008;77(1): 47-52.

Zitelli BJ, McIntire SC, Nowalk AJ. *Zitelli and Davis' Atlas of Pediatric Physical Diagnosis*. Philadelphia, PA: Saun-ders/Elsevier; 2012.

Be Prepared to Manage the Common Pediatric Rashes

Kayla McManus, DO and Todd Wylie, MD

Skin disorders are among the top reasons for pediatric emergency department visits. When evaluating patients with rashes, it is easy to "miss the forest for the trees" as a rash may be so distracting that one forgets to evaluate the overall disease process. Key historical components include initial rash appearance, progression, exposures, medical history, medications, associated signs/symptoms, and immune status since immune-compromised patients are at risk for significant morbidity and mortality. It is also essential to evaluate all areas of the skin, including the palms, soles, and mucous membranes. Focus on the major skin signs and recognize that prior therapeutic interventions may alter the rash appearance. (see Table 120.1).

Though not a comprehensive list, some common rashes and their management are described below and in Table 116-1.

Contact Dermatitis

Contact dermatitis is a localized, pruritic, erythematous rash following contact with an external material. It is divided into irritant and allergic dermatitis. Irritant dermatitis is secondary to non–immune-modulated skin irritation. Symptom onset may be immediate. Allergic contact dermatitis is due to a cell-mediated delayed hypersensitivity reaction. Initial allergen exposure leads to sensitization, and re-exposure causes a T-cell–mediated inflammatory cascade resulting in erythema, papules, vesicles, and pruritus.

Common irritant dermatitides include diaper dermatitis and dry skin dermatitis. Treat by removing offending agents and restoring water to the skin surface with preservative, lanolin, and fragrance-free moisturizers.

Toxicodendron Dermatitis

Toxicodendron (*Rhus*) dermatitis results from contact with *Toxicodendron* plants, including poison oak, poison ivy, and poison sumac. The causative allergen, urushiol, may remain on clothing and skin, so patients should immediately shower and wash clothing following contact. In sensitized individuals, the rash usually develops within 2-3 days but may take up to 15 days in some patients. The rash is self-limited with resolution in 1-3 weeks. Wet compresses, oral antihistamines, and calamine lotion may improve itching. Early topical corticosteroids may reduce symptoms. Reserve systemic corticosteroids for severe cases or those involving vital structures (eg, eyes).

Nickel Dermatitis

Nickel allergic contact dermatitis presents as a local or systemic reaction. Local nickel dermatitis results from contact with jewelry, buttons, or other nickel containing items. Common sites include the umbilicus (buttons), fingers (rings), and earlobes (earrings). Systemic nickel reactions are uncommon and are associated with nickel ingestion from dietary sources (eg, chocolate, canned foods) and present with a generalized dermatitis. Treatment requires removal of nickel allergens and treating symptoms such as pruritus and local rash with antihistamines and topical corticosteroids. Oral corticosteroids are an option but may have significant side effects. Alternatively, topical immunomodulatory and anti-inflammatory agents (eg, tacrolimus) are effective against nickel dermatitis. UVB phototherapy may be indicated for patients with refractory nickel dermatitis.

Table 116-1 ■ Characteristics of Common Pediatric Rashes

Medical Diagnosis	Initial Presentation	Type of Lesion	Distribution	Progression of Rash
Contact Dermatitis (Irritant)	Erythema and pruritus; localized to skin contact site	Erythematous papules	Localized to site of contact; commonly affects hands	Dry skin, fissured skin, less distinct borders
Contact Dermatitis (Allergic)	Erythema and pruritus; localized to exposed skin	Erythematous papules	Localized to site of allergen/skin contact; distinct borders, lines, and patterns	Acute—erythema, edema, vesicles Chronic—erythema, lichenification, excoriations
Toxicodendron Dermatitis	Erythematous, pruritic eruption—linear or streak-like distribution where plant contacted skin	Erythematous papules	Distribution related to area(s) of skin contact	Progress to vesicles, and in severe cases, bullae
Nickel Dermatitis	Grouped, erythematous papules at contact site; pruritus	Erythematous papules—vesicles	Local reaction at site of skin contact	Chronic exposure—erythema, fissures, lichenification, excoriations
Scabies	Small red papules; intense pruritus	Erythematous papules; excoriation, scabbing	Interdigital spaces, buttocks, axillary folds, wrists, elbows; possibly palms/soles in infants	Commonly spread to those in close living quarters
Pityriasis Rosea	Initial "herald patch" (erythematous patch; fine scale collarette)	Oval lesions; scale collarette	Trunk and proximal extremities	Initial "herald patch," followed by oval lesions (lesion long axes follow skin lines)

Scabies

Scabies is caused by *Sarcoptes scabiei* var. *hominis*. Infestation causes intense pruritus due to mite antigen hypersensitivity. Scabies is diagnosed clinically. Visualizing the mite under microscopy using skin scrapings confirms the diagnosis. First-line treatment consists of topical permethrin 5% for 8-12 hours with reapplication 1 week later. Washing clothing, linens, and towels in hot water or storing in an airtight bag is necessary to eradicate scabies. Patients are not contagious 1 day after treatment, but pruritus may continue for weeks.

Pityriasis Rosea

Pityriasis rosea (PR) is a pruritic rash of adolescents and young adults. Although a viral etiology has been proposed, the definitive etiology is unknown. Presence of a "herald patch" and "Christmas tree" distribution of the rash strongly suggests the diagnosis. In sexually active individuals, rapid plasma reagin (RPR) testing is necessary to rule out secondary syphilis due to similar appearance of the rashes. PR is self-limited and treatment is not necessary, although topical corticosteroids may decrease pruritus. The rash may not subside for several months, so appropriate anticipatory guidance is needed.

KEY POINTS

- History and physical is key to identify common rashes.
- Follow-up is recommended following ED diagnosis and treatment.
- Provide anticipatory guidance based on the known clinical progression of a rash.

Suggested Readings

Allmon A, Deane K, Martine KL. Common skin rashes in children. *Am Fam Physician*. 2015;92:211-216.
Kliegman R, Stanton B, St. Geme JW, Schor NF, Behrman RE. *Nelson Textbook of Pediatrics*. 20th ed. Philadelphia, PA: Elsevier; 2016:1594-1596, 1570, 3221-3226.
Usatine RP, Riojas M. Diagnosis and management of contact dermatitis. *Am Fam Physician*. 2010;82:249-255.

Be Prepared to Manage Common Pediatric Infectious Rashes

James Buscher, MD and Madeline Joseph, MD, FACEP, FAAP

Pediatric rashes can be anxiety provoking for parents and often leads to families seeking care in the emergency department (ED). In 2015, 1.4 million pediatric patients were seen for skin and subcutaneous tissue disorders. While a rash may be a sign of potential serious illness, many are common infectious rashes that are self-limited and resolve with supportive care or simple treatment. ED clinicians must recognize benign rashes and avoid extensive workups and reassure families.

Viral

Molluscum contagiosum is caused by a poxvirus. Mollusca are small, raised, smooth, firm, and flesh colored with central umbilication. They can occur anywhere on the body and are spread by contact. The rash self-resolves in 6-12 months but can remain for up to 4 years. Referral can be made to a dermatologist if in a sensitive location or for family concern to expedite resolution.

Erythema infectiosum (Fifth disease) is caused by Parvovirus B19. Symptoms consist of fever, rhinorrhea, and headache followed by the rash, which is a typically erythematous area on the cheeks ("slapped cheek") but can be a reticular rash on the body that lasts 7-10 days. Once the rash develops, the patient is no longer contagious. Although there is no treatment, providers should be aware of complications such as aplastic anemia, which can occur in immunocompromised patients including pregnant women.

Roseola (exanthema subitum or sixth disease) is caused by HHV-6 and less commonly HHV-7 commonly HHV-7 and most often affects children 1-5 years of age. The rash is comprised of small, pink, or red papules 2-5 mm and starts on the trunk and spreads to the neck, extremities, and face. The rash is preceded by mild URI symptoms and high fever (up to 104°F) for 3-5 days with abrupt defervescence as the rash starts. Up to 15% of children may experience febrile seizures. Treatment is standard supportive care.

Hand-foot-and-mouth disease is caused by enteroviruses, with coxsackievirus A16 being the most common. Patients are most contagious during the first week of illness and develop fever and red spots in the mouth that can blister and become painful (herpangina). Lesions can also be found on the body, with the hands and feet being most common but can occur anywhere. Treatment is supportive care, but pain should be addressed since it can limit oral intake causing dehydration.

Fungal

Tinea is caused by dermatophytes, and the nomenclature is based on location: capitis (head), corporis (body), cruris (groin), pedis (feet), unguium (nails), barbae (beard/mustache), and manuum (hands).

Tinea capitis primarily impacts school-aged children, and is characterized by annular patches in the scalp with areas of alopecia with black dots within the patch. Due to the dermatophytes living within the hair follicle, oral therapy is required. First-line therapy consists of griseofulvin with alternatives including itraconazole and terbinafine.

Tine corporis (ringworm) presents on the body, and typically presents with a circular, erythematous plaque with a demarcated border. Treatment usually is topical, but oral therapy can be considered with diffuse lesions.

Bacterial

Scarlet fever is due to a toxin produced by group A streptococcus. The rash is characterized by fine, erythematous macules and papules with a "sandpaper" texture. The rash appears after 1-2 days of illness on the neck, axillae, or groin and then spreads over the body. Desquamation of the fingertips, groin, and toes may be present and persist for up to several weeks. First-line treatment consists of single dose of intramuscular or oral penicillin.

Impetigo is a rash commonly caused by group A streptococci or *Staphylococcus aureus* and can be classified as either bullous or nonbullous. Bullous impetigo is almost universally caused by *S. aureus* and begins with small vesicles that become flaccid bullae. With nonbullous impetigo, the vesicles rupture and form a secondary yellow crust (honey crusting). Treatment is antibiotics, either topical or oral depending on the extent of the lesions.

KEY POINTS

- Be sure to expose the patient as the rash may only be present in the groin or oropharynx.
- Not all rashes require medication as many only need supportive care.
- Most fungal infections can be treated topically with one exception being tinea capitis requiring oral dosing.

Suggested Readings

Kliegman R, Stanton B, St. Geme JW, et al. *Nelson Textbook of Pediatrics.* 20th ed. Philadelphia, PA: Elsevier; 2016:1594-1596, 3221-3226.

Liu C, Bayer A, Cosgrove SE, et al. Clinical practice guidelines by the Infectious Diseases Society of America for the treatment of methicillin-resistant *Staphylococcus aureus* infections in adults and children: executive summary. *Clin Infect Dis.* 2011;52:285-292.

The Fits and Starts of Atopic Dermatitis: Strategies to Adjusting Treatment

Sami K. Saikaly, MD and Jennifer J. Schoch, MD

Atopic dermatitis (AD), commonly known as eczema, occurs in 10%-20% of children and is typically more severe at younger ages. Children with AD flares often seek treatment in the emergency departments (EDs). Clinicians must be aware of treatment for AD flares and connect patients with appropriate follow-up to relieve symptoms.

Treatment

Replacement and repair of the defective skin barrier is critical in AD treatment. Sensitive skin care is recommended, including daily bathing with lukewarm water and nonfragranced bar soap. Emollient therapy with thick lubricants results in an improved skin barrier and blocks the downstream inflammatory cycle and subsequent itching.

Once this inflammatory cycle has begun, topical corticosteroids are the first-line therapy. A lower potency corticosteroid is typically used for the face and skin folds such as hydrocortisone 2.5% ointment. For the trunk and extremities, higher potency corticosteroids may be utilized, such as triamcinolone 0.1% ointment. These are typically utilized twice daily until the skin clears. AD is a chronic disease, so ED physicians should emphasize the need for the patient to follow-up for maintenance therapy-both to improve the patient's quality of life and avoid repeated ED visits.

For moderate to severe AD patients, local care involves applying topical corticosteroids to AD areass, wearing a damp dressing layer (ie, socks, gloves, or pajamas), and covering this damp dressing with a dry layer (ie, dry clothing, towels, or blankets) to maintain moisture.

In severe pediatric AD that is uncontrolled by topical therapy, patients should be referred to dermatology for consideration of phototherapy or systemic therapy. Systemic corticosteroids are not recommended due to long-term adverse effects and frequent flares once treatment is withdrawn.

Other Considerations

Impaired barrier function and trauma from scratching may result in open skin, which can lead to superinfection and worsening inflammation. Triple antibiotic creams and neomycin should be avoided due to increased risk of contact dermatitis. Control of the eczema should be the primary goal in treating superinfected AD. Systemic antibiotics should be used only in acute episodes with clear evidence for bacterial infection. In case of recurrent bacterial infection, application of intranasal mupirocin twice a day for 10 days and/or bathing in diluted bleach may limit recurrence. Other preventive measures include washing bedding weekly, and avoiding sharing toiletries.

Other infections complicating AD can occur, such as infection with herpes simplex virus (eczema herpeticum, Kaposi varicelliform eruption). Children with eczema herpeticum require treatment with acyclovir as early as possible and often hospital admission. In teenagers or others with AD localized to the head and neck that does not respond to therapy, the presence of a fungal infection (Malassezia) should be considered and treated with a topical or oral antifungal.

AD has been shown to significantly affect patient and family quality of life, due to frequent topical therapy applications, social stigmatization, and sleep disturbances. Treating concurrent dermatographism (if present) with nonsedating antihistamines such as cetirizine or fexofenadine may reduce pruritus.

KEY POINTS

- Treatment of AD includes sensitive skin care, moisturization, assessment for superinfection, and controlling inflammation and pruritus.
- Treatment of AD with an appropriately short course of potent topical corticosteroid provides less cumulative corticosteroid exposure than long-term nonefficacious use of less potent topical corticosteroids.
- AD is a chronic disease, and maintenance therapy with lower potency topical steroids 2-3 times weekly helps prevent relapse.
- Oral corticosteroids are not recommended in routine care of AD.

Suggested Readings

Brar KK, Nicol NH, Boguniewicz M. Strategies for successful management of severe atopic dermatitis. *J Allergy Clin Immunol Pract*. 2019;7(1):1-16.

Galli E, Neri I, Ricci G, et al. Consensus conference on clinical management of pediatric atopic dermatitis. *Ital J Pediatr*. 2016;42:26.

Leung DYM. Why is eczema herpeticum unexpectedly rare? *Antiviral Res*. 2013;9:153-157.

Mayba JN, Gooderham MJ. Review of atopic dermatitis and topical therapies. *J Cutan Med Surg*. 2017;21(3): 227-236.

Takahata Y, Sugita T, Kato H, et al. Cutaneous Malassezia flora in atopic dermatitis differs between adults and children. *Br J Dermatol*. 2007;157:1178-1182.

Travers JB, Kozman A, Yao Y. Treatment outcomes of secondary impetiginized pediatric atopic dermatitis lesions and the role of oral antibiotics. *Pediatr Dermatol*. 2012;29:289-296.

Be Prepared to Recognize and Manage the "Bad" Rashes

Akhila Reddy Mandadi, MD and Madeline M. Joseph, MD, FACEP, FAAP

The majority of the skin conditions presenting to the pediatric emergency department (ED) are benign. It is important for ED physicians to recognize the following red flags that represent conditions that need emergent interventions.

- Erythroderma (redness of skin involving more than 90% body surface area)
- Desquamation
- Allodynia
- Petechial rash/purpura

Several skin conditions present with all or some of the above red flags. Conditions that present with erythroderma, fever, and multiorgan involvement (such as hepatic and renal failure, DIC, and hypotension) include toxic shock syndrome (TSS), DRESS syndrome (drug rash and eosinophilia and systemic symptoms), Steven-Johnson syndrome (SJS), toxic epidermal necrolysis (TEN), and staphylococcal scalded skin syndrome (SSSS). SJS, TEN, and SSSS additionally present with severe allodynia.

TSS and SSSS are staphylococcal toxin-mediated illnesses from existing wounds. SSSS is seen in young children and in renally impaired patients. TSS is seen in adolescents (such as secondary to prolonged tampon use), nasal packing, and in adults from surgical or other wounds.

TEN/SJS and DRESS syndrome are all drug reactions, most commonly secondary to sulfonamides, anticonvulsants allopurinol, dapsone, or NSAIDs. The drug ingestion precedes the rash by 1-3 weeks.

Certain distinguishing features can help diagnose these rashes. SSSS presents as superficial thin-walled blisters, while TSS typically presents with maculopapular or petechial rash that is worse in flexural areas with desquamation seen from trunk toward palms and soles. DRESS syndrome presents with a distinctive scaly generalized rash and lymphadenopathy. Lastly, SJS presents with <10% body surface area epidermal sloughing in contrast to TEN, which has more than 30% epidermal sloughing. TEN also presents with targetlike lesions, desquamation, characteristic epidermal necrosis, and more than two mucosal surfaces involved. Severe eye involvement requires emergent ophthalmologic evaluation.

All the above conditions are diagnosed clinically, but lab testing could be pursued to detect associated complications. For example, SJS/TEN can be associated with lymphopenia, neutropenia, and thrombocytopenia, and DRESS syndrome is associated with eosinophilia. Transaminitis and electrolyte disturbances are seen in all these conditions. Blood and fluid cultures maybe negative, but nasopharyngeal cultures in TSS and cultures from fluid in blisters in SSSS are often positive. Skin biopsy will definitively help differentiate all the above conditions if the clinical picture is not clear.

Treatment is typically supportive with care similar to burn treatment with careful fluid and electrolyte management. Antibiotics are only indicated in SSSS and TSS. Vancomycin is used for severe cases and clindamycin for theoretical antitoxin and synergistic effects. Steroids in DRESS syndrome and IVIG in SJS/TEN may be beneficial.

There are several skin conditions that present with local skin manifestations that can have serious complications such as necrotizing fasciitis (NF) and cellulitis when it involves eye, hand, and perineum. In NF, patients have pain out of proportion to findings on the physical examination that may precede the necrotic hemorrhagic bullae by 24-48 hours. Crepitation, bullae, burgundy coloration, and frank gangrene spreading rapidly are characteristic. Consider calculating a Laboratory Risk Indicator for Necrotizing Fasciitis (LRINEC) score (CRP, Na, WBC, hemoglobin creatinine, and glucose) or Pediatric LRINEC (only CRP and Na) to distinguish patients with severe cellulitis/abscess vs necrotizing fasciitis. A LRINEC score ≥6 is a reasonable cut-off to rule in necrotizing fasciitis, but a LRINEC <6 does not rule out the diagnosis. Patients with highly suspicious NF need emergent surgical management and IV antistreptococcal antibiotics.

An ill-appearing child with fever, multiorgan involvement, and petechial and purpuric rash should raise suspicion for sepsis, meningococcemia secondary to *Neisseria meningitidis*, or Rocky Mountain spotted fever secondary to *Rickettsia rickettsii*. Meningococcemia presents with abrupt onset of fever, rapidly progressing purpura, DIC, altered mental status, and shock. Cultures should be obtained and antibiotics (such as a third-generation cephalosporin such as ceftriaxone) given along with aggressive sepsis management. Death occurs rapidly without the prompt administration of third-generation cephalosporins. Rocky Mountain spotted fever presents with rash within first 2 weeks after tick exposure. The rash starts on wrists and ankles and spreads to palms, soles, and lastly on trunk and face. Labs will often show thrombocytopenia and hyponatremia. Treatment includes immediate tick removal and prompt antibiotic administration with the first choice being doxycycline regardless of the age of the child.

KEY POINTS

- Rashes associated with erythroderma, desquamation, allodynia, or petechial/purpura require immediate attention to rule out life-threatening diseases.
- An ill-appearing child with fever and petechial and purpuric rash should raise suspicion for sepsis. Cultures should be obtained and antibiotics given along with aggressive sepsis management.

Suggested Readings

Aronson PL, Florin TA. Pediatric dermatologic emergencies: a case-based approach for the pediatrician. *Pediatr Ann.* 2009;38(2):109-116.

Kress KW. Pediatric dermatology emergencies. *Curr Opin Pediatr.* 2011;23:403-406.

Usatine RP, Sandy N. Dermatologic emergencies. *Am Fam Physician.* 2010;82(7):773-780.

120

Do Not Be Tricked Into Missing a Diagnosis of Henoch-Schönlein Purpura

Ankita Taneja, MD, MPH and Todd Wylie, MD

Henoch-Schönlein purpura (HSP) is the most common childhood vasculitis with an incidence of ~20 cases per 100 000 children annually. Though HSP more commonly occurs in the fall and winter and often follows an upper respiratory infection, no causal association between infectious agents and HSP has been clearly demonstrated. The peak age range is 3-15 years of age. It is more common in white and Asian children and in males (2:1 predominance).

HSP classically involves the skin, gastrointestinal (GI) tract, joints, and kidneys. Skin manifestations may begin with petechiae but ultimately develop into the classic palpable purpura rash of HSP. Purpura predominantly occurs in gravity-dependent areas, particularly the lower extremities and buttocks. Nonambulatory children may develop manifestations on the face, upper extremities, and trunk. GI symptoms generally follow onset of the rash and typically trail by ~1 week. Symptoms range from nausea, vomiting, and abdominal pain to intussusception, bowel ischemia, gastrointestinal bleeding, and rarely, bowel perforation. Intussusception is the most common GI complication of HSP, occurring in up to 3.5% of cases.

Joint symptoms of arthritis and arthralgia are often transient, migratory, and principally involve large joints of the lower extremities. Ambulation during the illness may be limited due to pain, but joint involvement does not lead to permanent articular damage or chronic disability. Symptomatic treatment is indicated for pain management.

Renal manifestations usually present within the first month following onset of systemic symptoms but may be delayed up to 3 months. Manifestations range from microscopic hematuria and mild proteinuria to nephrotic syndrome and renal failure. Hypertension may develop at the onset or during recovery from HSP. Most renal complications associated are mild, and the chances of recovery are good.

Other organ systems are affected less commonly. Males may experience scrotal or testicular pain with swelling and tenderness. Rarely, patients may have central nervous system involvement (eg, seizures and encephalopathy).

Extensive laboratory and imaging studies are generally not required but may help exclude other diagnostic considerations and evaluate for possible complications. For an example, normal platelets count and coagulation studies exclude thrombocytopenia and coagulopathy as an etiology for the purpura. At a minimum, however, a screening urinalysis should be obtained in all patients with suspected HSP to evaluate for renal involvement. If intussusception is suspected clinically, an abdominal ultrasound is the initial diagnostic study of choice.

Treatment is primarily symptomatic (pain control, hydration) in the absence of renal pathology or significant gastrointestinal complications. Nonsteroidal anti-inflammatory drugs (NSAIDs) are helpful for joint pain. However, NSAIDs should not be used if glomerulonephritis or gastrointestinal bleeding is present.

Abdominal and joint pain are reported less frequently in patients receiving glucocorticoids, but treatment with glucocorticoids is generally reserved for patients with abdominal pain that affects oral intake or is not improved by NSAIDs. It is critical to confirm that the etiology of abdominal pain is not secondary to intussusception or bowel perforation prior to initiating therapy.

There is no consensus on treatment of significant renal complications. Some experts advocate early pulse dose steroids for patients with nephrotic syndrome or glomerulonephritis followed by oral steroids. Decisions on this treatment should be made in conjunction with a nephrologist for long-term management.

Hospital admission is required for patients requiring intravenous fluids, those with significant gastrointestinal complications (eg, intussusception, GI bleeding), renal involvement, or for severe pain control due to arthritis.

KEY POINTS

- Think of the diagnosis of HSP with
  - Purpura, classically palpable, nonpruritic, and starting on buttocks and lower extremities.
  - Absence of thrombocytopenia.
  - Arthritis associated with HSP most commonly involves the knees and ankles and is self-limited.
- Check urine for hematuria and proteinuria to rule out renal involvement.
- Be in the lookout for any signs or symptoms of intussusception.

Suggested Readings

Gedalia A. Henoch-Schönlein purpura. *Curr Rheumatol Rep*. 2004;6(3):195-202.

Hetland LE, Susrud KS, Lindahl KH, Bygum A. Henoch-Schönlein purpura: a literature review. *Acta Derm Venereol*. 2017;97(10):1160-1166.

Tizard EJ, Hamilton-Ayres MJJ. Henoch Schonlein purpura. *Arch Dis Child Educ Pract Ed*. 2008;93(1):1-8.

Be Prepared to Accurately Diagnose and Support Your Patients With Erythema Multiforme

Corey W. Dye, MD and Madeline M. Joseph, MD, FAAP, FACEP

Erythema multiforme (EM) accounts for 1% of dermatologic outpatient visits. EM is an immune-mediated response to a variety of antigens both infectious and iatrogenic. The reaction is considered to be a type 4 T-cell–mediated immune response. The most common infectious agents responsible include herpes simplex virus (HSV) and mycoplasma pneumonia. The most common drugs associated with the condition include penicillins, sulfonamides, anticonvulsants, and NSAIDs.

Erythema multiforme presents as acrofacial target lesions. EM has historically been considered to be an inclusive spectrum of disease ranging from mild manifestations referred to as erythema multiforme minor to severe, life-threatening manifestations referred to as erythema multiforme major. This terminology has since fallen out of favor as research has shown significantly different pathogenesis between erythema multiforme and Stevens-Johnson syndrome (SJS) or toxic epidermal necrolysis (TEN), which were previously classified under erythema multiforme major.

Presentation and Defining Characteristics

Diffuse red targetoid lesions are the hallmark of EM, but depending on the stage of the disease process in which the patient presents, the rash can look very different. It can start as erythematous macule or sharply marginated wheal, in the center of which a papule or vesicle develops, thus creating the multiformity of lesions. This central lesion later clears forming the hallmark targetoid lesions. New lesions can continue to erupt and evolve over a course as long as 2-3 weeks thus allowing for a wide spectrum of presentations. With this in mind, a patient could present with only wheals mimicking urticaria, a mixture of differently staged lesions, or only targetoid lesions making accurate diagnosis difficult. When targetoid lesions do predominate, the rash most closely resembles erythema annulare centrifugum. Close examination with the use of a magnifying glass of dermoscope can help differentiate the two as erythema multiforme will have small petechiae within the eruption whereas erythema annulare centrifugum will not.

Erythema multiforme is typically a symmetrical eruption and can affect any part of the body although the hands and feet (including the palms and soles) and extensor surfaces of the upper and lower extremities are most common. Mucosal involvement is also common. However, there is rarely ever more than a single mucosal surface involved and the presence of multiple mucosal sites should raise the index of suspicion for early SJS or TEN. Mucosal lesions can present isolated or in conjunction with cutaneous lesions, and the oral mucosa is the most commonly involved. When involved, oral lesions seldom involve the gingiva, a characteristic that can help distinguish between erythema multiforme and gingivostomatitis secondary to HSV.

Management

There is no proven definitive treatment for EM, and the mainstay of treatment is supportive care. Specific recommendations include

- Specific etiologies:
  - If an offending pharmacological agent is identified, it should be stopped immediately.
  - If secondary to mycoplasma, treatment with an appropriate antibiotic is indicated.
  - If the patient has a history of EM attributed to HSV infection, acyclovir or another appropriate antiviral is indicated.
- Symptomatic treatment of pain and pruritus
  - Topical steroids
  - Antihistamines
  - NSAIDs
- If oral lesions present
  - Careful assessment of the patient's ability to tolerate oral intake to maintain nutritional and hydration status (may require admission)
  - Consider antiseptic/analgesic oral rinses
- If conjunctival/ocular lesions present, immediate ophthalmology consultation as this can lead to scarring and blindness.
- Systemic corticosteroids are NOT routinely indicated and have been shown to increase recurrence rates after cessation and prolong disease course.

KEY POINTS

- EM is a type 4 T-cell–mediated immune response to a variety of antigens.
- Hallmark rash is symmetric targetoid lesions but a wide variation exists as lesions continually develop and evolve over clinical course.
- Be wary and maintain a high degree of suspicion for early SJS or TEN.
- Treatment is primarily supportive, systemic steroids may worsen condition and lead to recurrence.

Suggested Readings

Gruskin KD. Rash—maculopapular. In: Fleisher GR, Ludwig S, Bachur RG, et al., eds. *Textbook of Pediatric Emergency Medicine*. 6th ed. Philadelphia, PA: Wolters Kluwer Health/Lippincott Williams & Wilkins; 2010:Chapter 62.

Hurwitz S. *Clinical Pediatric Dermatology*. 2nd ed. Saunders; 1993.

Read J, Keijzers GB. Pediatric erythema multiforme in the emergency department: more than "just a rash". *Pediatr Emerg Care*. 2017;33(5):320-324.

Sokumbi O, Wetter DA. Clinical features, diagnosis, and treatment of erythema multiforme: a review for the practicing dermatologist. *Int J Dermatol*. 2012;51(8):889-902.

Weller M, Clingenpeel J. *Erythema Multiforme*. Evanston, IL: PEPID, LLC; 2019. http://www.pepid.com

122

DKA: Being Overly Concerned About IV Fluids

Nadira Ramkellawan, MD and Frederick Place, MD, FACEP, FAAP

One of the rare but devastating causes of morbidity and mortality in patients with diabetic ketoacidosis (DKA) is cerebral edema. Although a number of theories exist, the exact mechanism remains elusive. One long-held theory was the hyperosmolar theory, fueled by studies in the 1980s that suggested patients treated with greater intravenous fluid volumes were at increased risk of cerebral edema and worsened outcomes. The hyperosmolar theory hinges on the understanding that DKA causes dehydration and high intracellular osmolarity in the brain. Rapid fluid administration could then results in a drop in the extracellular osmolarity, driving free water into the cell, thereby causing cellular swelling and cerebral edema.

For hemodynamically stable pediatric patients in the emergency department, the generally accepted initial bolus volume is 10 cc/kg of isotonic fluids (eg, normal saline), up to 0.5 L over 1 hour. A fluid deficit is calculated based on the reasonable assumption of 5% dehydration with mild acidosis and replaced slowly over the following 24-48 hours, while a 10% deficit is assumed for moderate to severe acidosis. Half-normal saline is traditionally used for replacement after the initial bolus, but normal saline may be continued and then changed to ½ NS based on trended sodium values. Hemodynamically unstable patients should receive a standard 20 cc/kg bolus or more until stable, followed by the slower deficit replacement. An insulin drip (0.05-0.1 units/kg/h) is started to correct acidosis only after completion of initial fluid resuscitation and establishing that the potassium is not low. Dextrose is titrated into the maintenance replacement fluids once the serum glucose is below 250-300 to prevent hypoglycemia while the patient is on an insulin drip.

Given the infrequency of cerebral edema in DKA, it has been difficult to adequately power studies to assess the true effect of our interventions in this at-risk population. However, within the last two decades, a number of studies and case series have been published that seem to reject the hyperosmolar theory and propose other more plausible mechanisms responsible for cerebral edema that do not implicate intravenous fluids.

The PECARN FLUID (2018) study to date is the only large-scale prospective, randomized controlled trial on the subject of fluid administration and cerebral edema in DKA. The study looked for differences in neurologic outcomes from giving fluids at different rates and/or different sodium concentrations. In the emergency department, every patient received an initial 10 cc/kg normal saline bolus. In the "fast" group, physicians were allowed to give one additional 10 cc/kg bolus, up to 1 L total, as deemed necessary. After the initial bolus, subsequent fluid administration was provided through four randomized arms: fluid deficit replacement either "slowly" or "quickly," with either normal or half-normal saline. The "fast" group assumed a deficit of 10% upfront, correcting half of the fluid deficit in the first 12 hours, delivering the remaining over the next 24 hours. The "slow" group assumed a deficit of 5%, replaced evenly over 48 hours. Although no statistically significant results were demonstrated between any groups, suggesting no difference between rate of rehydration or sodium concentration, there was a minimal trend observed with the "slow" rehydration exhibiting worse neurologic outcomes. While emergency department management was essentially the same as current recommended management, this study may further inform fluid deficit replacement practices within the first 24-48 hours.

The PECARN FLUID study revealed that some DKA patients presented with evident neurologic deficits prior to fluid replacement, supporting a newer theory that clinical or subclinical neurotoxicity may already be present on arrival and not due to subsequent fluid administration practices. Using newer radiographic imaging techniques, one large case series showed that up to 39% of patients with objective neurologic deficits had no apparent abnormality on brain imaging, with edema developing much later, subsequent to the initial clinical findings, suggesting that cerebral edema may be a downstream effect and not necessarily linked to intravenous fluid administration. Furthermore, sophisticated MRI studies have evidenced accumulation of water in extracellular spaces in patients with DKA, not intracellularly as posited by the hyperosmolar theory.

KEY POINTS

- In the emergency setting, judicious use of intravenous fluid resuscitation in hemodynamically stable patients in DKA may be safely administered.
- In the hemodynamically unstable patient, aggressive fluid resuscitation as necessary is still recommended.
- Fluid deficit replacement within the first 24–48 hours after initial resuscitation may be managed somewhat more aggressively than previously thought.
- Cerebral edema may actually be a primary manifestation of the neurotoxic effects of DKA and not secondary to fluid administration practices as previously feared.

Suggested Readings

Codner E, Acerini CL, Craig ME, et al. ISPAD clinical practice consensus guidelines 2018: limited care guidance appendix. *Pediatr Diabetes.* 2018;19(suppl 27):328 338. doi:10 1111/pedi.12767.

Glaser N, Barnett P, McCaslin I, et al. Risk factors for cerebral edema in children with diabetic ketoacidosis. The Pediatric Emergency Medicine Collaborative Research Committee of the American Academy of Pediatrics. *N Engl J Med.* 2001;344(4):264-269.

Kuppermann N, Ghetti S, Schunk JE, et al. Clinical trial of fluid infusion rates for pediatric diabetic ketoacidosis. *N Engl J Med.* 2018;378(24):2275-2287.

Muir A, Quisling R, Yang M, et al. Cerebral edema in childhood diabetic ketoacidosis. *Diabetes Care.* 2004;27(7):1541-1546.

Allowing Hypoglycemia to Surprise You in the Pediatric Patient Presenting With Gastroenteritis

Lindly A. Theroux, DO   and Scott W. Sutton, MD

Gastroenteritis is frequently encountered in the emergency department. Hypoglycemia can easily be an associated complication and needs to be considered. Understanding why this occurs and when to investigate further for alternative causes is paramount for emergency physicians.

Definition of Hypoglycemia

Historically, hypoglycemia was defined as a plasma glucose (PG) concentration of <40–50 mg/dL, but hypoglycemia is mainly a clinical diagnosis. First, the threshold for specific brain responses to hypoglycemia occurs at a variety of PG concentrations. Secondly, there is no specific PG concentration that can be defined as when brain injury will occur. Furthermore, while adult literature suggests basing diagnosis on symptomatic diagnosis, this can be challenging for young patients who cannot articulate signs and symptoms. Common symptoms of hypoglycemia include sweating, tachycardia, irritability, weakness, lethargy, nausea, vomiting, confusion, slurred speech, tremor, and seizures.

Etiologies of Hypoglycemia

The most common type of hypoglycemia is ketotic hypoglycemia. The typical presentation is a child 1-3 years of age who has been eating poorly, missed a meal, or has a gastrointestinal illness. The child is either difficult to arouse the next morning or begins exhibiting symptoms of lethargy or irritability. At the time of documented hypoglycemia (typically <50 mg/dL), high levels of ketones are found in the urine and plasma. During fasting, the main source for ongoing gluconeogenesis is skeletal muscle. The theory is that these patients are typically smaller for age, with low glycogen stores and limited muscle mass, coupled with high brain metabolism demands, which leads to hypoglycemia.

Most children with this diagnosis can have recurrent episodes but typically grow out of it with age. Other etiologies for hypoglycemia include inborn errors of metabolism, hyperinsulinism, hypopituitarism, adrenal insufficiency, and accidental ingestion (insulin, sulfonylureas, beta blockers).

Workup

Ketotic hypoglycemia is the most common etiology, and if urine ketones and acidosis is present, this is likely the cause. But, if a patient has had more than one episode and/or there are additional clues with the history and physical, this may warrant further investigation. One study by White et al. in 2018 suggests that all patients should have further studies to determine the etiology of their hypoglycemia as they cited an associated high-risk disorder in 10% of their 160 patients with hypoglycemia. The most important step is to obtain a "critical sample" to investigate the underlying cause. It is paramount that this is sent at the time of hypoglycemia to obtain accurate results. Critical sample includes serum electrolytes, insulin, C-peptide, cortisol, growth hormone, FFAs, lactate, beta-hydroxybutyrate (BHOB), and ammonia.

Treatment

Risk factors for hypoglycemia in association with gastroenteritis include female sex, neurologic symptoms of hypoglycemia, greater duration of vomiting than diarrhea, and use of water for rehydration (instead of glucose containing liquids). Once a child is found to be hypoglycemic, you must give dextrose. In mild cases of hypoglycemia (mildly low PG, few symptoms), patients can be trialed with PO dextrose containing fluids. Concerning more severe cases, the mainstay of treatment is IV dextrose. The "rule of 50" is commonly used to determine the amount and type of dextrose to use and is applied as such: the concentration of dextrose (10%, 25%, 50%) multiplied by the volume (5, 2, and 1 mL/kg) should always equal 50. The patient should have frequent glucose checks with repeat dextrose boluses as needed and or placed on a continuous infusion of IV dextrose.

KEY POINTS

- Have a low threshold to check a point of care glucose or plasma glucose in a child with gastroenteritis.
- Children at highest risk for hypoglycemia with gastroenteritis include toddlers that are small for age, with prolonged vomiting in the setting of gastroenteritis.
- Ketotic hypoglycemia is the most common etiology of hypoglycemia in conjunction with gastroenteritis.
- If a child presents with hypoglycemia on multiple occurrences, consider a broader diagnostic workup.

Suggested Readings

Heeley-Ray T, Nemeth J, Mitchell J. The prevalence of hypoglycemia in children with vomiting or decreased oral intake and irritability. *Pediatr Emerg Care*. 2012;28(4):333-335.

Levasseur KA, Tigchelaar H, Kannikeswaran N. Persistent hypoglycemia. *Pediatr Emerg Care*. 2013;29(7): 838-841.

Thornton PS, Stanley CA, De Leon DD, et al. Recommendations from the pediatric endocrine society for evaluation and management of persistent hypoglycemia in neonates, infants, and children. *J Pediatr*. 2015;167(2): 238-245.

White K, Truong L, Aaron K, Mushtaq N, Thornton PS. The incidence and etiology of previously undiagnosed hypoglycemic disorders in the emergency department. *Pediatr Emerg Care*. 2018. doi:10.1097/PEC.0000000000001634.

Do Not Forget the Stress-Dose Steroid in Hypopituitarism!

Jonathan Lee, MD, FAAP and Vivian Hwang, MD, FACEP, FAAP

Problem list: Panhypopituitarism. The thought of it can send providers' minds reeling trying to recall all the hormones, their pathways, feedback mechanisms, and implications on the patient in front of them. While every hormone is important, in the acute setting, do not forget the steroids!

A Brief Overview of Hypopituitarism

The pituitary gland is a midline structure sitting at the base of the brain responsible for the storage, excretion, and/or production of multiple hormones including the following: growth hormone, luteinizing hormone, follicle-stimulating hormone, thyroid-stimulating hormone, adrenocorticotropin, vasopressin, and oxytocin. While there can be single hormone deficiencies, reduced or absent levels of multiple hormones will lead to panhypopituitarism. There are many causes of panhypopituitarism and include genetic etiologies, cancer, sequelae from surgery/radiotherapy/chemotherapy, trauma, vascular events (Sheehan syndrome), autoimmune disorders (sarcoidosis, histiocytosis X, lymphocytic hypophysitis), infections (TB, neurosarcoidosis), and more.

Presentation

Depending on the deficient or absent hormone as well as degree of insufficiency, presentations can be variable. The specific presentation and diagnosis of each separate hormonal deficiency is beyond the scope of this chapter. However, clinicians treating ill-appearing patients with known panhypopituitarism, adrenal insufficiency, or on steroids long term must consider adrenal crisis.

Like all other hormonal regulation, ACTH secretion is mediated by positive and negative feedback loops. Corticotropin-releasing hormone (CRH) from the hypothalamus stimulates the anterior pituitary to release ACTH, which stimulates the adrenal gland to increase synthesis of steroid hormones. The cortisol released inhibits the secretions of CRH and ACTH. Cortisol is involved in many systems from cardiac, renal, to metabolism.

Lack of cortisol leads to decreased cardiac output and HYPOtension through its modulation of catecholamine response, HYPOnatremia through its regulation of free water balance, and HYPOglycemia through its regulation of glucose metabolism. With ACTH deficiency, HYPERkalemia may not be seen as the renin-aldosterone-angiotensin system is intact.

Do Not Forget to Stress Dose Steroids!

Patients with panhypopituitarism must be given STRESS-DOSE steroids to supplement the cortisol insufficiency during times of stress seen with any illness.

These patients are typically on daily replacement steroid regimens at the following doses:

Pediatrics: Hydrocortisone 7.5 mg to 15 mg/m^2/d divided into 3-4 doses.
Adults: Hydrocortisone 15-25 mg or cortisone acetate 20-35 mg, divided into 2-3 doses.

During times of stress, patients will need the following STRESS doses:

Pediatrics IM/IV: Hydrocortisone initial 50-100 mg/m2 once, max dose 100 mg. Followed by 100 mg/m2/d q6h.
Adults IV: Hydrocortisone 100 mg IV followed by infusion 200 mg/24 hours or 50 mg q6h.

STRESS dosing without concern for adrenal insufficiency:

Pediatrics IV/IM/PO: Hydrocortisone 30-50 mg/m2/d divided TID (~3-4 times usual daily dose) during illness with fever, diarrhea, vomiting, decreased intake or 100 mg/m2/d divided q6h for major illnesses and surgery
Adults: 2-3 times replacement dose for minor illnesses until recovery. For major illness/trauma/surgery, hydrocortisone 100 mg IV followed by infusion of hydrocortisone 200 mg/24 hours or 50 mg q6h IV/IM.

Commonly, patient will have an IM dose of hydrocortisone to self-administer prior to presentation in the ED. Do not forget to ask!

Not All Steroids Are Created Equal!

The preferred steroid for replacement is hydrocortisone due to its decreased side effect profile, mineralocorticoid effect, and ability to titrate vs prednisone and dexamethasone. Also remember that endogenous steroids have different effects! Putting aside sex hormones, the corticosteroids can have glucocorticoid effects—involved in the stress response—or mineralocorticoid effects—for maintaining blood volume and electrolyte balance. The steroid you choose to stress dose will affect these paths differently!

KEY POINTS

- Do not forget to stress dose patients who have adrenal insufficiency during times of illness.
- Stress dosing is ~3 times their normal dose for minor illness, higher for sepsis or major trauma/surgery.
- Signs of cortisol deficiency secondary to panhypopituitarism include HYPOtension, HYPOnatremia, and HYPOglycemia.
- HYPERkalemia may be present with primary adrenal insufficiency.

Suggested Readings

Bornstein SR, Allolio B, Arlt W, et al. Diagnosis and treatment of primary adrenal insufficiency: an endocrine society clinical practice guideline. *J Clin Endocrinol Metabol.* 2016;101(2):364-389. doi:10.1210/jc.2015-1710.
Capatina C, JAH W. Hypopituitarism. *Endocrinol Metab Clin North Am.* 2015;44(1):127-141. doi:10.1016/j.ecl.2014.11.002.
Park J, Didi M, Blair J. The diagnosis and treatment of adrenal insufficiency during childhood and adolescence. *Arch Dis Child.* 2016;101(9):860-865. doi:10.1136/archdischild-2015-308799.

125

Not Using Hydrocortisone for Treating Congenital Adrenal Hyperplasia (CAH)

Mahmoud Hamdan, MD, CDE, ABCL

"Is that baby a little girl or a little boy?" If you ever finish examining a baby and ask that question, your next question should be "Is this a child with congenital adrenal hyperplasia (CAH)?"

CAH is the most common cause of adrenal insufficiency in infancy. It is caused by enzymatic deficiency in the pathway that converts cholesterol to adrenal steroid hormones—including aldosterone, cortisol, and androgens. The three most common deficiencies that can cause CAH are 21-hydroxylase deficiency (90% of cases), 11-hydroxylase deficiency, and 17-hydroxylase deficiency. While CAH 21-hydroxylase deficiency newborn screening is routine, there are reported false-negative newborn screens. So keep CAH on your differential.

Of 21-hydroxylase deficiency cases, 70% are salt wasting because the body is unable to make aldosterone, leading to **hyponatremia** and **hyperkalemia**. Do NOT disregard this hyperkalemia. Metabolism then shunts these precursors toward cortisol production, but the 21-hydroxylase enzyme is also involved in that, so the child is unable to make cortisol—resulting in associated **hypoglycemia**. The precursors are then shunted on toward androgens, which is why female infants often have ambiguous genitalia. While easy to overlook in a sick infant, do not forget to do a quick genitourinary examination. Males do not display this characteristic change in external genitalia and are therefore more likely to present late with "salt-losing" features at age 1–2 weeks (vomiting, dehydration, and failure to thrive [FTT]). Less common types of CAH (11-hydroxylase deficiency and 17-hydroxylase deficiency) differ in that they result in excess mineralocorticoid production and therefore present with hypertension rather than hypotension.

The clinical presentation for CAH can be striking, with infants presenting with vomiting, dehydration, weakness, poor weight gain, poor feeding, and FTT—especially within the first 2 weeks of life in salt-losing CAH. Children may be hypotensive (21-hydroxylase deficiency) or hypertensive (11-hydroxylase deficiency) and may truly be lethargic. In females, the genitalia are ambiguous, and with more severe enzyme deficiency, more virilization is present. Most males have normal-appearing genitalia. Some may present with underdeveloped genitalia as in 17-hydroxylase deficiency.

These children may often present in extremis, and basic circulation, airway, and breathing (CABs) need to be addressed. They commonly have altered mental status, so remember the acutely reversible causes of altered mental status of hypoxia, hypoglycemia, and hyponatremia. These children will likely have hypoglycemia and hyponatremia. Whether CAH is on your differential or not at this point during your initial assessment, these children will likely have electrolytes checked and be given a 10–20 mL/kg IV fluid bolus for their hypotension. Reassess hydration. A quick look at their heart with ultrasound may give important information on cardiac squeeze.

On labs, hyponatremia, metabolic acidosis ($\downarrow$ HCO_3^-), and hyperkalemia will probably be seen. **Do NOT assume that hyperkalemia is a hemolyzed specimen**. Treat it appropriately with calcium for membrane stabilization, insulin, and glucose. You will probably be simultaneously evaluating sepsis, congenital heart disease, and other inborn errors of metabolism too. After stabilizing the patient and recognizing CAH, consultation with a genetics/metabolism/endocrinology service is ideal as well as involvement of a PICU team. Labs that may be ordered in consultation are adrenal hormones 17-OH progesterone, DHEAS, and cortisol. You may or may not have time to get an abdominal ultrasound looking for large adrenal glands.

When you have an increased suspicion for CAH and adrenal crisis, give hydrocortisone but not dexamethasone, methylprednisolone, or another steroid. Give hydrocortisone after drawing a baseline serum cortisol level. Hydrocortisone is the only parental steroid with mineralocorticoid activity for adrenal crisis. Start with 50-100 mg/m². If the body surface area cannot be calculated or is not available, use simplified age-based dosages:

- 0-3 years—25 mg
- 3-12 years—50 mg
- 12 years—100 mg

Then continue with the same dose divided every 6 hours for the next 24-48 hours.

KEY POINTS

- For any newborn that presents to the ED with vomiting, FTT, and poor weight gain, consider CAH in your differential diagnosis.
- Hydrocortisone is the only parenteral steroid with mineralocorticoid activity for suspected adrenal crisis secondary to CAH. No other steroid will more acutely help with an adrenal crisis.
- Do not disregard the associated CAH findings of hypoglycemia, hyponatremia, and hyperkalemia.

Suggested Readings

Chan CL, McFann K, Taylor L, et al. Congenital adrenal hyperplasia and the second newborn screen. *J Pediatr.* 2013;163(1):109-113.
Speiser PW, Arlt W, Auchus RJ, et al. Congenital adrenal hyperplasia due to steroid 21-hydroxylase deficiency: an endocrine society clinical practice guideline. *J Clin Endocrinol Metab.* 2018;103(11):4043-4088.

Overlooking the Clinical Scenarios That Place a Child at Risk for SIADH

Joseph Abraham Tanga, MD and Matthew Neal, MD, MBA

Introduction

Antidiuretic hormone (ADH) aids the kidney in water resorption by increasing the number of water transport channels in the distal tubule and collecting duct. The syndrome of inappropriate ADH secretion (SIADH) results in fluid retention and as a consequence, plasma osmolality and serum sodium [Na⁺] are inappropriately lowered. Excessive free water causes hyponatremia, which may lead to seizure, obtundation, coma, and potentially fatal cerebral edema with subsequent brainstem herniation. Multiple conditions found in the pediatric population can be associated with SIADH.

Pathophysiology

Increased tonicity of the fluid surrounding receptors in the left atrium and the hypothalamus coupled with signaling from cortical centers increases ADH. The lungs also have vestigial capacity to secrete ADH. As ADH increases, an increased number of water channels are formed in the collecting duct of the kidneys leading to increased water retention and diluted plasma.

Pathologic conditions causing SIADH in pediatric patients are broad but can be generally divided into four categories; CNS disorders, thoracic disorders, medication induced, and other causes. It is essential for the clinician to pay special attention to the possibility of SIADH stemming from these disease states. The most clinically relevant are listed below:

- **CNS:**
  - Infections: meningitis (>50% of patients), encephalitis
  - Prolonged hypoxia
  - Intracranial hemorrhage, tumor, head trauma
- **Thoracic:**
  - Infections: pneumonia, empyema, bronchiolitis,
  - Positive-pressure ventilation (20% of patients)
  - Asthma, cystic fibrosis, and pneumothorax
- **Medications:**
  - Psychoactive medications: carbamazepine, sodium valproate, and lamotrigine
  - Chemotherapeutics: cyclophosphamide, vincristine, and methotrexate
  - Pain medications: morphine, acetaminophen, indomethacin
- **Other causes:**
  - Pain, nausea, neuroblastoma, extreme hypothyroidism
  - Rocky Mountain spotted fever (70% of patients)

Diagnosis

Symptoms are usually evident as the plasma [Na$^+$] approaches 125 mmol/L. Symptoms range from the relatively benign such as headache, nausea, vomiting, muscle cramps, and tremors to the progressively more severe such as confusions, hallucinations, altered mental status, seizures, coma, and subsequent death.

The diagnostic approach to SIADH combines the interpretation of the clinical picture, diagnostic studies, and response to therapy. The patient's overall hydration status and edema are important factors to note on physical exam. Lab evaluation involves checking both serum urine tests. In the serum, sodium and osmolality will be low. In the urine, osmolality and urinary sodium will be high. Urine osmolality typically will be >100 mOsm/kg and urinary sodium >18 mmol/L.

Treatment and Management

Significantly ill patients with SIADH may present with severe lethargy, coma, or seizures. These effects are more likely to be seen in patients having acute rather than chronic hyponatremia. In correcting hyponatremia, we must always be mindful that a very aggressive correction may cause osmotic demyelination and severe neurologic consequences. However, patients with symptomatic and severe hyponatremia require action, and the risk of cerebral edema from hyponatremia is more significant than the risk of osmotic demyelination. Most children with acute-onset hyponatremia have not had time to develop cerebral adaption. Hypertonic saline (3%) is the most appropriate way to correct severe hyponatremia. Typical dosing patterns are 3 mL/kg administered approximately every 15 minutes. Each 1 mL/kg of 3% saline would be expected to increase the [Na$^+$] by 1 mmol/L. Seizures from hyponatremia can be difficult to control. They should be treated in conjunction with hyponatremia correction and will likely not fully abate until the sodium levels begin to rise.

KEY POINTS

- Clinicians may want to employ phenytoin or fosphenytoin in this clinical scenario as both have been shown to be inhibitors of ADH release.
- SIADH produces low plasma sodium and osmolality as a result of fluid retention. Urine as a result is concentrated demonstrating high urinary sodium and osmolality levels.
- SIADH is commonly associated with CNS, thoracic disorders, and some medications.
- Most strongly associated with SIADH are meningitis, pneumonia, head trauma, positive-pressure ventilation, and RMSF.
- Use 3% saline for correction of severe, symptomatic hyponatremia.

Phenytoin or fosphenytoin may be helpful in managing seizures associated with SIADH through their suppression of ADH release.

Suggested Readings

Fleisher GR, Ludwig S. *Textbook of Pediatric Emergency Medicine*. 6th ed. Philadelphia, PA: Willams & Wilkins; 2010:773-774.

Hasegawa H, Okubo S, Ikezumi Y, et al. Hyponatremia due to an excess of arginine vasopressin is common in children with febrile disease. *Pediatr Nephrol*. 2009;24:507.

Rose BD, Post TW. *Clinical Physiology of Acid-Base and Electrolyte Disorders*. 5th ed. New York, NY: McGraw-Hill; 2001:703.

Somers MJG. Fluid and electrolyte therapy in children. In: Avner ED, Harmon WH, Niaudet P, Yoshikawa N, eds. *Pediatric Nephrology*. 6th ed. Berlin, Germany: Springer-Verlag; 2009.

Forgetting Thyrotoxicosis in Patients With Vague Complaints

Mahmoud Hamdan, MD, CDE, ABCL

Most simply stated, thyrotoxicosis refers to excessively high thyroid hormone action in tissues. Hyperthyroidism, more specifically, is the most common cause of thyrotoxicosis and is a disease or condition that causes an increased production and secretion of thyroid hormone from the thyroid. Other causes of thyrotoxicosis exist, such as exogenous overadministration (eg, an intentional overdose or inadvertently taking too much levothyroxine), painless thyroiditis, and subacute thyroiditis. Both painless and subacute thyroiditis cause thyrotoxicosis by the release of previously formed thyroid hormone after the thyroid becomes inflamed. Painless thyroiditis is commonly caused by drugs. Subacute thyroiditis is often viral and commonly has associated fever. While these other causes of thyrotoxicosis exist, we are going to focus on hyperthyroidism for this discussion.

Graves disease is the most common cause of hyperthyroidism, accounting for more than 95% of all cases. It is more common in females (6:1, female:male ratio) and more common in adolescents. It is an autoimmune disease characterized by the increased production of autoantibodies that stimulate thyroid-stimulating hormone (TSH) receptors, leading to an increased secretion of thyroid hormone.

Symptoms of hyperthyroidism involve about every organ system and are often vague and nonspecific. There are often general symptoms of fatigue, weakness, weight loss, and heat intolerance. Cardiovascular symptoms include palpitations and hypertension. From the GI perspective, hyperthyroidism can cause nausea, vomiting, and diarrhea. Neurologically, the patient may have nonspecific findings of muscle weakness, fine tremor, or headaches. In general, these patients can have all sorts of nonspecific symptoms affecting about every organ system—so it is important to keep hyperthyroidism on your differential. In addition, an important thing to note is that hyperthyroidism can cause psychiatric/mood disorders, including hyperactivity, labile emotion, anxiety, and agitation, so do not just assume that an emotionally labile child is just a primary psychiatry issue. It may be hyperthyroidism. The earliest manifestations of the disease include changes in personality and anxiety without other symptoms.

If symptoms of hyperthyroidism are reported, ask about a past medical history/family history of other autoimmune diseases, not just thyroid disease. Other important questions to ask are regarding recent viral illnesses, a history of a painful neck, and a dietary history of consumption of thyroid supplements. Interestingly, there have even been reported cases of community outbreaks of "hamburger thyrotoxicosis" from contaminated hamburger meat with thyroid tissue.

Hyperthyroidism demonstrates a number of physical findings. Simple things that may be most easily noticed include tachycardia and mild proptosis and possibly hair loss, goiter, and fine tremor. These are not all the signs that can be observed. There can be chorea, hyperreflexia, café au lait spots, and lid lag, to name a few. Be sure not to glaze over the neck examination and miss a goiter. In Graves disease, the thyroid goiter should be homogenously enlarged, while in toxic multinodular goiter, there are irregular swellings.

Diagnostic screening for thyrotoxicosis is rather simple: assess a TSH level. If your suspicion is really high for thyrotoxicosis, then you may want to add a free T4 and free T3. If these tests are significantly abnormal, then additional labs/imaging tests might be desired after consultation with an endocrinologist, including TSI (thyroid-stimulating immunoglobulin), thyroid peroxidase, and radioiodine uptake on radiology.

So now you have thyrotoxicosis. How do you treat it?

1) Beta-blocker (propranolol or atenolol), for symptomatic treatment and to slow the heart rate, preferably prior to the start of antithyroid treatment
2) Antithyroid medications: methimazole once daily or propylthiouracil
3) If thyroid storm is present—meaning there is additionally fever and altered mental status—it should be managed in the PICU. You may also add potassium iodide drops and steroids at the request of the endocrinologist.

KEY POINTS

- Symptoms of thyrotoxicosis are often vague, so do not forget to keep thyrotoxicosis on your differential diagnosis.
- It is importance to check a TSH for a child who presents with new-onset psychological/psychiatric symptoms.
- Do a thorough neck examination on every patient who presents with new psychiatric or cardiac symptoms.

Suggested Readings

Lazar L, Kalter-Leibovici O, Pertzelan A, et al. Thyrotoxicosis in prepubertal children compared with pubertal and postpubertal patients. *J Clin Endocrinol Metab*. 2000;85(10):3678-3682.

Ross DS, Burch HB, Cooper DS, et al. 2016 American Thyroid Association guidelines for diagnosis and management of hyperthyroidism and other causes of thyrotoxicosis. *Thyroid*. 2016;26(10):1343-1421.

Not Considering Rickets as a Cause of New-Onset Seizures in Young Children

Joyce Granger, MD, FAAP

Rickets

Rickets is a well-described disorder caused by extreme vitamin D deficiency or resistance. Rickets is most commonly characterized by its skeletal abnormalities arising from poorly calcified bones. Children with rickets may exhibit bone pain, bowed legs, susceptibility to fractures, frayed and widened metaphyses, rachitic rosary on chest x-ray, or craniotabes.

Vitamin D deficiency rickets occurs due to impaired bone mineralization resulting from a lack of 1,25-dihydroxyvitamin D (the active vitamin D metabolite). Vitamin D obtained from dietary sources is synthesized from cholesterol via a pathway requiring interaction of a precursor molecule with sunlight. Further hydroxylation in the liver and kidney results in the active 1,25-dihydroxy vitamin D. Rarely, rickets can occur due to an inherited deficiency of 1-alpha-hydroxylase in the kidney (type 1 vitamin D–dependent rickets) or end-organ resistance to 1,25-dihydroxyvitamin D (type 2 vitamin–dependent rickets).

Fortunately, widespread vitamin D supplementation in cow's milk and infant formula led to a significant decrease in the incidence of rickets in the early 1900s. Vitamin D deficiency is still a real concern for certain individuals. Risk factors include breast-feeding infants without supplementation with formula or vitamin D, dark skin individuals, inadequate exposure to sunlight, prematurity, malabsorption disorder, liver disease, and renal disease. In fact, case reports and chart reviews have reported an increase in rickets cases in recent years.

In 2008, in response to a rising concern over vitamin D deficiency in infants, the American Academy of Pediatrics increased its recommendations for vitamin D supplementation in breast-fed infants from 200 to 400 IU/d.

Rickets-Associated Hypocalcemia

Though rickets is often identified by its skeletal characteristics, vitamin D is essential for the absorption of calcium and phosphorus from the intestines and their mobilization from bone. Calcium homeostasis is tightly regulated by the interactions of PTH, vitamin D, and bone metabolism. A failure of this regulation due to severe vitamin D deficiency can lead to hypocalcemia.

Neurologic manifestations of hypocalcemia occur when *ionized* calcium levels are <2.5 mg/dL (0.63 mm/L) and result from over excitation of neuronal membranes due to increased permeability of sodium. Initial signs of hypocalcemia may include perioral or peripheral paresthesia, muscle cramps, tremor, twitching, hyperreflexia, laryngospasm, stridor, or tetany. Although severe hypocalcemia (serum calcium <7 mg/dL) is unusual in rickets, these patients still warrant careful attention during initial vitamin D treatment. Treatment can lead to "hungry bone syndrome" where rapid bone recalcification results in a significant decrease of serum calcium levels and symptomatic hypocalcemia.

Treatment of Hypocalcemic Seizures

Unlike in older children, vitamin D deficiency in neonates and infants often present in an atypical fashion and may initially demonstrate severe symptoms of hypocalcemia such as seizures, tetany, and apnea. Therefore, it is important for EM providers to consider rickets and hypocalcemia in any pediatric patient presenting with an afebrile seizure.

Anticonvulsant medication is not an adequate treatment for hypocalcemic seizures. For children presenting with severe symptoms of rickets such as seizure, the preferred treatment is IV calcium infused over 5-10 minutes. Calcium gluconate is preferred over calcium chloride because it is less likely to cause tissue necrosis if extravasation occurs. However, calcium gluconate requires hepatic metabolism and may not be ideal in patients with hepatic failure or in low blood flow states. Continuous ECG monitoring is necessary during IV calcium infusion as it has been associated with bradycardia and asystole.

KEY POINTS

- Rickets (vitamin D deficiency) is on the rise and should be considered in pediatric patients with skeletal pain, fractures or abnormalities.
- Though rare, vitamin D deficiency can lead to severe hypocalcemia causing complications such as seizures, particularly in neonates and infants.
- EM providers should consider hypocalcemia in pediatric patients presenting with afebrile seizures and is treated with IV calcium gluconate when appropriate.

Suggested Readings

Bellazzini MA, Howes DS. Pediatric hypocalcemic seizures: a case of rickets. *J Emerg Med*. 2005;28(2):161-164.

Bloom E, Klein EJ, Shushan D, Feldman KW. Variable presentations of rickets in children in the emergency department. *Pediatr Emerg Care*. 2004;20(2):126-130.

Lazol JP, Cakan N, Kamat D. 10-year case review of nutritional rickets in Children's Hospital of Michigan. *Clin Pediatr*. 2008;47(4):379-384.

NEUROLOGY

Not So Simple, or Is It? Prepare to Care for Febrile Seizures in Children

James (Jim) Homme, MD, FACEP

Febrile seizures (FS) occur in 2%–5% of children ages 6 months to 5 years of age, with a peak incidence at 18 months of age. Presentation prior to 6 months (6%) or after 3 years of age (4%) is uncommon. Temperature of ≥38.0°C at the time of the seizure is required for the diagnosis, and FS are subcategorized as either simple or complex. A diagnosis of a simple febrile seizure (SFS) is made in neurologically normal children without history of prior afebrile seizures presenting with a generalized tonic and clonic seizure lasting <15 minutes, without evidence of focality or recurrence within 24 hours. Therefore, this diagnosis is presumptive at the time of initial evaluation unless the patient presents in a delayed fashion. Complex febrile seizures (CFS) are defined by any individual or combination of the following features: recurrence within 24 hours, duration longer than 15 minutes, witnessed focality at onset, or postictal temporary neurologic abnormality such as a Todd paralysis. Febrile status epilepticus (FSE) is a unique subset of FS where the seizure duration exceeds 30 minutes. Approximately 5% of cases of FS present as FSE. Two-thirds of FS encountered in the ED are SFS. Genetics clearly play a role in the development of FS as 10% of parents and 20% of siblings of a patient presenting with a FS will have a history of FS.

Regardless of the underlying diagnosis, any patient seizing for 3–5 minutes should receive abortive therapy in the form of a benzodiazepine. Prolonged FS are managed similarly to nonfebrile seizures until seizure termination.

Evaluation of a suspected FS requires a thorough history focusing on preceding events, seizure characteristics, and any past history of neurologic disorders that would disqualify the patient from the diagnosis. A head to toe physical examination with special attention to any focal or persistent neurologic abnormalities, signs of underlying CNS infection, and investigation for the source of the febrile illness is obligatory. Less sensitive temperature measurement techniques may miss lower-grade fevers, so rectal thermometry is recommended in young children with a suspected FS in whom tympanic, axillary, or temporal devices fail to record a fever. Workup of an SFS is targeted towards detection and management of the underlying cause of the febrile illness as the majority of patients with SFS will have no laboratory, lumbar puncture, neuroimaging, or electroencephalography (EEG) abnormalities. Lumbar puncture *should* be done in patients where clinical examination is suggestive of meningitis and *considered* in patients 6-12 months of age unvaccinated against *Hib* or *Pneumococcus* or on antibiotics at time of seizure. For patients presenting with a CFS, additional testing may be indicated based on seizure characteristics.

A great dissonance exists between the disquieting experience of the caregiver(s) and the commonplace response of the health care provider(s) to FS. Therefore, counseling of caregivers regarding the relatively benign nature of the FS, recurrence risk and actions to purse in the event of another seizure is a *critical* component of optimal care. There is no evidence of neurologic morbidity from FS (except in patients with prolonged FSE) and lifetime risk for epilepsy is only slightly increased over the baseline population, concentrating in higher risk subgroups. Approximately one-third of patients will experience a second FS, 15% a third, and <5% will have greater than three events. Risk factors for recurrence include family history of FS, younger age at onset, lower peak temperature, and short duration of fever prior to seizure. Patients with none of the risk factors have very low recurrence risk (~4%), while those with all four risk factors have much higher rates (~76%). Aggressive caregiver attention to fever management *does not* impact recurrence rates and potentially *increases anxiety,* and consequently it should be stressed that antipyretics are given for patient comfort only and not as a prevention strategy. Side effects of daily or intermittent antiepileptic agents greatly outweigh benefits and are not recommended. Discharge with abortive therapy can be considered for patients presenting in prolonged FSE or those at high risk for recurrence, but special caution is needed to ensure that caregivers know how to correctly administer and respond to side effects of these agents. Follow-up with a neurologist is generally not necessary except in cases of "outliers" such as extremes of age at initial presentation, high number of recurrences, FSE, or CFS with both focality and prolonged duration.

KEY POINTS

- Thorough history and physical examination focused on detection of source of the fever is typically the only workup necessary for patients with SFS.
- Caregiver education is a critical component of optimal care of FS.
- Subspecialty follow-up should be reserved for the "outliers" and not a routine part of FS care.

Suggested Readings

Kimia AA, Bachur RG, Torres A, Harper MB. Febrile seizures: emergency medicine perspective. *Curr Opin Pediatr.* 2015;27(3):292-297.
Subcommittee on Febrile Seizures, American Academy of Pediatrics. Neurodiagnostic evaluation of the child with a simple febrile seizure. *Pediatrics.* 2011;127:389-394.
Whelan H, et al. Complex febrile seizures—a systematic review. *Dis Mon.* 2017;63:5-23.

Status Epilepticus: The Most Common Neurologic Emergency in Children

Brittany Tyson, MD and Emily Rose, MD, FAAP, FAAEM, FACEP

Status epilepticus is the most common neurologic emergency in children with an estimated mortality rate of 3%. Status epilepticus treatment algorithms should be initiated in seizures lasting ≥5 minutes. Seizures are more difficult to stop when prolonged and serious permanent neurologic sequelae increase with increased duration and type of seizure. Status includes continuous seizure activity or recurrent activity without return to baseline.

Convulsive Status

Convulsive seizures may be generalized tonic-clonic with global motor activity and loss of consciousness or more subtle. Partial seizures have focal motor or sensory activity without loss of consciousness (simple) or altered consciousness (complex). Seizures in neonates can have quite subtle signs manifested by abnormal eye movements, lip smacking, rhythmic movements (eg, leg "bicycling"), or automatisms.

Nonconvulsive Status

Nonconvulsive seizures typically manifests as alteration in consciousness with negative symptoms (aphasia, amnesia, mutism) and/or positive symptoms (ocular movements, rhythmic twitching). EEG confirms clinical suspicion. Nonconvulsive status is difficult to recognize and diagnose. Permanent sequelae rises significantly after 60 minutes.

Management

Initial management priorities of the patient in status focus on avoidance of hypoxia and hypoventilation along with termination of the seizure. Glucose and electrolytes should be obtained on all altered patients and those with persistent seizures.

First Line

Benzodiazepines are the recommended first-line agents due to rapid onset of action. Lorazepam at 0.1 mg/kg (max 4 mg/dose) is preferred with IV access due to a longer duration of action (4-6 hours). Midazolam (0.1-0.4 mg/kg; buccal, intranasal, intramuscular, or intraosseous) can be given without IV access. Diazepam (2-5 years old, 0.5 mg/kg; 6-11 years old, 0.3 mg/kg; and >12 years old, 0.2 mg/kg) or lorazepam (0.1 mg/kg) may be administered rectally, but absorption is erratic. Repeat a second benzodiazepine dose at 5 minutes if seizure persists.

Second Line

Persistent seizures despite two appropriate doses of benzodiazepines (defined as refractory status) receive second-line antiepileptic agents. Options include phenytoin/fosphenytoin, levetiracetam, valproic acid, or phenobarbital. Initial dosing for all second-line agents is ~20 mg/kg. If a patient continues to seize, a second agent may be used and/or levetiracetam may be dosed up to 60 mg/kg. Phenobarbital remains the preferred agent for neonates in status. Valproate should not be used in children <2 years old or in those with metabolic disorders.

Third Line

Seizures that are persistent despite benzodiazepines and two second-line agents requires continuous antiepileptic infusion. Patients should be intubated at this point due to high rates of apnea. Infusion options include midazolam, propofol, or barbiturates (pentobarbital or thiopental). Successful treatments with ketamine administration (intermittent bolus or infusion) have also been reported in case reports/series.

Additional Treatment Considerations

IV pyridoxine should be strongly considered in patients with refractory status epilepticus particularly in young infants and those with potential INH toxicity. Pyridoxine-dependent seizures may occur in young infants and has been described in older children.

Hypoglycemia and hyponatremia require emergent treatment as seizures will not stop without correction. Glucose can be simply dosed with 2.5-5 mL/kg D10W. Hyponatremic seizures are treated with 3% NaCl at 5 mL/kg over 20 minutes just until seizure termination. If 3% NaCl is not readily available, 0.9% NaCl is an inferior but available alterative until hypertonic saline is obtained. Avoid overcorrection of the hyponatremia to decrease the risk of central pontine myelinolysis.

Patients with congenital causes of hypocalcemia such as DiGeorge's may also present with status epilepticus. These patients should be treated with 10% calcium gluconate at 1 mL/kg or 100 mg/kg over 5-10 minutes. Inborn errors of metabolism causing elevated ammonia levels can also cause refractory seizures with morbidity and mortality directly related to ammonia level and duration of altered mental status. Rapid removal through scavenging agents and dialysis is critical to optimize outcomes.

Antibiotics/antivirals should be administered for seizures with a suspected infectious etiology. Emergent neuroimaging is indicated only when intracranial mass, hemorrhage, or cerebrovascular event is suspected or in the persistently altered and/or seizing patient. EEG is imperative in the intubated and paralyzed patient or when nonconvulsive status is suspected to confirm the presence or absence of ongoing seizure activity.

KEY POINTS

- A status epilepticus protocol should be initiated within 5 minutes of seizure onset.
- Delayed treatment of seizures increases morbidity and mortality.
- Benzodiazepines given IV, IN, IM, or IO are first-line therapy for status.

Suggested Readings

Au CC, et al. Management protocols for status epilepticus in the pediatric emergency room: systematic review article. *J Pediatr (Rio J)*. 2017;93:84-94.

Glauser T, et al. Evidence-based guideline: treatment of convulsive status epilepticus in children and adults: report of the guideline committee of the American Epilepsy Society. *Epilepsy Curr*. 2016;16:48-61.

Minardi C, et al. Epilepsy in children: from diagnosis to treatment with focus on emergency. *J Clin Med*. 2019;8:39.

Santillanes G, et al. Emergency department management of seizures in pediatric patients. *Pediatr Emerg Med Pract*. 2015;12:1-28.

131

A Lower Threshold to Seize: Understand First-Time Seizure in Pediatric Patients

Nicholas Orozco, MD, MS and Emily Rose, MD, FAAP, FAAEM, FACEP

Seizures are relatively common in children with about 1% of children having an afebrile seizure by adolescence and up to 5% experiencing a febrile seizure before the age of 6 years. Over half of patients with epilepsy have their first seizure during childhood. Children have a lower threshold for seizures, and they can occur more frequently with acute events compared to adults. Identifying life-threatening causes of seizure and determining appropriate workup, treatment, prognosis, and follow-up are essential components of management.

Evaluation and Diagnosis

Broadly, seizures represent heightened excitability in the brain resulting in alterations in consciousness, motor, sensory, and autonomic function. There are many potential seizure mimics in children, and at times, the definitive diagnosis of seizure may be difficult to elucidate.

Seizures can be categorized as provoked or unprovoked. Provoked seizures include those arising from central nervous system (CNS) infections, metabolic derangement or toxic exposure, structural abnormalities, and head trauma. Provoked seizures are less likely to recur as long as the inciting event/condition is avoided. Unprovoked seizures frequently do not recur but may represent the beginning of epilepsy.

Unprovoked seizures have an unknown etiology during the initial evaluation.

CNS infections include meningitis, encephalitis, and abscess/empyema. Lumbar puncture is indicated with toxic appearance, meningeal signs, persistent altered mental status, or when an infectious etiology is suspected. Empiric treatment with antibiotics and antivirals should be initiated.

Metabolic derangements including hyponatremia, hypocalcemia, and hypoglycemia can also provoke seizures. Glucose should be checked immediately with any seizure to rule-out hypoglycemia as an etiology. Formula-fed infants may have hyponatremia from overdilution of formula. Labs should be considered to evaluate for an inciting cause in patients with metabolic disorders, diabetes, or those receiving intravenous fluids.

Head trauma in the setting of prolonged or persistent seizures raises the concern for intracranial hemorrhage or clinically significant contusion.

Indications for emergent imaging include seizures in patients with persistent altered mental status or focal neurologic deficits. Additional high-risk conditions include infants, those with malignancy, coagulopathy, sickle cell disease, ventricular shunt, cardiac disease, or prior stroke. Focal seizures are more commonly associated with abnormalities on imaging compared to generalized convulsions.

Seizures in neonates are often the presenting clinical sign of a CNS disorder and require imaging, septic workup, and admission. Additionally, approximately half of all infants <6 months have a clinically significant abnormality on imaging so more thorough evaluation should occur after a seizure in infancy.

Treatment

Active seizures should be treated with benzodiazepines and status epilepticus protocol initiated if seizures persist >5 minutes. If the seizure is provoked, treatment is targeted toward treating CNS infection, correcting metabolic derangement or toxic elimination, and managing the central structural lesion or injury. If the seizure is unprovoked and the patient is not an infant, has a normal mental status, and normal neurologic examination, then no emergent evaluation is required. Urgent outpatient follow-up should be arranged including EEG and possibly neuroimaging, ideally a magnetic resonance imaging (MRI).

Anticonvulsant medications are not initiated for the vast majority of first-time, brief seizures due to a relatively low recurrence risk balanced against medication side effects.

Prognosis

Patients with unprovoked afebrile seizure have a 20%-30% chance of recurrence within the first year. Those with developmental delay or CNS lesions have a 35%-40% recurrence rate. The risk of seizure recurrence is highest in patients with focal seizures or an abnormal MRI or EEG.

KEY POINTS

- Most children with a normal mental status and neurologic examination do not require emergent imaging or laboratory evaluation.
- All patients with an unprovoked seizure require follow-up EEG.
- Imaging and laboratory evaluation are required after a seizure with persistent altered mental status or focal neurologic deficits.
- Emergent imaging should be considered in high-risk conditions including infancy and those at risk for bleeding or intracranial complications.
- Anticonvulsant therapy is not initiated after a first afebrile seizure in the vast majority of patients.
- Seizure recurrence is more likely with focal seizures or an abnormal MRI or EEG.

Suggested Readings

Berg CD, Schumann H. An evidence-based approach to pediatric seizures in the emergency department. *Pediatr Emerg Med Pract*. 2009;6(2):1-26.

Chelse AB, Kelley K, Hageman JR, Koh S. Initial evaluation and management of a first seizure in children. *Pediatr Ann*. 2013;42(12):244-248.

Santillanes G, Luq Q. Emergency department management of seizures in pediatric patients. *Pediatr Emerg Med Pract*. 2015;12(3):1-28.

Sidhu R, Velayudam K, Barnes G. Pediatric seizures. *Pediatr Rev*. 2013;34(8):333-341. 342.

132

Pediatric Headache

Amy Briggs, MD and Emily Rose, MD, FAAP, FAAEM, FACEP

Headache is common in children; >90% of 18-year-olds have reported headaches. The prevalence of headaches among children increases with age and is most common between 16 and 18 years of age. In children <3 years, headache is uncommon; more serious etiologies should be considered and investigated.

Diagnosis

Headaches are broadly divided into two categories: primary and secondary. Primary headaches include migraine, tension, cluster, and chronic headaches. These types are generally of less emergent concern as they rarely represent a headache caused by a potentially life-threatening etiology. Alternately, secondary headaches have a wide range of causes that range from benign (eg, viral illness) to serious (eg, intracranial abscess or mass). History and physical examination guide the differential diagnosis. Patients with a history of coagulopathy, hemoglobinopathy, or vascular malformations are at higher risk for intracranial hemorrhage and thrombosis. Immunosuppressed or immune compromised individuals are at increased risk for infection. Neurofibromatosis is associated with intracranial masses. Severe hypertension suggests hypertensive crisis from secondary causes such as renovascular or aortic structural abnormalities, pheochromocytoma, or most commonly a toxic ingestion. Carbon monoxide poisoning should be considered with possible exposure, especially when household members experience similar symptoms.

The evaluation of atraumatic pediatric headache patients focuses on historical or physical examination red flags suggestive of an intracranial infection, vascular process, or mass lesion (Table 132.1). These red flags should prompt consideration of imaging. Pediatric patients presenting after a traumatic head injury should be risk stratified for clinically important injuries through utilization of a clinical decision rule. A detailed physical examination and a complete neurological examination (including visual fields and evaluation for papilledema) should be performed.

Imaging modalities include CT and MRI. MRI is superior in evaluating the posterior fossa and avoids ionizing radiation but is less available, takes longer, and may require sedation in young children. CT is preferred when emergent imaging is required.

Table 132.1 ■ Red Flags for Atraumatic Pediatric Headache That Should Prompt Consideration for Neuroimaging	
History	Physical Examination
Wakes patient from sleep or is worse with lying down	Ataxia[a]
Worse with Valsalva or exertion	Focal neurologic deficit (including visual fields)[a]
Occipital location	Abnormal eye movements[a]
Worsening over time (chronic progressive)	Papilledema[a]
Nausea or vomiting	Altered mental status[a]
Sudden or maximal in onset (thunderclap)	Seizure
Unresponsive to medical therapy	Fever
Duration <6 months	Nuchal rigidity
Age <3 years	Photophobia

[a]Patients with these findings should have neuroimaging in the ED.

Lumbar puncture should be performed when there is clinical concern for meningitis, encephalitis, idiopathic intracranial hypertension, or subarachnoid hemorrhage. Obtaining an opening pressure is critical for establishing a diagnosis of intracranial hypertension. CT prior to lumbar puncture is indicated in patients with altered mental status, signs of increased ICP, focal neurologic examination findings, VP shunts, or other neurosurgical history.

Treatment

Treatment of pediatric primary headache involves pain control and lifestyle modification counseling. Medications for primary headache include ibuprofen, ketorolac, prochlorperazine, triptans, valproate, magnesium, and dihydroergotamine. Steroids are commonly used for adults with headache in the ED, but evidence is lacking to support their use in pediatric patients. Opioids are not recommended.

Treatment of secondary pediatric headache is directed towards the underlying cause. Antipyretics may be used for fever.

KEY POINTS

- History and physical should focus on the red flags of pediatric headache.
- Severe unexplained headache in children under age 3 requires investigation.
- Patients with papilledema or abnormal neurologic examination should have emergent neuroimaging.
- Lumbar puncture should be performed when there is suspicion for meningitis, encephalitis, or idiopathic intracranial hypertension.
- MRI is the generally preferred headache imaging modality when available with CT utilized for suspected hemorrhage, hydrocephalus, or large mass lesions.

Suggested Readings

American College of Radiology. ACR appropriateness criteria. Headache—child. https://acsearch.acr.org/docs/69439/Narrative/

Lewis DW, Ashwal S, Dahl G, et al. Practice parameter: evaluation of children and adolescents with recurrent headaches. Report of the Quality Standards Subcommittee of the American Academy of Neurology and the Practice Committee of the Child Neurology Society. *Neurology.* 2002;59(4):490-498.

Little RD. Emergency department evaluation and management of children with headaches. *Clin Pediatr Emerg Med.* 2017;18(4):298-302.

Sheridan DC, Meckler GD, Spiro DM, et al. Diagnostic testing and treatment of pediatric headache in the emergency department. *J Pediatr.* 2013;163(6):1634-1637.

Pediatric Stroke Is Routinely Missed on Initial Presentation: Do Not Be Routine!

Danielle Wickman, MD and Emily Rose, MD, FAAP, FAAEM, FACEP

Pediatric stroke is a leading cause of childhood mortality. Additionally, stroke carries a risk of persistent neurological deficits, recurrent seizures, and/or recurrent stroke. Childhood stroke represents a true neurologic emergency, for which prompt diagnosis can affect treatment considerations and outcome. Unfortunately, most pediatric stroke is not diagnosed until >24 hours after onset. Despite potential neuroplasticity, two-thirds of children will have persistent neurologic deficits after a stroke.

Arterial ischemic stroke (AIS) comprises 50% of pediatric strokes and occurs secondary to arteri-opathy, cardiac etiology, prothrombotic states, or systemic disorders (such as sickle cell disease, sepsis, genetic disorders). Hemorrhagic stroke is relatively more common in children and has higher mortality compared to ischemic events (25% vs 10%). Common etiologies for hemorrhagic stroke include AVM (most common cause), cavernous malformations, aneurysms, tumors, and bleeding disorders. Athero-sclerosis (the most common cause of stroke in adults) plays almost no role in pediatric stroke.

Clinical Presentation

Signs and symptoms of pediatric stroke can be difficult to appreciate, contributing to diagnostic delay and poor outcomes. A key distinguishing feature is sudden onset of symptoms. Children are more likely than adults to have seizures and altered mental status as presenting symptoms. Focal neurologic deficits may be subtle, particularly in young children and may present as preferential arm use, limp, or loss of balance. Headache is present in approximately half of pediatric stroke and does not help differentiate from other diagnoses. Additional common symptoms include hemiplegia, unilateral weakness, sensory disturbances, dysarthria, aphasia, and dysphagia. Less common symptoms include mood or behavior changes.

The most common stroke mimics are migraines, seizures with Todd paralysis, peripheral CN VII paralysis, and conversion disorder. Other neurologic emergencies that are commonly found in potential stroke patients include meningoencephalitis, brain tumors, and traumatic brain injury.

Diagnosis

Diagnostic expediency can be improved with the implementation of a stroke protocol and consistent performance of a detailed neurologic examination on every child with focal neurological complaints, seizure, altered mental status, or behavioral changes. Laboratory studies including glucose, electrolytes, and coagulation profiles should be obtained. MRI is the most valuable imaging modality but may not be emergently available. MRI/MRA (especially with the addition of neck angiography) is more sensi-tive for acute ischemia, better evaluates the posterior fossa, and more effectively evaluates the etiology of stroke (or diagnoses common stroke mimics) in children compared to CT. Alternately, a noncontrast CT with a CT angiography if hemorrhage is demonstrated may be obtained if MRI is not emergently available.

Treatment

Current recommendations for therapy are based on adult studies and remain controversial due to both the lack of robust trials in children as well as the differing pathophysiology of stroke in children com-pared to adults. Acute antithrombotic therapy decreases mortality in ischemic stroke, but it is unclear if antiplatelet or anticoagulation therapy is superior. Hemorrhagic stroke should be managed with surgical intervention if indicated and reversal of bleeding diathesis. Emergent exchange transfusion decreases both morbidity and mortality from stroke in patients with sickle cell disease. Hemodynamic and neurologic supportive care is also important. Thrombolytics are controversial and not currently recommended routinely in children, particularly in children <12 years old.

KEY POINTS

- Pediatric stroke is a significant cause of childhood mortality and morbidity.
- Diagnostic delay is common and contributes to worse outcomes.
- Long-term consequences occur in the majority and include permanent sensorimotor deficits, language impairment, intellectual disability, behavior problems, and epilepsy.
- Early recognition and institution of neuroprotective measures is crucial to improving outcomes in children with stroke.

Suggested Readings

Felling RJ, Sun L, Maxwell E, et al. Pediatric arterial ischemic stroke: epidemiology, risk factors, and management. *Blood Cells Mol Dis.* 2017;67:23-33.

Kim H, Shoval H, Kim N. Pediatric neurologic disorders. In: Mitra R, ed. *Principles of Rehabilitation Medicine.* New York, NY: McGraw-Hill; 2019.

Rivkin M, Bernard T, Dowling M, et al. Guidelines for urgent management of stroke in children. *Pediatric Neurology.* 2016;56:8-17.

Ropper A, Samuels M, Klein J. *Adams and Victor's Principles of Neurology.* New York, NY: McGraw-Hill; 2014.

Schreiner TL, Yang ML, Martin JA, et al. Neurologic & muscular disorders. In: Hay WW Jr, Levin MJ, Deterding RR, et al., eds. *Current Diagnosis & Treatment: Pediatrics.* 24th ed. New York, NY: McGraw-Hill; 2018.

134

"Flaming Hot Pediatric Brains"—Anti-NMDA and Other Forms of Encephalitis

Anna Darby, MD, MPH and Emily Rose, MD, FAAP, FAAEM, FACEP

Encephalitis is inflammation of the brain parenchyma, which causes neurologic dysfunction. Presentation varies and depends on both the etiology and area of brain involvement. Patients may present with coma, altered mental status, seizures, focal neurologic deficits (motor or sensory), behavior or personality chances, and/or movement disorders. Encephalitis can be self-limited or may be an acute, life-threatening emergency where the cause must be identified and appropriate treatment initiated.

Etiologies

Encephalitis has many causes including an acute infection, postinfectious autoimmune dysfunction, and toxic or metabolic etiologies. Viruses (including enteroviruses, Herpesviridae, influenza, West Nile, and CMV) account for the majority of infectious cases, but bacteria, fungi, and parasites are also potential agents. Postinfectious autoimmune encephalitis (eg, acute disseminated encephalomyelitis/ADEM) frequently occurs 2-4 weeks after an often unidentified viral infection. Encephalitis may also be a presenting symptom of underlying malignancy. Ovarian teratomas are found in approximately half of adult females with anti-NDMA receptor encephalitis but in <10% of girls under 14 years of age.

Anti-NMDAR encephalitis has surpassed any other cause of encephalitis, including viral, as the most prevalent single cause of encephalopathy in the pediatric population, with the youngest reported case occurring in an 8-month-old. Diagnostic delay is common. Patients may have headache, fever, or a viral prodrome. Psychiatric/behavioral symptoms are predominant in the early stages and include mood, behavior or personality changes, visual or auditory hallucinations, and anxiety/agitation. Movement disorders, insomnia, and alterations of speech are common. Seizures, autonomic instability (less common in children compared to adults), and hypoventilation may also occur.

Diagnosis

Suspected cases of encephalitis should have a thorough neurological examination, basic laboratory studies, neuroimaging, and lumbar puncture with CSF Gram stain, culture, and viral PCR studies. Anti-NMDAR encephalitis is definitively diagnosed with either serum and/or CSF antibodies. Many cases of anti-NMDAR encephalitis have been documented preceding HSV infection. Approximately

60% of children with encephalitis have CSF pleocytosis. Neuroimaging abnormalities are seen in 60%-70% of cases. MRI is more sensitive than CT for abnormalities. EEG is abnormal in ~90% of patients and may have characteristic patterns to aid diagnosis.

Treatment

Treatment for encephalitis varies based on etiology. Most viral encephalitis is treated with supportive care without specific medication therapy. HSV encephalitis is an important exception as it is a devastating infection with significant sequelae. Acyclovir decreases mortality rate, but even with treatment, two-thirds of children have permanent neurologic sequelae.

Definitive diagnosis is difficult to obtain emergently, and typically, therapy should be initiated for HSV (with acyclovir) and broad-spectrum antimicrobial therapy (vancomycin + third-generation cephalosporin) until cultures are negative and a bacterial etiology is excluded.

A regimen of methylprednisolone, intravenous immunoglobulin (IVIG), and/or plasmapheresis is effective in the majority of cases of autoimmune encephalitis. If a concomitant malignancy is discovered, tumor resection should be performed in conjunction with the above treatments. Refractory cases may require other immunomodulating agents such as cyclophosphamide or rituximab.

Complications of encephalitis include status epilepticus, cerebral edema, and fluid and electrolyte disturbance. Seizures should be aggressively treated, but routine prophylaxis is not recommended. Patients with severe encephalitis are at high risk for acute neurologic and cardiorespiratory decline, and therefore, intensive monitoring is required.

Approximately half of children recover without permanent sequelae. Developmental delay and behavioral problems are common. Rarely, persistent focal deficits occur, including hearing and vision loss.

KEY POINTS

- Consider an organic etiology of all new-onset psychosis/altered mental status in pediatric patients.
- Recognize the constellation of symptoms in anti–NMDAR encephalitis: mental status changes > movement disorders > autonomic instability.
- Anti–NMDAR encephalitis requires a specific serum or CSF antibody test for diagnosis.
- Have a low threshold to perform LP in pediatric patients with vague neurologic symptomatology.
- Encephalitis patients are at high risk for complications and sequelae.

Suggested Readings

Armangue T, Titulaer MJ, Málaga I, et al. Pediatric anti-N-methyl-D-aspartate receptor encephalitis—clinical analysis and novel findings in a series of 20 patients. *J Pediatr.* 2013;162(4).

Bronstein DE, Shields WD, Glaser CA. Encephalitis and meningoencephalitis. In: Cherry JD, Harrison GJ, Kaplan SL, et al., eds. *Feigin and Cherry's Textbook of Pediatric Infectious Diseases.* 7th ed. Philadelphia, PA: Elsevier Saunders; 2014:492.

Florence-Ryan N, Dalmau J. Update on anti-N-methyl-D-aspartate receptor encephalitis in children and adolescents. *Curr Opin Pediatr.* 2010;22:739-744.

Lebas A, Husson B, Didelot A, et al. Expanding spectrum of encephalitis with NMDA receptor antibodies in young children. *J Child Neurol.* 2009;25(6):742-745.

Pediatric Vertigo: Differentiating Life-Threatening From Benign Etiologies

Daniel L. Johnson, MD, MSEd

Symptoms of dizziness and vertigo are often difficult to elucidate and differentiate, particularly in the young child. The differential diagnosis is broad and includes both benign and life-threatening etiologies.

History

It is first essential to distinguish between vertigo and pseudovertigo (also referred to as disequilibrium). The latter refers to complaints of "dizziness" without a rotary component, such as "light-headedness" or "floating" type sensations. Vertigo involves the perception of movement relative to the environment. These symptoms arise from a disturbance in the vestibular system and can be further classified into peripheral or central in etiology. Symptoms such as ataxia, vomiting, irritability, a desire to remain immobile, or nystagmus may be the only clue to vertigo in young or nonverbal children.

Other important historical elements to explore include the time course, onset, singularity or recurrence of symptoms, any recent head or ear trauma, fever or infectious symptoms, altered mental status, vomiting, ataxia, and medications or potential ingestions.

Examination

Vital sign abnormalities should be noted and addressed. Fever and/or hypotension may suggest infectious etiology such as central nervous system (meningitis/encephalitis/abscess) or peripheral (ear infections). Hypertension and bradycardia may occur with increased intracranial pressure, mass, or traumatic bleed. Imaging should be considered with traumatic injury. Altered mental status increases the likelihood that a central or life-threatening etiology is present.

Comprehensive ear and neurologic examinations should be performed. The ear may have evidence externally of vesicles suggesting Ramsay Hunt syndrome. Swelling, erythema, and tenderness over the mastoid suggest a diagnosis of mastoiditis. Within the ear, a bulging tympanic membrane with decreased mobility can be found in otitis media and hemotympanum. Otorrhea or tympanic membrane perforation may occur with trauma. Hearing loss or endorsed tinnitus is often associated with a peripheral cause of vertigo.

The neurologic examination includes mental status, evaluation of the cranial nerves, evaluation and characterization of any nystagmus, and assessment of cerebellar function. Nystagmus is the most common physical finding in vertigo. Unidirectional horizontal nystagmus suggests a peripheral cause, whereas bidirectional or vertical nystagmus more commonly indicates a central cause. Abnormal cerebellar tests or true gait abnormalities are also concerning for central etiologies of vertigo.

Differential

The most common etiologies of peripheral vertigo vary by age. Congenital causes and anatomic anomalies usually present early in life. Otitis media is more common in younger children than is benign paroxysmal vertigo of childhood (BPVC). BPVC occurs in children <5 years. Patients have severe symptoms of vertigo often with nausea/vomiting for brief episodes triggered by movement. Family history of migraines is commonly seen in this condition. Nearly 20% of children with classic migraines have aura with vertigo. Basilar migraines are also often accompanied by vertigo.

Labyrinthitis (inflammation of the vestibular apparatus) presents with sudden-onset hearing loss and vertigo. Vestibular neuritis has more severe vertigo but not hearing loss. Ménière disease (ear fullness, vertigo, and sensorineural hearing loss) is often associated with congenital malformations of the ear. Vertigo occurs in 30%–50% of patients with multiple sclerosis and may be of either peripheral or central involvement and is neurologic in nature. Central vertigo in children may be caused by CNS tumors (including acoustic neuromas), infections, inflammation, and less commonly stroke.

Treatment

When a cause is identified, appropriate treatment and evaluation should ensue. Symptomatic otitis media is treated with analgesics and antibiotics. Evaluation for meningitis or mastoiditis when clinically suggested should occur and treatment should be initiated. Concern for CNS infection warrants empiric antibiotic and antiviral therapy, advanced imaging, and emergent lumbar puncture. Traditional adult treatments for peripheral vertigo such as meclizine are generally avoided in children under 12, although they can be considered for severe cases. The Epley maneuver is useful in children with BPVC. Standard migraine therapies are effective treatment for migrainous vertigo.

KEY POINTS

- Differentiating true vertigo vs pseudovertigo can be difficult in children by history alone and requires caregiver corroboration and a detailed physical examination.
- Signs of severe infection or trauma should prompt appropriate workup and treatments.
- Peripheral vertigo may have otic complaints including tinnitus. Gait abnormalities and cerebellar findings are concerning for central etiologies.

Suggested Readings

Callebrant ML, Mandel EM. Balance disorders in children. *Neurol Clin*. 2005;23(3):807-829.
Gioacchini FM, et al. Prevalence and diagnosis of vestibular disorders in children: a review. *Int J Pediatr Otorhinolaryngol*. 2014;78:718.
Goldstein A. Child Neurology Foundation. Vertigo. https://www.childneurologyfoundation.org/disorders/vertigo/.
Raucci U, et al. Vertigo/dizziness in pediatric emergency department: five years' experience. *Cephalgia*. 2016;36(6):593.
Ravid S, et al. A simplified diagnostic approach to dizziness in children. *Pediatr Neurol*. 2003;29:317.

Be Able to Scrutinize the Causes of Pediatric Ataxia

Kelsey Ford Bench, MD and Emily Rose, MD, FAAP, FAAEM, FACEP

Ataxic children have impaired coordination and balance commonly due to cerebellar pathway dysfunction. An unsteady or wide-based gate is common. Etiologies range from benign, self-limiting processes to progressive degenerative diseases. History and detailed physical examination frequently determine the likely cause.

Life Threatening

Many serious etiologies of ataxia cause mass effect or increased intracranial pressure (ICP). Common associated symptoms are vomiting, headache, and papilledema.

Infection

Typically, ataxia caused by infection will have other systemic signs of illness. Rarely, ataxia can be the first sign of developing infection. Cerebellar abscesses often progress from untreated otitis media or mastoiditis. Fever, increased ICP, and meningismus may be present. Brainstem encephalitis and cerebellitis (2% of ataxia) may develop rapid posterior fossa edema and associated high morbidity and mortality. Patients with cerebellitis have abnormal CSF and EEG changes.

Acute Disseminated Encephalomyelitis
Acute disseminated encephalomyelitis (ADEM) is a postinfectious inflammatory demyelinating disease (2% of ataxia). Most patients have multifocal neurological signs on examination.

Intracranial Hemorrhage
Rapidly progressive symptoms occur with bleeding into the posterior fossa. Vascular malformations, hemorrhage within a tumor, and trauma are the most common causes.

Tumors
Approximately half of all childhood tumors arise in the cerebellum or brainstem. Symptoms of ataxia are gradual and accompanied by signs of increased ICP, including morning headaches and nausea and vomiting. Concomitant papilledema and other neurological deficits are common.

Opsoclonus-Myoclonus-Ataxia
This condition presents with severe ataxia, opsoclonus (chaotic ocular movements), and myoclonus. It is commonly a paraneoplastic disorder associated with neuroblastoma.

Stroke
Ataxia may occur with stroke in at-risk patients if the cerebellum or vertebrobasilar vessels are involved.

Benign Etiologies
Benign causes of ataxia are by far more common than life-threatening etiologies. These conditions are often brief and self-limiting.

Acute Cerebellar Ataxia
Acute cerebellar ataxia is an autoimmune postinfectious focal encephalitis. It is the most common cause of pediatric ataxia accounting for ~50% of cases. The condition occur most commonly in children <6 years. Children often have lack of coordination, alteration in tone, sensory loss, and/or involuntary movements. Notably, these patients are otherwise well appearing, alert, and without signs of infection. Symptom resolution occurs in 2 weeks to 2-3 months without treatment.

Guillain-Barre Syndrome
Guillain-Barre syndrome (GBS) is an acute postinfectious demyelinating disorder. Symptoms are primarily ascending motor weakness though sensory involvement may occur. The Miller Fisher variant presents with the triad of ataxia, areflexia, and ophthalmalgia. Symptoms will often progress over several days.

Toxins
Many medications and illicit drugs cause pediatric ataxia, accounting for 10%-30% of cases. Mental status changes (confusion, lethargy) and slurred speech are common. Antiepileptic medications, alcohol, illicit drugs, lead, and carbon monoxide are important culprits of accidental and intentional ingestions.

Migraines
Ataxia may occur with specific migraine syndromes such as basilar or familial hemiplegic migraines. Headache need not be present.

Labyrinthitis and Benign Paroxysmal Vertigo
Vertigo-inducing conditions may present as ataxia, particularly in the young child.

Evaluation

Physical Examination

Mental status evaluation and detailed neurologic assessment of each patient should occur. Evaluate for concomitant focal deficits, nystagmus, speech disturbances, coordination, and signs of increased ICP.

Laboratory

Blood glucose and metabolic panels should be obtained in all ataxic patients. Alcohol and toxicology screens may assist diagnosis. Cerebrospinal fluid should be obtained if acute infection is suspected. Many demyelinating conditions may have elevated CSF protein (though 20% may be normal, and lumbar puncture is not always required).

Imaging

Neuroimaging should be obtained in children with ataxia plus altered levels of consciousness, cranial neuropathies, focal neurological deficits, signs of elevated ICP, or a history of trauma. MRI is the best modality, better visualizing the posterior fossa and at demonstrating findings of demyelinating diseases and encephalitis.

KEY POINTS

- Most commonly, pediatric ataxia is benign and self-limited.
- Acute cerebellar ataxia accounts for 50% of pediatric ataxia.
- Posterior fossa tumors typically present with focal neurologic deficits and symptoms of increased ICP.
- Toxins are an important cause of ataxia in children.
- Abrupt onset in symptoms may be due to traumatic, infectious, postinfectious, or toxic etiology.

Suggested Readings

Casselbrant ML, et al. Balance disorders in children. *Neurol Clin.* 2005;23:807.
Dinolfo E. Evaluation of ataxia. *Pediatr Rev.* 2001;22(5):177-178.
Friday JH. Ataxia. In: Fleisher GR, Ludwig SL, eds. *Textbook of Pediatric Medicine.* 6th ed. Philadelphia, PA: Lippincott Williams & Wilkins; 2010:164.
Ryan MM, et al. Acute ataxia in childhood. *J Child Neurol.* 2003;18:309.

Muscular Dystrophy

Carlee Carranza, DO and Emily Rose, MD, FAAP, FAAEM, FACEP

Muscular dystrophy (MD) is a heterogeneous group of degenerative muscle disorders characterized by progressive weakness. Males are predominantly affected. The age of presentation varies by subtype; most present with progressive muscular weakness and/or hypotonia. The majority involve an absence or deficiency of dystrophin, which is necessary for stabilization of skeletal and cardiac muscle fibers. Without stabilization, these fibers cannot sustain normal contraction forces and undergo necrosis and replacement with adipose and connective tissue. This reorganization affects multiple organ systems and results in diminishing pulmonary function, progressive heart failure, dysphagia, and musculoskeletal weakness.

Respiratory

One of the hallmarks of MD is progressive weakness of respiratory musculature, contributing to hypoventilation, hypercarbia, ventilation/perfusion mismatch, decreased cough and mucous clearance, atelectasis, and respiratory distress. The patient's baseline respiratory status/function helps guide management. Early consultation is useful though intubation may be required emergently prior to the ability to mobilize resources.

Tachypnea may be subtle or absent despite significant respiratory distress. During acute illness, children with MD have weak pulmonary musculature and are frequently not be able to mount an adequate respiratory response with increased work of breathing. Even a small degree of hypoxemia (eg, oxygen saturation <95%) should trigger immediate intervention. Consider noninvasive positive pressure ventilation (NIPPV) early in the setting of respiratory distress. Rapid desaturation may occur due to poor reserve and hypoventilation, and therefore, aggressive preoxygenation methods should be utilized prior to intubation, including high-flow nasal cannula and NIPPV if necessary. If intubation is required, a nondepolarizing paralytic must be used (eg, rocuronium) as depolarizing agents (eg, succinylcholine) may induce life-threatening hyperkalemia and rhabdomyolysis.

Cardiac

In Duchenne's and some other forms of MD, cardiac musculature undergoes necrosis and replacement with fibrofatty tissue, resulting in cardiomyopathy and congestive heart failure (CHF). With disease progression, CHF is a common etiology of significant morbidity and mortality. Most patients are non-ambulatory when the cardiac ejection fraction decreases limiting clinical clues of CHF exacerbation. Dyspnea can be a predominant yet nonspecific symptom of heart failure. Life-threatening arrhythmias are also common, including ventricular tachycardia and fibrillation. Many patients require automatic internal cardiac defibrillators (AICD).

Endocrine

Glucocorticoid therapy forms the cornerstone of MD management to prevent disease progression and prolong ambulation. Treatment is initiated in the majority of patients within the first decade of life. In the setting of an acute illness, trauma, fracture, or fulminant respiratory distress, stress dose steroids should be administered to compensate for relative adrenal insufficiency. Hydrocortisone should be given: 50 mg for those <2 years and 100 mg for older children.

Musculoskeletal

MD patients frequently fall as weakness progresses and the ability to ambulate declines. Chronic steroid use and repeated trauma significantly increase the risk of both long bone and vertebral fractures. Even seemingly low-energy mechanisms such as transferring patients from vehicle to wheelchair can precipitate a fracture. Consider spinal or long bone radiography in the setting of back pain or bony tenderness regardless of the mechanism. These patients are also at risk for posttraumatic embolic events.

KEY POINTS

- Muscular dystrophy results in dysfunction of multiple organ systems, particularly pulmonary, cardiac, and musculoskeletal.
- MD creates a vulnerability to any respiratory illness and typical warning signs of respiratory distress may be lacking. Therefore, utilize respiratory support early as symptoms or respiratory distress may be subtle.
- Avoid depolarizing neuromuscular blocking agents such as succinylcholine as these can result in hyperkalemia and rhabdomyolysis.
- MD patients frequently have cardiac arrhythmias and complications of heart failure.
- Due to chronic corticosteroid use, stress dose steroids should be administered to MD patients with acute infections or trauma.

Fractures are common and may occur with minimal or no trauma. Maintain a low threshold for imaging.

Suggested Readings

Buddhe S, et al. Cardiac management of the patient with Duchenne muscular dystrophy. *Pediatrics*. 2018;142(suppl 2):S72–S81.

Manzur AY, Kuntzer T, Pike M, Swan AV. Glucocorticoid corticosteroids for Duchenne muscular dystrophy. *Cochrane Database Syst Rev.* 2008;1:CD003725.

Noritz G, et al. Primary care and emergency department management of the patient with Duchenne muscular dystrophy. *Pediatrics*. 2018;142(suppl 2):S90–S98.

Sheehan DW, et al. Respiratory management of the patient with Duchenne muscular dystrophy. *Pediatrics*. 2018;142(suppl 2):S62–S71.

Skull Fractures: When Do We Really Need to Know They Are There?

Mark S. Mannenbach, MD

Skull fractures are common after injury events in children. Infants and young children are at increased risk due to the presence of more membranous bone, which is thin relative to that of older children. Skull fractures in infants result mainly from falls but may represent physical abuse. Older children and adolescents suffer skull fractures usually as result of motor vehicle crashes or sports-related injuries.

Fractures occur in any bone of the skull although the parietal bone is most often involved. Children with skull fracture typically present with soft tissue swelling or hematoma overlying the fracture site. The scalp hematoma may become progressively more evident overlying the fracture site leading to an apparent delay in seeking care as many children including infants will have little in the way of symptoms with an isolated injury resulting from short-distance falls. However, scalp hematomas have been found in multiple studies to be sensitive but not specific in predicting skull fractures.

Decisions regarding imaging of infants and children with head injury should be based upon reliable decision-making aids such as the PECARN head injury study or whether there is specific concern for physical child abuse. Skull fractures can be discovered as incidental findings with head CT imaging or with dedicated plain skull radiographs as part of a complete skeletal survey.

Linear skull fractures are the most common type of fracture seen in pediatric patients accounting for up to 90% of all fractures. Most linear skull fractures require no specific intervention. If there is no associated intracranial hemorrhage, abnormal neurologic exam, or concern for physical trauma abuse, outpatient management with a reliable caregiver is appropriate.

The depressed skull fracture includes any skull fracture in which the bone fragment is depressed below the inner table of the skull. Typically management involves operative elevation of the depressed skull fragment if there is a 1-cm or greater depression or the depth is greater than the thickness of the skull.

One potential complication of a skull fracture is the development of a leptomeningeal cyst or "growing" fracture. These fractures result from a tear in the dura underlying the fracture followed by herniation of meningeal tissue into the fracture line. These fractures are more likely to occur in patients with depressed or larger and more widely diastatic fractures at presentation. Growing fractures can present weeks or months after the initial injury and can be visualized as a "boggy" or pulsatile soft tissue mass. The concern for the development of a growing fracture is often the rationale for recommended follow-up with a neurosurgeon.

Fractures to the skull base are unique in that they may lead to an increased risk for the development of intracranial infection. Basilar skull fractures account for up to 20% of all pediatric skull fractures and often have the classic presentation of periorbital ecchymosis ("raccoon eyes"), postauricular mastoid ecchymosis ("Battle sign"), hemotympanum, or CSF rhinorrhea or otorrhea. Controversy exists regarding the need for antibiotic prophylaxis for basilar skull fractures with proponents arguing for a reduced risk of infection and skeptics raising concern for the possible development of subsequent meningitis due to resistant bacteria. Similar to children with isolated linear skull fractures, patients with basilar skull fracture who have a normal neurologic exam, no associated intracranial pathology on head CT imaging, and no evidence of CSF leak may be safely discharged to home with reliable caregivers. Decision-making regarding acute management including potential surgical intervention and the use of antibiotics as well as a plan for follow-up should be made in collaboration with a neurosurgeon.

KEY POINTS

- Skull fractures are common injuries to children and especially infants after falls.
- Imaging studies should be obtained for patients with concern for associated intracranial pathology or for physical child abuse.
- Many children with isolated skull fractures can be safely discharged home with reliable caregivers if there are no associated intracranial abnormalities, abnormal neurologic findings, or concerns for physical abuse.
- Children with isolated linear skull fractures should have a follow-up plan established in the event that a "growing" fracture or leptomeningeal cyst develops.

Suggested Readings

Einhorn A, Mizrahi EM. Basilar skull fractures in children: the incidence of CNS infection and the use of antibiotics. *Am J Dis Child*. 1978;132:1121-1124.
Kuppermann N, Holmes JF, Dayan PS, et al. Identification of children at very low risk of clinically-important brain injuries after head trauma: a prospective cohort study. *Lancet*. 2009;374:1160-1170.
Powell EC, Atabaki SM, Wootton-Gorges S, et al. Isolated linear skull fractures in children with blunt head trauma. *Pediatrics*. 2015;135:e851-e857.
Woestman R, Perkin R, Serna T, et al. Mild head injury in children: identification, clinical evaluation, neuroimaging, and disposition. *J Pediatr Health Care*. 1998;12:288-298.

When a River Does Not Run Through It—Prepare to Manage Pediatric Hydrocephalus

Flavien Leclere, MD, MA and Emily Rose, MD, FAAP, FAAEM, FACEP

Hydrocephalus is the most common surgically correctable neurologically disorder in children. An imbalance between cerebrospinal fluid (CSF) production and absorption leads to excessive fluid within the cerebral ventricles and/or subarachnoid spaces. This, in turn, produces ventricular dilation and increased intracranial pressure (ICP).

Two broad subsets exist: (1) communicating hydrocephalus, where CSF is inadequately absorbed without obstruction and, most commonly, (2) noncommunicating/obstructive hydrocephalus, where CSF flow from the ventricles to the subarachnoid spaces is obstructed.

Hydrocephalus develops from both congenital and acquired etiologies. Most cases are congenital and present at birth or soon after. Postinfectious and posthemorrhage hydrocephalus are, respectively, the single most common causes internationally and in the United States.

Diagnosis

Signs and symptoms of hydrocephalus vary according to age, etiology, and speed of development. In children <2 years of age, the cranial sutures remain open leading to head enlargement as the main presenting sign. Other clinical features include irritability, lethargy, vomiting, abnormal head shape, bulging anterior fontanelle, splaying of cranial sutures, prominent scalp veins, downward displacement of eyes ("setting sun" sign), optic nerve atrophy, nystagmus and random eye movement, increased lower extremity deep tendon reflexes and muscle tone, and growth retardation. Symptoms increase in severity with disease progression. Older children with fused sutures present with signs of increased ICP such as morning headache, visual complaints, and seizures. Physical examination shows evidence of increased ICP including papilledema, spasticity of lower limbs, hyperreflexia, abnormal hypothalamic functions, and other cranial nerve (III, IV, VI) abnormalities.

The diagnosis of hydrocephalus can be suspected based on symptoms but must be confirmed with imaging (CT or MRI). While CT is typically more available, both provide accurate assessment of ventricular size, extracerebral spaces, and site of obstruction. MRI is the preferred modality, providing radiation sparing increased anatomic detail.

Management

Hydrocephalus is a surgical disorder, and acute obstruction represents a surgical emergency. Surgical intervention is occasionally initially deferred in young, asymptomatic children. Urgent CSF diversion procedures should be performed on patients with persistent head growth, neurological deficits, or symptoms attributable to hydrocephalus. In patients with acute rapidly progressive hydrocephalus, external ventricular drainage (EVD) catheters can be emergently placed at bedside as a lifesaving procedure. Drugs such as isosorbide, which produce hyperosmotic diuresis, and acetazolamide, which decrease the secretion of CSF, are less effective therapies that may be used as temporizing measures to decrease ICP and for patients too unstable for surgery. Diuretics in newborn infants with posthemorrhagic hydrocephalus should not be used as they are associated with complications and generally not effective at decreasing ICP.

Complications

In patients with indwelling shunts, the presentation of shunt malfunction is similar to the presentation of hydrocephalus and can develop rapidly. Malfunctions occur at any segment of the shunt with mechanical failure most common during the first year after placement. The majority of obstructions occur at the ventricular catheter site. Fractured tubing accounts for ~15% of shunt malfunctions. Shunt migration and excessive CSF drainage are other common complications. Shunt infections may also occur (~5%-15% of patients), most commonly in the first 6 months after placement.

Imaging is required in all symptomatic patients, and an emergent neurosurgery consult should be placed early in the evaluation. A shunt tap with fluid removal may be performed as a temporizing measure to relieve increased ICP due to malfunction before operative intervention. Inability to draw fluid from the shunt reservoir may indicate proximal shunt hardware malfunction. Febrile or toxic-appearing patients with indwelling hardware should also be evaluated and treated for meningitis.

KEY POINTS

- Most cases of hydrocephalus in children are due to obstruction of CSF flow.
- Common signs and symptoms of hydrocephalus include headaches, irritability, behavior changes, developmental delays, vomiting, and lethargy.
- The diagnosis of hydrocephalus is established with neuroimaging.

- CSF diversion procedures are lifesaving and the current gold standard treatment for patients with hydrocephalus.
- Shunt malfunction and infection are the most common complications after surgical intervention for hydrocephalus.

Suggested Readings

Flannery AM, Mitchell L. Pediatric hydrocephalus: systematic literature review and evidence-based guidelines. Part 1: introduction and methodology. *J Neurosurg Pediatr.* 2014;14(suppl):3-7.

Kahle KT, Kulkarni AV, Limbrick DD Jr, Warf BC. Hydrocephalus in children. *Lancet.* 2016;387:788-799.

Rizvi R, Anjum Q. Hydrocephalus in children. *J Pak Med Assoc.* 2005;55(11):503-507.

Wright Z, Larrew TW, Eskandari R. Pediatric hydrocephalus: current state of diagnosis and treatment. *Pediatr Rev.* 2016;37(11):478-490.

Be Prepared to Troubleshoot and Manage Shunts

Seema Shah, MD

Medically complex children present unique challenges to physicians, especially with implantable devices such as cerebroventricular shunts. Hydrocephalus may develop from a variety of different causes, and shunts serve as a primary treatment modality. However, these devices can pose significant risk and result in serious complications such as shunt infection, obstruction, breakage, or migration. Any of these conditions may become life threatening, warranting prompt recognition and intervention.

Shunt Infection

Most shunt infections are felt to occur through contamination during placement. Thus, when evaluating a child with a shunt, it is imperative to determine when it was placed or the last revision date. Most infections occur within the first 6 months of placement. Presenting symptoms may be acute or subacute and nonspecific. Fever, headache, nausea, vomiting, subtle behavioral changes, or overt meningeal signs can all signal an infection. On examination, there may be redness, swelling, or induration along the shunt tubing, but this is not common. Most times there are no external signs of infection. An abdominal pseudocyst (cerebrospinal fluid collection) may also cause infection. Peritoneal signs on abdominal examination may be present. Infectious organisms are also different from postsurgical contamination. Skin flora, staphylococcus or streptococcus, predominate in postsurgical, whereas pseudocysts may be caused by *Propionibacterium acnes*. Initial work-up includes complete blood count, c-reactive protein, and blood culture. The positive and negative predictive values of these tests are not sufficient to rule in or rule out the condition. Therefore, a diagnostic tap is the definitive test and should be considered especially in a community setting without access to neurosurgical consultation. With or without the shunt tap, if an infection is highly suspected, empiric antibiotics directed at likely organisms followed by prompt neurosurgical referral for possible surgical intervention is imperative.

Shunt Malfunction

Along with infection, fracture of the shunt tubing, clogging of the tract, migration of the tubing, and low flow state from a programmable valve are all potential causes of malfunction. The clinical presentation of obstruction overlaps with infection with the exception of fever and association with time since surgical placement. Caretakers should be asked about changes in behavior as alteration in mental status may be a subtle but early clue. Initial evaluation includes emergent imaging and prompt neurosurgical consultation.

X-ray along the course of the shunt ("shunt series") is obtained to assess location of shunt placement and continuity of tubing. Ventricular size also must be determined. Computed tomography (CT) scans of the brain traditionally have been the imaging study of choice. More recent attention to the potential risk of repeated exposures to ionizing radiation has resulted in utilization of "low-dose" CT scans or a rapid sequence magnetic resonance imaging (MRI) of the brain. These options have emerged as potentially safer options without compromising sensitivity. Ultrasound in children with open fontanelles can also be used to determine worsening hydrocephalus. In addition, ultrasound assessment of optic nerve sheath diameter has also been utilized. Measurements > 4.0 mm in children <12 months of age or >4.5 mm in children > 12 months of age should raise concerns for increased intracranial pressure.

Temporization through a therapeutic tap can be considered if definitive revision/replacement of the shunt is unavailable. Cushing triad (bradycardia, bradypnea with respiratory fluctuations, and hypertension with a widened pulse pressure) indicates a need for immediate surgical intervention. Pharmacologic intracranial pressure management with hypertonic saline or mannitol may be considered. These interventions typically work better for increased intracranial pressure due to edema.

KEY POINTS

- Consider subtle behavioral changes when evaluating patients who may have shunt malfunction or infection.
- Shunt infection most commonly presents within the first 6 months after surgery.
- Prompt neurosurgical consultation should be obtained in shunt malfunction or infection.
- Imaging for malfunction includes an x-ray shunt series and CT or MRI to assess ventricular size.

Suggested Readings

Lin SD, Kahne KR, El Sharif A, et al. The use of ultrasound-measured optic nerve sheath diameter to predict ventriculoperitoneal shunt failure in children. *Pediatr Emerg Care*. 2019;35(4):268-272.

Piatt JH, Garton J. Clinical diagnosis of ventriculoperitoneal shunt failure among children with hydrocephalus. *Pediatr Emerg Care*. 2008;24(4):201-210.

Trost MJ, Robison N, Coffey D, et al. Changing trends in brain imaging technique for pediatric patients with ventriculoperitoneal shunts. *Pediatr Neurosurg*. 2018;53(2):116-120.

Wright Z, Larrew TW, Eskandari R. Pediatric hydrocephalus: current state of diagnosis and treatment. *Pediatr Rev*. 2016;37(11):478-490.

141

Be Prepared to Manage Pediatric Neurologic Technology

Christopher S. Amato, MD, FAAP, FACEP

Pediatric patients with neurologic conditions are presenting with increased frequency to the acute care setting with implantable or wearable technology. In addition, new blood tests and even service animals are utilized to detect neurologic disease. Clinicians must have a basic understanding of this "neurotech" in order to initiate evaluation and management of an increasing number of patients.

Vagal Nerve Stimulator/Deep Brain Nerve Stimulator

Implantable nerve stimulators have found application in large number of clinical conditions. Most commonly utilized for patients with intractable epilepsy, other pediatric indications include chronic pain, cluster headache, narcolepsy, dystonia, essential tremor, neurodegenerative disease, stroke recovery, Tourette syndrome, traumatic brain injury, and other psychological diagnosis including addiction, bulimia, major depression, obsessive-compulsive disorder, and addiction. The frequency, amplitude, and duration of the stimulation pulses in the devices are all adjustable and tailored to treatment effect. For the vagal nerve stimulator (VNS), an external magnet can be placed over the VNS to initiate extra stimulation to help abort seizures or, if kept in place, to turn the unit off. Side effects of a VNS include cough, sore throat, anorexia, hoarseness, dysphasia, torticollis, and urinary retention. VNS typically are MRI safe with the major risk being excessive heating of leads. Safety is improved when a modified MRI protocol is followed, but the device requires interrogation pre-MRI/post-MRI to ensure settings are maintained.

Baclofen Pump

Baclofen pumps are battery-operated, implantable titanium pumps with a refillable reservoir, which provide continuous intrathecal delivery of baclofen for chronic muscular tone issues. The pump requires refilling approximately every 1-6 months while complete replacement occurs every 5-7 years. Programming the pump is done via a handheld device placed over the pump. They are safe for metal detectors, CT, and MRI but should be interrogated after an MRI to ensure correct settings.

Baclofen overdose primarily presents with altered mentation initially as drowsiness, which can progress to loss of consciousness and finally coma. Milder symptoms include light-headedness, dizziness, nausea, headache, weakness, and respiratory depression. Baclofen withdrawal may present with fever, increase in muscle spasticity, change in mental status, and severe muscle breakdown and organ failure. Treatment of withdrawal includes supporting the ABCs and use of benzodiazepines.

Wearable and Mobile Applications

A wearable device utilizes integrated sensors to monitor physical and chemical signals to provide real-time information on a patient's health and wellness. Current applications are geared toward physical fitness, blood sugar monitoring, and improving brain health. Studies are showing promise associated with decreasing the cognitive deficits associated with chemotherapy in breast cancer survivors. The use of these devices will likely be part of scientific research and require rigorous standardization.

Neurofeedback, utilized in cognitive and emotional health, can be used to improve attention providing the wearer with a visual readout of their beta wave (active thinking), which allow the subject to see and then modify their brain activity. This may help manage stress/anxiety, improve concentration, and alter sleep patterns, among other effects.

Blood Test for Closed Head Injuries

Serum level of proteins such as brain-derived neurotrophic factor (BDNF), S-100B serum protein biomarker or, glial fibrillary acidic protein (GFAP) may correlate with the severity of traumatic brain injury (TBI) and supersede the need for CT and exposure to ionizing radiation, predict recovery, and may help pinpoint which patients need further specialized treatments. Due to these limitations, testing for these proteins is not considered part of the standard care for a head trauma patient at this time.

Current limitations are the time required to obtain these results, as well as the potential need for a baseline level of the serum protein for each patient prior to any injury. As such, this may be viewed as part of preparticipation testing in athletes someday.

Service Animals

Service animals are being used for many disorders since the institution of their use for visually disabled patients. The list of diagnosis used in is growing but include multiple sclerosis, muscular dystrophy, rheumatoid degeneration, ALS, cerebral palsy, spinal cord injuries, and many other conditions affecting a person's mobility or strength. They can also be trained to assist with tasks related to a seizure disorder or hearing loss.

KEY POINTS

- **Vagal nerve stimulators:** Wave magnet over device to stimulate it or tape magnet over device to deactivate the device.
- **Baclofen pump:** Safe for MRI but will need interrogation and possible reprogramming afterward.
- **Neurologic blood tests and wearable devices** will be more available in the near future and will impact the care of a wide variety of neurology-affected patient.

Suggested Readings

Byrom B, McCarthy M, Schueler P, Muehlhausen W. Brain monitoring devices in neuroscience clinical research: the potential of remote monitoring using sensors, wearables, and mobile devices. *Clin Pharmacol Ther.* 2018; 104(1):59-71.

Deep brain Stimulators. https://www.aans.org/en/Patients/Neurosurgical-Conditions-and-Treatments/Deep-Brain-Stimulation

ORTHOPEDICS

142

Fingertip Injuries: Keep It SIMPLE, Do Not Forget to Check the Tendons, and Use Glue

Daniel Scholz, MD, MPH and James (Jim) Homme, MD

Besides the head, the hand is the most commonly injured pediatric body part. Fingertip injuries make up one-third of all hand injuries in the pediatric population—which makes sense as the fingertips are often the first part of the body to interact with our environment and also the last to get away from the threat of the closing door.

A thorough examination is important for all fingertip injuries. Normal two–point discrimination ranges from 2 to 5 mm but is not a reliable test until 6 years of age. Capillary refill provides essential information about blood flow to the distal finger. Active flexion and extension at the distal interphalangeal joint (DIP) is essential to evaluate for tendon injuries. Often due to anxiety or pain, complete examination of the affected digit is impossible until these issues are addressed.

One simple way to improve the examination is through utilization of a **SIMPLE** (Subcutaneous Injection in the Midline of the Phalanx with Lidocaine and Epinephrine) block. Up to 2 mL of 1% lidocaine and epinephrine 1:100 000 is administered in the volar subcutaneous space at the level of the proximal digital flexion crease in the midline just deep to the skin (NOT intradermal and NOT within the nerve sheath). Use of epinephrine in the digital block provides hemostasis and increased duration of anesthesia without any increased risk of digital necrosis in the absence of any preexisting vascular insufficiency (rare in the pediatric population).

The most common fingertip injury encountered is the extraphyseal fracture of the distal phalanx via a crushing mechanism often with associated soft tissue injury and/or nail bed involvement. Traditional teaching was that fingernail injuries with associated distal phalanx fractures and/or a subungual hematoma >50% of the nail bed should have the nail removed and the nail bed explored for possible repair. Today, regardless of size of the hematoma or presence of a distal phalanx fracture, evidence supports simple trephination for pressure management in the absence of nail or nail border disruption. With nail or nail fold disruption or displaced fracture fragments, nail removal and primary repair of the laceration is still recommended. Dermabond (Ethicon, Inc., Somerville, NJ) can be used both for repair of the nail bed laceration as well as to secure the nail plate under the eponychial fold and has been shown to save more than 18 minutes with no change in cosmetic appearance or functional outcomes. The distal phalanx and DIP are splinted in extension for protection up to 3-4 weeks, although clinical healing often proceeds radiographic healing. Prophylactic antibiotics are not routinely indicated after these repairs but consider their use with gross contamination, an immunocompromised patient, or delayed presentation to care.

Mallet finger is the most common closed tendon injury affecting the third digit most frequently. Forced flexion of the extended fingertip results in avulsion of the extensor tendon with or without an avulsed bony fragment from the dorsum of the base of the distal phalanx. Assuming appropriate reduction and <50% involvement of the articular surface, these injuries are managed conservatively with the DIP splinted in slight hyperextension leaving the PIP free for 6 weeks. Warning! The 6-week time period must be restarted if the DIP goes into flexion at any point during healing. Do not overlook a Seymour fracture when you see a mallet finger. This is technically a Salter-Harris type I or II injury or juxtaepiphyseal fracture with the proximal edge of the nail plate displaced superficial to the eponychial fold. This results in the clinical finding of the nail appearing longer than the contralateral uninjured digit. Seymour fractures require immediate care by hand surgery with irrigation, debridement, antibiotics, and exploration.

Flexor digitorum profundus (FDP) avulsion, more commonly known as a jersey finger, is caused by forced extension of a flexed DIP joint. This injury is rarely seen in younger children but does occur in adolescents, often in the setting of sports. If suspected, the finger should be splinted with the DIP and PIP in slight flexion with prompt referral to a hand surgeon as tendon retraction and scarring can be irreversible within 1 week depending on the extent of injury.

KEY POINTS

- SIMPLE blocks are an easy and effective digital block technique.
- Trephination may be the only treatment necessary for extensive nail bed hematomas.
- Seymour fractures are high-risk injuries that may masquerade as a mallet finger or proximal nail fold displacement.

Suggested Readings

Eiff MP, Hatch R, Higgins MK. *Fracture Management for Primary Care*. Philadelphia, PA: Elsevier Saunders; 2003.

Lee DH, Mignemi ME, Crosby SN. Fingertip injuries: an update on management. *J Am Acad Orthop Surg*. 2013;21:756-766.

Lin B. Closing the Gap, Wound Closure for the Emergency Practitioner. https://lacerationrepair.com/.

Supracondylar Fractures

Joseph Arms, MD

Introduction

Supracondylar fractures are common in children with high potential for significant long-term complications if not identified and treated quickly. The practitioner can rapidly assess high-risk fractures through a brief physical examination and utilization of simple radiographs. Same-day orthopedic consultation is usually required for more severe fractures.

History

The typical presentation is an early school-age child (peak 5 years of age, range 3-10 years) who has fallen on an outstretched hand ("FOOSH") with and extended elbow. Falls from the monkey bars is typical, though impact from a patient's own height often generates enough force to cause injury. Forces drive the proximal radius and ulna into the distal humerus, causing a disruption of the humeral cortex. The degree of cortical disruption, along with the neurovascular exam, guides management.

Physical Examination

The patient is typically in a significant pain. Intravenous or intranasal opioids and support of the extremity with a sling or pillows are usually required. Physical examination findings suggestive of high-risk fracture are poor hand perfusion, absent radial pulse, severe swelling/deformity, bruising of anterior elbow, open fracture, and neurologic injury.

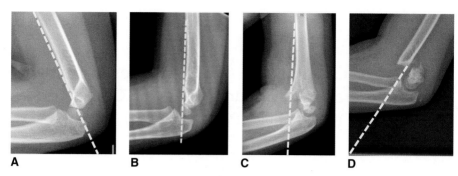

Figure 143.1 Gartland classification. **A. Normal:** Anterior Humeral line should intersect the middle portion of the capitellum. Look for effusions, especially posterior to humerus. **B. Type 1:** Non-displaced. Typically requires long arm splint and referral to orthopedics within one week. CMS abnormalities will require immediate orthoconsult. **C. Type 2:** Anterior humerus displaced with intact posterior. Will Require OR, usually with pin placement. Contact Ortho on call to discuss timing of OR management. Delayed reduction is common unless neurovascular exam is abnormal. **D. Type 3:** Posterior humerus displaced. Will Require OR, Usually the same day. Contact Ortho on call for acute plan.

Motor neuron function is rapidly assessed by asking the patient to make hand maneuvers from the game "rock, paper, scissors," and an "A-OK" sign. These maneuvers provide evaluation of the median ("rock"), radial ("paper"), ulnar ("scissors"), and anterior interosseous ("A-ok") nerves, respectively ("A-OK" is to circle thumb and first finger with tips in opposition and to hold the circle tight). Younger children and patients in a high degree of pain may not be capable of compliance with these maneuvers, complicating an accurate neurologic assessment.

Imaging

Failure to adequately manage pain makes obtaining adequate radiographs and development of a treatment plan challenging. A true lateral film of the elbow is essential to avoid missing subtle fractures. An AP view should be performed as well. Imaging the entire forearm prevents missed distal fractures.

Gartland Classification

The degree of cortical disruption to the humerus on radiographs determines Gartland classification, which, along with physical examination, guides determination of need for immediate surgical attention vs splinting with delayed surgery or casting. Gartland (Fig. 143.1) is the most efficient and commonly used nomenclature utilized for classification communication with orthopedic surgeon.

KEY POINTS

- Rapid pain control is essential for accurate assessment.
- True lateral radiographs are required.
- Both the anterior humeral and radiocapitellar lines should intersect with the middle portion of the capitellum.
- Concomitant distal forearm fractures occur in 10%–15% of patients.

Suggested Readings

Dabis J, Daly K, Gelfer Y. Supracondylar fractures of the humerus in children—review of management and controversies. *Orthop Muscular Syst* 2016;5:206. doi:10.4172/2161-0533.

Ladenhauf HN, Schaffert M, Bauer J. The displaced supracondylar humerus fracture: indications for surgery and surgical options: a 2014 update. *Curr Opin Pediatr.* 2014;26(1):64–69.

Shaw KN, Bachur RG, eds. *Fleisher & Ludwig's Textbook of Pediatric Emergency Medicine/Senior.* Philadelphia, PA: Wolters Kluwer; 2016:1209–1211.

It Is Not Just a Sprain: Do Not Miss Cases of Slipped Capital Femoral Epiphysis and Idiopathic Osteonecrosis (Legg-Calve-Perth Disease)

Jonathan Nielson, MD and Kelly R. Bergmann, MD

Background

Slipped capital femoral epiphysis (SCFE) and idiopathic osteonecrosis (Legg-Calve-Perth disease—LCP) are common orthopedic conditions encountered in the pediatric emergency department. SCFE tends to occur in older children and young adolescents, with a mean age of 12-13 years and overall incidence of ~1:1000-10 000. When compared to Caucasian children, African American children have a four times higher risk and Hispanic children have a three times higher risk. Additional risk factors include obesity, renal failure, endocrine disease, and genetic diseases. In contrast, LCP generally occurs in a younger population with a mean age at diagnosis of 5-7 years and estimated incidence of 0.2-19/100 000. Males predominant with a 3-4:1 rate compared to females and Caucasian have higher rates than African Americans. Obesity and autoimmune disease are known risk factors with no clearly identified genetic predisposition. The younger the diagnosis occurs, the higher the likelihood of a good outcome, with 60%-70% healing spontaneously with no functional impairment.

Both SCFE and LCP have similar clinical presentations, with pain or limp the most common presenting symptom. While both conditions localize to the hip, up to 15% of patients with SCFE report referred pain to the knee or thigh, necessitating a high index of suspicion to facilitate diagnosis and treatment. Although slight trauma may precipitate a slip of the femoral head, many children with SCFE have no history of trauma and some children present with subacute or chronic pain.

A few simple examination findings and radiological tests can be obtained to narrow the differential. Pain with internal or external rotation of the hip or inability to complete full range of motion, passively or actively, increases concern for either disease. Also on the differential for leg/joint pain suggestive of SCFE or LCP are septic arthritis, transient synovitis, fracture, dislocation, neoplastic disease, and juvenile idiopathic arthritis.

Assessment

SCFE is bilateral in up 60% of children, and there is a slight left predominance. The mainstay of diagnosis is AP and frog leg lateral radiographs. The classic finding is posterior displacement of the epiphysis, often referred to as "ice cream slipping off the cone." Klein lines are useful in diagnosis extending along the superior aspect of the femoral neck in the AP view and along the anterior femoral neck in a frog leg lateral projection intersecting the epiphysis. In patients with SCFE, the epiphysis is displaced posteriorly causing Klein lines to not intersect the epiphysis or intersect less than it should. Contralateral views are obtained for comparison and detection of bilateral involvement.

The history of LCP can be quite variable, especially given the age range of the patients who present with the disease. AP and frog leg lateral views of both hips are first-line imaging as LCP occurs bilaterally in 10%-20% of patients. Radiographic findings classically include sclerosis, articular collapse, and/or cortical depression of the femoral head. Magnetic resonance imaging (MRI) and bone scintigraphy provide more definite imaging but have limited utility in the emergency department.

Management

While the pathophysiology differs between SCFE and LCP, diagnosis of either warrants orthopedic consultation. Management of SCFE includes prompt surgical fixation to prevent further slip and allow for continued joint growth. If there is no surgical consultation available, transfer to a facility where orthopedics is available should be arranged. In some instances, the orthopedic surgeon may arrange for outpatient surgical repair while keeping the patient nonweight bearing to prevent worsening slip. Most children with LCP are managed with nonweight bearing and nonsteroidal anti-inflammatories. Most children with LCP can be discharged from the ED.

KEY POINTS

- Image bilateral hips in patients with concern for SCFE or LCP with AP and frog leg lateral views.
- Use Klein lines when interpreting x-rays to identify subtle changes for SCFE and avoid missing symmetric bilateral disease.
- Have a low threshold for imaging, even in patients with reassuring examinations, as histories and examinations vary and early identification can facilitate better outcomes.

Suggested Readings

Gholve PA, Cameron DB, Millis MB. Slipped capital femoral epiphysis update. *Curr Opin Pediatr.* 2009;21(1):39-45.
Gekeler J. Radiology of adolescent slipped capital femoral epiphysis: measurement of epiphyseal angles and diagnosis. *Oper Orthop Traumatol.* 2007;19(4):329-344.
Murphey MD, Roberts CC, Bencardino JT, et al. ACR appropriateness criteria osteonecrosis of the hip. *J Am Coll Radiol.* 2016;13(2):147-155.

Big Problems in Little Bones: Do Not Miss Physeal Fractures

Jana L. Anderson, MD and Mark S. Mannenbach, MD

Growth plates make pediatric bones unique. The adage, "that kids fracture and do not sprain," is fairly true until the end of puberty. In infancy, the epiphysis is all cartilage and acts as a "shock absorber." As the child ages and ossifies, more and more force is transmitted through the bone leading to fractures. Understanding bone development will help clinicians to avoid the common errors of (1) calling the injury a "sprain" when it is a growth plate fracture and (2) not arranging orthopedic follow-up.

Within the growth plate, cartilage hypertrophies and calcifies leading to lengthening of the bone. This zone of proliferation creates a weak point in the bone predisposing to fractures. The most commonly utilized fracture classification system was developed by two Canadian physicians, Salter and Harris (SH), which divide fractures into five types. Higher numbers correlate to increased likelihood of growth arrest. One mnemonic to remember SH classification system utilizes the plane of fracture or "SALT(E)R" (Fig. 145.1).

> S = Same or Slip = type I
> A = Away from joint = type II
> L = Lower into joint = type III
> T = Through both (lower and away) = type IV
> R = the Rest of it = type V

The most common locations for physeal fractures are the fingers (40%), distal radius (18%), distal tibia (11%), and distal fibula (7%). Overall, SH type II is the most common (75%) followed by types III (10%), IV (10%), and type I (5%). Type V is very rare.

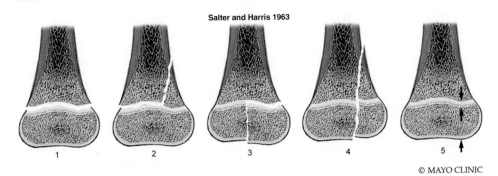

FIGURE 145.1 Pediatric Growth Plate Fractures – Salter-Harris Classification.

SH type I fractures may be radiographically occult with plain film findings ranging from completely normal or slight asymmetry of the growth plate cartilage to the extreme of a complete displacement or "slip" through the physis. The key to not missing these injuries is deliberate examination of each child. Any child with tenderness to palpation at the level of the growth plate should be treated as if they have a fracture even without specific radiographic evidence. This type of fracture typically occurs in younger children because of the thicker growth plate and periosteum. One exception to this is a slipped capital femoral epiphysis (SCFE), occurring in older and often heavier children. These patients frequently complain of knee pain rather than specific hip pain. Generally, treatment of the SH type I fracture involves placing the child in a removable splint and having them follow-up in 1–2 weeks. If there is any asymmetry or true displacement at the physis, or suspicion for SCFE, consultation with orthopedics is indicated.

SH type II fractures are the most common type of physeal fractures. The fracture line goes through the growth plate and then exits through the metaphysis. The metaphyseal fragment is called a Thurston-Holland fragment. The distal tibia is at particularly high risk of growth arrest with SH type 2 fractures correlating with millimeters of initial displacement.

In types III and IV, the fracture line exits through the joint surface, making them at increased risk of chronic joint issues. Type V SH fractures result from axial compression; the x-ray may reveal no true fracture pattern initially, just marked swelling of the surrounding soft tissue. Diagnosis is usually made retrospectively after growth arrest occurs.

Management of all displaced physeal fracture require pediatric orthopedic consultation for reduction, splinting, and follow-up. Type I and nondisplaced type II fractures can be managed by primary care, but if any concern, pediatric orthopedics referral would be appropriate.

KEY POINTS

- Tenderness to palpation at the level of the growth plate should be treated as a fracture even when the x-ray is negative.
- In nondisplaced Salter-Harris type I, place the child in a removable splint and have them follow-up with primary care in 1–2 weeks for repeat examination and radiographs.
- Any growth plate fracture that has displacement should have pediatric orthopedics consultation.

Suggested Reading

Cepela DJ, Tartaglione JP, Dooley TP, Patel PN. Classifications in brief: Salter-Harris classification of pediatric physeal fractures. *Clin Orthop Relat Res.* 2016;474(11):2531-2537.

146

Be Prepared for an Easy ED Fix: Subluxed Radial Head—The Nursemaid's Elbow

Jana L. Anderson, MD

Nursemaid's elbow, radial head subluxation, and pulled-elbow all refer to the most common pediatric orthopedic "dislocation": annular ligament displacement (ALD). Classically, the child will have a pulling mechanism on a pronated forearm with immediate disuse. The child will hold the arm in a "puppy paw" position with the elbow slightly flexed and the forearm pronated and held close to the body.

Common errors that clinicians should avoid are (1) obtaining x-rays to have the nursemaid's "reduced" by the radiology tech and (2) accidently "reducing" a supracondylar fracture. To avoid radiographs and misadventures in reduction, one must astutely use the child's age, presentation, and examination as a guide.

The anatomy of the pediatric elbow predisposes it to ALD. The annular ligament is made up of two bundles that wrap around the head of the radius. The radial head is about the same size of the neck until age 7. The proximal annular fibers connect with the lateral complex ligaments of the elbow not only making it more stable but also anchoring it to the humerus making more prone to slip into the joint space. These anatomical and developmental factors combine for a median age of 2.1 years (interquartile range, 1.5-2.8 years) for ALD. Conversely, these factors make it rare for kids older than 5 to have ALD.

The classic mechanism for ALD is sudden, axial traction of a pronated arm. When the forearm is in pronation, the ovoid radial head is 30% smaller. This allows the proximal annular ligament bundle to displace up over the radial head and become entrapped in the radial-capitellar space. Typically, the history will be of arm pulling or swinging, but almost 20% of children have either a report of a fall or unknown mechanism.

During examination, start with the unaffected side and palpate slowly down from the clavicles to the hand, comparing to the affected side. Then specifically, palpate simultaneously both elbows; move from the olecranon fossa and then down and around the medial and lateral epicondylar areas. There should be no swelling or asymmetry. If any swelling or asymmetry exists, obtain appropriate radiographs to evaluate for fracture or joint effusion.

ALD reduction is one of the most satisfying procedures in all of pediatrics. Many studies have been performed comparing hyperpronation to supination-flexion. Overall, hyperpronation is considered more successful on first attempt and less painful than supination-flexion. Sit facing the child, grasp the child's wrist using the hand of your same extremity as the child's affected side (ie, use your left if their left). Then place your other hand such that your thumb is resting over the radial head and the remaining portion of your hand is gently cradling the child's elbow. Rotate the child's wrist so that the thumb goes "down and around," using moderate force until you meet firm resistance. A "pop" should be felt with your thumb resting at the elbow. If the "pop" was not felt, then perform the supination-flexion maneuver. Re-grasp the wrist, then with the arm extended, bring the child's forearm into full supination and flex the arm until it touches the humerus. Generally, the longer the ALD has been present, the longer it takes for the child to regain normal use of the affected limb after reduction. Normal use of the extremity should be observed prior to discharge of the patient.

KEY POINTS

- Nursemaid's elbow is due to displacement of the proximal annular ligament bundle into the radio-capitellar space.
- Examination reveals no palpable asymmetry about the child's elbows.
- Hyperpronation is more successful and less painful method of reduction.
- Normal use of the affected extremity provides proof of ALD reduction.

Suggested Readings

Bexkens R, Washburn FJ, Eygendaal D, et al. Effectiveness of reduction maneuvers in the treatment of nursemaid's elbow: a systematic review and meta-analysis. *Am J Emerg Med.* 2017;35:159-163.

Diab HS, Hamed MM, Allam Y. Obscure pathology of pulled elbow: dynamic high-resolution ultrasound-assisted classification. *J Child Orthop.* 2010;4(6):539-543. https://doi.org/10.1007/s11832-010-0298-y.

Gottlieb M, Suleiman LI. Current approach to the management of forearm and elbow dislocations in children. *Pediatr Emerg Care.* 2019;35:293-298.

Rudloe TF, Schutzman S, Lee LK, et al. No longer a "nursemaid's" elbow: mechanisms, caregivers, and prevention. *Pediatr Emerg Care.* 2012;28:771-774.

147

Ankle Fracture—Triplane and Juvenile Tillaux Fracture

Rahul Kaila, MD

Pediatric ankle fractures are the second most common fractures in children. Physeal injuries are of particular concern in growing children as physis are weak as compared to its surrounding structure. During adolescent growth spurt, which is around age 10-15 years of age, there is a period prior to physeal closure when physeal fracture can easily occur. It takes 18 months for the distal tibial physis to close, first centrally and then medially and finally laterally. During this period the unfused portion of the physis is at risk of fractures called juvenile Tillaux and triplanar fractures. Tillaux are Salter-Harris (SH) III fracture (Fig. 147.1) of distal anterolateral part of distal tibia occurring more often in children

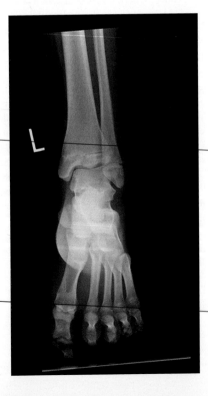

Figure 147.1 Tillaux Fracture.

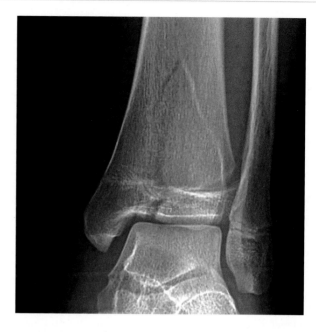

Figure 147.2 Triplane Fracture.

12-14 years of age. Mechanism of injury is generally by lateral rotation of the foot or by medial rotation of the leg on the fixed foot. Long-term risk includes growth problems and intra-articular involvement causing joint incongruity and hence CT scan is the preferable imaging modality when suspecting SH-3 Tillaux fracture on radiography. Conservative management if <2 mm displacement requires posterior leg splint and immobilization. If >2 mm displacement is noted, then open reduction internal fixation (ORIF) is the preferable modality of the treatment.

The triplane fracture is a multiplanar fracture with three classically defined fracture fragments. It involves (1) the epiphysis fractured on the lateral aspect (same as Tillaux fracture) seen on the AP radiograph (Fig. 147.2), (2) the metaphysis fractured on the posterior aspect seen on the lateral radiograph, and (3) the physis seen separated in the axial plane. The triplanar fracture is typically seen in children 12-15 years of age and slightly higher in boys than in girls. Mechanism of injury is generally external rotational force on a supinated foot. As it involves the physis, epiphyses, and metaphyses, it is consistent with a Salter-Harris type IV. Initial radiography of the ankle demonstrates a Salter-Harris type III fracture on anteroposterior radiographs and a Salter-Harris type II fracture on lateral radiographs. CT scan of ankle is highly recommended for fracture alignment and surgical needs. Orthopedics consult in the ED is highly recommended for both fractures. Conservative management is recommended if there is <2 mm displacement with posterior leg splint and immobilization, and if there is >2 mm displacement, then ORIF is recommended.

KEY POINTS

- Juvenile Tillaux and triplane fractures are physeal fracture during adolescent growth spurt.
- Tillaux is SH-III and triplane is a SH-IV fracture.
- The tibial physis close first centrally, then medially, and finally laterally.
- In both fractures, orthopedics consult and CT scan of ankle are highly recommended.

Suggested Readings

Kay RM, Matthys GA. Pediatric ankle fractures: evaluation and treatment. *J Am Acad Orthop Surg.* 2001;9(4):268.
Olgun DZ, Maestre S. Management of pediatric ankle fractures. *Curr Rev Musculoskelet Med.* 2018;11(3):475-484.
Schnetzler K, Hoernschemeyer D. Pediatric triplane ankle fracture. *J Am Acad Orthop Surg.* 2007;15(12):738-747.
Wuerz TH, Gurd DP. Pediatric physeal ankle fracture. *J Am Acad Orthop Surg.* 2013;21(4):234-244.

148

Pediatric Cervical Spine Trauma: The Biggest Pain in the Neck Would Be to Miss One

Atim Uya, MD and Michael Hazboun, MD

The incidence of pediatric cervical spine injury is low; however, a lack of familiarity with these injuries can lead to missed diagnosis, overuse of imaging studies, and potentially devastating outcomes.

Pediatric Cervical Spine Anatomy and Risk Factors for Injury

Children have large heads compared to their bodies, a higher fulcrum than adults, underdeveloped paraspinous muscles, greater ligamentous laxity, and incompletely ossified vertebrae. This leaves the pediatric cervical spine more susceptible to shearing forces, flexion/extension injuries, higher cervical injuries, and injuries without radiographic abnormalities compared to adults. Cervical spine injury should be assumed in any pediatric patient involved in a multisystem blunt trauma as well as any patient who is altered, has neurologic deficits, or who complains of neck or back pain. Additionally, certain pediatric patients are at additional risks due to congenital abnormalities, especially those with Down syndrome, Chiari malformations, and rheumatoid disease among many others.

Initial Management and Stabilization

Evaluation should begin with obtaining a history to identify risk factors for cervical spine injury. Children with suspected cervical spine injury should have immediate immobilization of the cervical spine while managing the ABCs of trauma resuscitation. This is best achieved with application of a hard cervical collar or use of manual in-line stabilization when a collar is unavailable or access to the patient's neck is required for airway management or procedural intervention. Secondary injuries should be anticipated and planned for.

Examination and Imaging

Following the primary survey and intervention to address any life-threatening injuries, a thorough examination of the cervical spine should be performed. Clearance of the cervical spine by physical examination should only be completed in patients with low-risk injury mechanisms who are awake, cooperative, and do not have a significant distracting injury.

Evaluation for cervical spine injury should include imaging in patients with high-risk mechanism of injury, neurologic deficits, intoxication, or altered mental status. Radiographic evaluation can begin with plain radiographs with a minimum of two views—anteroposterior (AP) and lateral. In older, more cooperative children, a third view through the mouth (odontoid view) may be attempted. Adequate imaging should include visualization of all of the cervical vertebrae including the C7-T1 junction on the lateral radiograph. These radiographs can help identify vertebral fractures or subluxations; however, soft tissue abnormalities are often the only signs of significant injury. These abnormalities include surrounding soft tissue edema or widening of the prevertebral space. The normal prevertebral space in a child is two-thirds or less of the AP width of the vertebral bodies at or above C3. At C4 or below, this space is roughly equal to the width of the associated vertebral body. Pseudosubluxation of C2 on C3 can often be seen in children under 7 years old and mistaken for a true injury. A true injury of the cervical spine should be assumed if the distance between the spinolaminar line and the posterior arch of C2 is >2 mm.

Computed tomography (CT) can be considered as a first-line screening tool in patients with significant altered mental status (Glasgow coma scale < 12), in younger children (<8 years old) at risk for higher cervical injuries CT (improved views of C1-C2), or as a secondary screen if radiographs are inadequate or unrevealing. Magnetic resonance imaging provides greater detail of ligamentous or soft tissue injury without the risk of ionizing radiation but is inferior to CT scan in the evaluation of the vertebrae themselves. Persistent neurologic deficits with normal imaging findings should raise concern for spinal cord imaging without radiographic abnormalities (SCIWORA) and patients should remain in a cervical collar until consultation with a specialist.

KEY POINTS

- Pediatric cervical spine injuries are uncommon; however, they can be devastating if missed or mismanaged.
- High index of suspicion, early immobilization, and systemic evaluation are key to prevention of secondary injury.
- Secondary injuries can be life threatening and should be anticipated and planned for.
- Evaluation for cervical spine injury should include imaging in any injured patient with neurologic deficits or altered mental status.
- When in doubt, maintain cervical immobilization and consult your pediatric subspecialist.

Suggested Readings

Hoffman J, Wolfson A, Todd K, et al. Selective cervical spine radiography in blunt trauma: methodology of the National Emergency X-Radiography Utilization Study (NEXUS). *Ann Emerg Med.* 1998;32(4):461-469.

Leonard J, Kupperman N, Olsen C, et al. Factors associated with cervical spine injury in children after blunt trauma. *Ann Emerg Med.* 2011;58(2):145-155.

Leonard J, Jaffe D, Kupperman N, et al. Cervical spine injury patterns in children. *Pediatrics.* 2014;133(5):1179-1188.

Tat S, Mejia M, Freishtat R, et al. Imaging, clearance, and controversies in pediatric cervical spine trauma. *Pediatr Emerg Care.* 2014;30(12):911-915.

Woodward GA, O'Mahony L. Neck trauma. In: Shaw KN, Bachur RG, eds. *Fleisher and Ludwig's Textbook of Pediatric Emergency Medicine.* 7th ed. Philadelphia, PA: Wolters Kluwer; 2016:1238-1277.

SCIWORA: Do You SCIWORA What I SCIWORA?

Ryan Ericksen, MD and Amanda L. Bogie, MD, FAAP, FACEP

Spinal cord injury without radiographic abnormality (SCIWORA) is a traumatic myelopathy characterized by neurological deficits in the setting of normal plain radiographs or computed tomography (CT) images. The phenomenon is rare in the adult population but reported to be as high as 20% in children with spinal cord injury, with younger children at higher risk. Motor vehicle crashes, sporting activities, and falls account for the majority of cases. The anatomic characteristics of the pediatric spinal cord likely contribute to this type of injury (Table 149.1). These injuries commonly occur from hyperextension or flexion mechanisms, but can also develop from rotational, lateral bending, vertical compression, or distractive forces. SCIWORA can also occur from spinal cord infarction.

Patients with SCIWORA have various signs and symptoms. Patients commonly have neck or back pain. Neurologic symptoms range from mild paresthesias or weakness, to more obvious findings, such as paralysis or spinal shock. The timing of symptoms is variable. Symptoms may be transient or persistent and can occur immediately or have a delayed presentation (up to a few days after injury).

Pediatric trauma patients with suspected spinal cord injury should have their spinal motion restricted while the airway, breathing, and circulation are addressed. Patients should then undergo

Table 149.1 ■ Anatomic Differences	
Anatomic Characteristics of the Pediatric Cervical Spine	
Anatomic differences in children compared to adults:	
Interspinous ligaments and joint capsules	More flexible
Vertebral bodies	Wedged anteriorly and tend to slide forward with flexion
Facet joints	Flat
Head and neck	Relatively large head compared with the neck Angular momentum is greater Fulcrum exists higher in the cervical spine (which accounts for more injuries at the level of the occiput to C3) Forces applied to the upper neck are relatively greater than in the adult
Growth plates	Opened, and growth centers are not completely formed

spinal imaging. Initial imaging includes plain radiographs of the spine, but by definition, patients with SCIWORA will not have x-ray abnormalities, such as fractures or subluxations. Advanced trauma life support guidelines do not recommend the routine use of CT as screening modalities of the pediatric cervical spine, but these modalities are indicated when plain films cannot adequately visualize the entire cervical spine; to help delineate abnormalities seen on plain films; when the patient has an altered mental status such as with a traumatic brain injury; or when a patient has neurologic deficits (either by history or on examination). Patients with suspected SCIWORA with normal x-rays and CT scans require MRI. Some patients who would have been previously diagnosed with SCIWORA based on normal x-ray and CT findings but abnormal exam will have abnormalities detected on MRI. However, an MRI can still be normal in patients with mild or incomplete neurological deficits. A spine surgeon should be consulted for patients with SCIWORA; definitive treatment depends on symptoms and imaging findings. Many patients with SCIWORA require hospital admission.

In summary, a normal cervical spine film or CT scan is not adequate to rule out a spinal cord injury in pediatric trauma patients when neurologic symptoms are present. These patients may or may not have MRI abnormalities, and a spine surgeon should be consulted on children suspected of having SCIWORA, regardless of imaging findings.

KEY POINTS

- SCIWORA occurs more commonly in pediatric trauma patients due to the unique anatomic and physiologic aspects of the pediatric spinal column.
- Normal plain radiographs or CT scans do not rule out spinal cord injury in the pediatric trauma patient.
- MRI may be used to identify pediatric spinal cord injuries that historically have been classified as SCIWORA.

Suggested Readings

American College of Surgeons Committee on Trauma. *Advanced Trauma Life Support Student Course Manual.* 10th ed. Chicago, IL: American College of Surgeons; 2018.

Babcock L, Olsen CS, Jaffe DM, et al. Cervical spine injuries in children associated with sports and recreational activities. *Pediatr Emerg Care.* 2018;34:677-686.

Mahajan P, Jaffe DM, Leonard JC, et al. Spinal cord injury without radiologic abnormality in children imaged with magnetic resonance imaging. *J Trauma Acute Care Surg.* 2013;75:843-847.

Shah BR, Lucchesi M. Spinal cord injury without radiographic abnormality (SCIWORA). In: Shah BR, ed. *Atlas of Pediatric Emergency Medicine*. 2nd ed. McGraw Hill; 2013:790-791.

Woodward GA, O'Mahony L. Neck trauma. *Textbook of Pediatric Emergency Medicine*. 7th ed. Wolters Kluwer/Lippincott Williams & Williams:1238-1279.

Overuse Syndromes: When a Good Thing Has Gone Too Far

David Soma, MD, CAQSM

Youth participation in sports provides significant value with physical, mental, and emotional benefits. However, overuse syndromes are on the rise. These injuries are the result of repetitive submaximal loading to various musculoskeletal structures in the absence of adequate recovery. It is important for all pediatric providers to recognize the location of bony growth centers and understand their relative vulnerability to injury. Key overuse syndromes are summarized here.

Apophysitis

An apophysis is a secondary ossification center where a ligament or tendon attaches. Apophysitis is pain as a result of repetitive traction over this area. Osgood-Schlatter, the most commonly diagnosed apophysitis, occurs at the patellar tendon insertion site on the tibial tubercle. Apophysitis typically occurs in young individuals 8-15 years of age, with earlier presentation in females. Apophysitis can occur across many sites, most notably the calcaneus, the inferior pole of the patella (Sinding-Larsen-Johansson syndrome), base of the fifth metatarsal, medial epicondyle, and pelvis. The condition is typically self-limited with the mainstay of treatment consisting of activity modification, nonsteroidal anti-inflammatory medication, and physical therapy. The natural history of these conditions is resolution with a minority of patients developing chronic pain if left untreated.

Stress Fractures

Stress reactions and fractures occur in children as they do in adults with similar risk factors. The majority of these heal with conservative measures, but some stress fractures are prone to delayed union, nonunion, or chronic pain. Sites that are at highest risk are the pars interarticularis, tension side of femoral neck, patella, anterior tibia, medial malleolus, talus, navicular, sesamoid, and junction of the metaphysis/diaphysis at the base of the fifth metatarsal. Medical providers need to have a high index of suspicion for these conditions, and advanced imaging may be necessary to establish the diagnosis. Examination reveals a focal area of bony tenderness and pain with load placed over area. Since the hip and spine are not as easily palpated, internal rotation of the hip and pain with hopping or extension of the spine provides clues to the diagnosis. Treatment usually requires removal of loading stress and varying degrees of immobilization.

Physeal Stress Injuries

Physeal and growth plate injuries caused by stress through repetitive rotational, compressive, or distracting forces are unique to the pediatric population. Little league shoulder, injury to the proximal humeral physis, and gymnast wrist, injury to the distal radial physis, are common examples. History typically consists of progressive pain with loading activity. Examination reveals pain with reproduction of offending stress or palpation over the physis. Treatment consists of removal from activity for 2-3 months with regulated reintroduction back to sports.

Osteochondritis Dissecans

Osteochondritis dissecans (OCD) is an injury to the subchondral bone and cartilage in active young individuals thought to be related to overuse and/or trauma. The most commons sites include the femoral condyles, talus, and capitellum, presenting with persistent joint pain followed by swelling and mechanical symptoms. Radiographs are required to make the diagnosis and magnetic resonance imaging (MRI) used to assess stability. Stable lesions can be treated nonoperatively. Initial treatment consists of removal from activities and referral to an orthopedic surgeon. Without appropriate treatment, there can be loss of cartilage and bone leading to chronic pain.

Effort Thrombosis

Effort thrombosis occurs in athletes performing strenuous and repetitive activities of the upper extremity and is often associated with thoracic outlet syndrome (TOS) causing compression of the axillary/subclavian vein. These patients typically present with pain, arm swelling, and sometimes discoloration. Ultrasonography is the preferred method of diagnosis. Management includes anticoagulation with increasing evidence that surgical interventions like first rib resection may help treat symptoms and prevent recurrence.

KEY POINTS

- Overuse injuries are common in pediatric patients, and understanding the location and vulnerability of growth centers is important for appropriate diagnosis.
- Bone-related overuse injuries are more common in young individuals, and imaging is often beneficial for diagnosis.
- Treatment for the majority of overuse syndromes is conservative; however, not identifying these conditions may have long-lasting effects.

Suggested Readings

Arnold A, Thigpen CA, Beattie PF, et al. Overuse physeal injuries in youth athletes: risk factors, prevention, and treatment strategies. *Sports Health.* 2017;9(2):139-147.

Bell DR, Post EG, Biese K, et al. Sport specialization and risk of overuse injuries: a systematic review with meta-analysis. *Pediatrics.* 2018;142(3):e20180657.

DiFiori JP, Benjamin HJ, Brenner JS, et al. Overuse injuries and Burnout in Youth Sports: A Position Statement from the American Medical Society for Sports Medicine. *Br J Sports Med.* 2014;48(4):287-288.

What to Know About Lumbago

Jonathan Strutt, MD, FAAP

Back pain in the pediatric emergency department (ED) is an uncommon complaint. For this reason, many providers often are concerned for a more sinister diagnosis. However, the most common causes of acute pediatric back pain are musculoskeletal strain or trauma. The most common infectious cause is pyelonephritis. The prevalence of back pain increases with age and is more common in females. History and physical examination are essential to differentiate between the wide range of benign and pathologic causes.

History

Several key historical features of back pain help identify a cause in the majority of patients. These include location, exacerbating symptoms, and duration. Description of the pain can help to localize the source. Neurologic pain is often described as sharp and/or burning, muscular/inflammatory pain is nonlocalizable, and fracture or bony lesions are focal. Red flag symptoms that warrant further investigation include fever, weight loss, pain that awakens the child from sleep, and progressively worsening pain. Additionally, chronic back pain lasting >4 weeks has a higher likelihood of a pathologic diagnosis.

Physical Examination

A thorough physical examination is useful in localizing the source of pain and can increase or decrease concern for pathology. A complete neurologic examination that includes lower extremity sensation, strength, and reflexes should be performed. Inspection of the back will allow assessment of any bruising, focal swelling, vertebral column deformity, signs of infection, trauma, or rash. Palpation for tenderness should include the vertebral bony landmarks, paraspinal muscles, costovertebral angle, iliac crests, and sacroiliac joints. Focal bony tenderness suggests infection or trauma. Paraspinal tenderness is often noted with muscular strain. Costovertebral angle tenderness suggests renal pathology. Range of motion testing is useful to assess for reproducible pain as well as functional limitations. Spondyloarthritis caused by inflammatory conditions such as ankylosing spondylitis will result in decreased lumbar lordosis during forward flexion. A positive stork test (reproduction of pain while standing on one leg with back hyperextension) helps to identify spondylolysis, a common overuse injury in young athletes.

Diagnostic Imaging and Laboratory Assessment

The majority of patients presenting to the pediatric ED with back pain are diagnosed by history and physical examination alone. There are instances where laboratory and/or imaging are needed. Suspicion for infectious, inflammatory, or malignancy as the cause necessitate obtaining a complete blood count and inflammatory markers. Focal tenderness or associated trauma should prompt further diagnostic evaluation with imaging. Radiographs of the spine are the initial imaging modality. The two-view posteroanterior and lateral examinations are all that are needed to identify most pathology. The oblique view offers little diagnostically. Radiographs may reveal acute fracture, primary bony tumors, subacute or chronic osteomyelitis, spondylolysis (pars interarticularis stress fracture), spondylolisthesis (vertebral dislocation), or Scheuermann kyphosis (rigid thoracic hyperkyphosis). A targeted noncontrast CT can further delineate fractures seen on radiographs and should be obtained in the setting of focal neurologic deficits. In acute back pain without focal neurologic deficits, normal laboratory findings, and normal radiographs, further imaging should be deferred until symptoms are present for at least 4 weeks. Emergent imaging is needed for any neurologic abnormalities not associated with trauma. The preferred modality is magnetic resonance imaging (MRI), with the addition of contrast when suspecting an infectious or neoplastic process.

KEY POINTS

- The most common pediatric ED causes of back pain are trauma and muscle strain.
- Red flag symptoms include fever, weight loss, pain that awakens the child form sleep, and progressively worsening pain.
- Chronic back pain lasting >4 weeks has a higher likelihood of a pathologic diagnosis.
- Emergent advanced imaging should be pursued in the setting of atraumatic focal neurologic deficits, fevers, weight loss suggestive of neoplasm, or elevated inflammatory markers.

Suggested Readings

Booth TN, Iyer RS, Falcone RA, et al. ACR appropriateness criteria back pain-child. *J Am Coll Radiol.* 2017;14(55):S13–S24.

Brooks TM, Friedman LM, Silvis RM, et al. Back pain in a pediatric emergency department: etiology and evaluation. *Pediatr Emerg Care.* 2018;34:e1–e6.

MacDonald J, Stuart E, Rodenberg R. Musculoskeletal low back pain in school-aged children. *JAMA Pediatr.* 2017;171(3):280–287.

INFECTIOUS DISEASE

Everything At Once—Obtain Cultures Quickly But Do Not Delay Antibiotics for Fever in the First 28 Days

Candace Engelhardt, MD, FAAP

Febrile neonates <28 days old are at high risk for serious bacterial infections, even when well appearing. This increased risk is partially due to increased susceptibility and partially due to a difficult and unreliable examination. Rochester criteria, historically, are the most used criteria for evaluation and management, yet a recent study showed a wide variety of management of well-appearing febrile infants in emergency departments (EDs) across the country.

Do Not Delay Antibiotic Administration

In a busy ED, neonates' antibiotic therapy is often delayed until diagnostic testing is complete; however, it is extremely important that antibiotic therapy begins promptly. It is well established that morbidity and mortality increase with every hour of delay of antibiotics in adults with sepsis. Weiss et al. demonstrated similar outcomes in pediatrics with the risk of mortality progressively increasing each hour until appropriate antibiotics were administered, up to 3 hours. Murray et al. demonstrated that the development of a clinical pathway for febrile neonates in a pediatric ED reduces the time to administration of antibiotics. It is important to identify the febrile neonate and complete all diagnostic testing as quickly as possible so antibiotics can be administered, even if the dose is given intramuscularly.

Avoid Administering Antibiotics Prior to Obtaining a Lumbar Puncture

While starting antibiotics is of the utmost importance, whenever possible it is important to perform the lumbar puncture first. Kanegaye et al. demonstrated complete sterilization of cerebral spinal fluid in the first 2-4 hours after administration of parenteral antibiotics. Lack of adequate culture material may result in false negatives, prolonged treatment, and inability to tailor therapy. This is especially true if there is a positive blood culture and cerebral spinal fluid pleocytosis is present on subsequent lumbar puncture. Pretreating lumbar punctures can lead to longer hospital stays. Once a febrile neonate is identified, it is important to perform all diagnostic tests and administer antibiotics as quickly as possible.

Do Not Use a Bag Urine for Culture

All urine cultures obtained need to be via a catheter. Bag urines are not sterile no matter how well the area is cleaned. Bag urines lead to many false-positive UTI diagnoses leading to prolonged or unnecessary hospital stays. Etoubleau et al. found that bag urine cultures lead to misdiagnosis or an impossible diagnosis in 40% of cases. Urine sample obtained via catheter is the only way to assure that the culture will not be contaminated. Additionally, consider obtaining this first, as a crying neonate undergoing IV placement for lumbar puncture testing will likely urinate, which may make subsequent straight catheter attempts unsuccessful.

Do Not Forget About Herpes Simplex Virus

Herpes simplex virus (HSV) is rare but can cause serious central nervous system infection in febrile neonates. Neonates do not commonly present with the typical vesicles that are the clinical feature of HSV infection. When evaluating a febrile neonate, if there are seizures, maternal history of HSV, or the neonate is toxic appearing, acyclovir should be started along with the parenteral antibiotics and cerebral spinal fluid PCR should be included in the workup. Other signs of HSV infection include cerebral spinal fluid showing lymphocytosis or presence of high amount of red blood cells in an atraumatic lumbar puncture, and possibly disseminated intravascular coagulation and elevated liver enzymes. In fact, some argue that testing and empiric treatment should be performed on neonates 21 days and younger.

KEY POINTS

- Do not delay administering antibiotics to febrile infants.
- Avoid pretreatment of CSF whenever possible.
- Always obtain urine cultures via catheter.
- Do not forget about HSV infection in the febrile infant <28 days old.

Suggested Readings

Etoubleau C, Reveret M, Brouet D, et al. Moving from bag to catheter for urine collection in non-toilet trained children suspected of having urinary tract infection: a paired comparison of urine cultures. *J Pediatr.* 2009;154:803-806.

Kanegaye JT, Soliemanzadeh P, Bradley JS. Lumbar puncture in pediatric meningitis: defining the time interval for recovery of cerebrospinal fluid pathogens after parenteral antibiotic pretreatment. *Pediatrics.* 2001;108:1169-1174.

McGuire JL, Zorc J, Licht D, et al. Herpes simplex testing in neonates in the emergency department. *Pediatr Emerg Care.* 2012;28:949-955.

Murray AL, Alpern E, Lavelle J, Mollen C. Febrile young infant clinical pathway in a pediatric emergency department. *Pediatr Emerg Care.* 2017;33:e33-e37.

Weiss S, Fitzgeral JC, Balamuth F, et al. Delayed antimicrobial therapy increases mortality and organ dysfunction duration in pediatric sepsis. *Crit Care Med.* 2014;42:2409-2417.

Risky Business: Know How to Approach the "What Ifs" in Neonatal Fever Risk Stratification

Clifford C. Ellingson, MD, FAAP

In the well-appearing febrile infants <90 days old, we aim to identify and treat those with serious bacterial infection (SBI) while avoiding overtesting and invasive procedures in those without. Over the last 30 years, clinical trial such as the Boston, Philadelphia, and Rochester criteria have tried to find the best approach in this situation. A newer, validated pathway called "Step by Step" incorporates C-reactive protein (CRP) and procalcitonin (PCT) without cerebrospinal fluid (CSF) testing and boasts a higher specificity and sensitivity. The "Step by Step" pathway identifies low-risk infants if age >21 days, well appearing, no pyuria, PCT < 0.5, CRP < 20, and absolute neutrophil count (ANC) <10 000. More recently, the Pediatric Emergency Care Applied Research Network group internally validated another pathway with excellent sensitivity for well-appearing febrile infants <60 days old. Patients with a negative urinalysis, ANC ≤ 4090, and PCT ≤ 1.71 were deemed low risk.

Risk stratification tools can be used to avoid invasive testing in well-appearing, low-risk febrile infants. Unfortunately, the febrile infant with an SBI often looks the same as those without SBI, thus the adage "never trust a neonate." Those <28 days old or with complex medical histories warrant a comprehensive workup. Complex medical histories include prematurity, prolonged hospital stays, antenatal exposure to maternal infections, or chronic medical conditions.

Well-appearing patients who are low risk for SBI are reasonable candidates for outpatient management. Discuss the workup with caregivers including tests performed and deferred and follow-up. Caregivers must be reliable with access to follow-up. All other patients require admission and empiric antibiotic therapy with ceftriaxone. Consider cefotaxime if <28 days, ampicillin to cover *Listeria monocytogenes and Enterococcus*, and acyclovir for HSV if concern exists. Consider adding vancomycin if signs of soft tissue infections or bacterial meningitis as *Streptococcus pneumoniae* strains can be resistant to cephalosporins.

"What Ifs" in Neonatal Fever Workup

What if there was a measured fever at home, but not on evaluation? Trust the caregiver and do the workup. Not only do these patients have the same historical rate of SBI but it is important to gain the trust of parents to facilitate an important discussion and/or evaluation.

What if there was a tactile fever at home, but no fever in the ED? This is a gray zone and warrants a risk-benefit discussion with the caregiver. Tactile temperatures do not carry the same risk of SBI so shared decision-making can be used to determine whether a workup will be pursued. Certainly provide education on measuring a temperature and return precautions if the patient is discharged.

What if I cannot obtain CSF in the well-appearing infant? Should I still give antibiotics? If <28 days old, yes. If the patient is not deemed low risk by your risk stratification instrument, consider having a discussion with the admitting pediatrician. A pretreated CSF culture may expose them to an unnecessary prolonged hospitalization and course of antibiotics though early antibiotic therapy is crucial for those with meningitis.

What if I cannot get an IV? A femoral vein stick with a butterfly needle is a quick option for blood cultures and studies. Antibiotics can then be given IM.

What if I cannot get urine, should I try a bag specimen? A bag specimen can be used for urinalysis but not for culture. Consider a straight catheterization before painful procedures as the infant will likely urinate during these procedures. Ultrasound can confirm urine in the bladder or guide a suprapubic catheterization if urethral approach fails.

What if the infant tests positive for a virus? Studies show that virus positive infants, such as RSV, >28 days old are at lower risk for SBI, but the risk remains, especially for a urinary tract infections. Therefore, urine testing is strongly recommended.

KEY POINTS

- Risk stratification tools can reduce testing and invasive procedures.
- Have a plan for the "what ifs" that occur during the neonatal fever workup.

Suggested Readings

Bonsu BK, et al. Identifying febrile young infants with bacteremia: is the peripheral white blood cell count an accurate screen? *Ann Emerg Med.* 2003;42(2):216-225.

Gomez B, et al. Validation of the "Step-by-Step" approach in the management of young febrile infants. *Pediatrics.* 2016;138(2):e20154381.

Kuppermann N, et al. A clinical prediction rule to identify febrile infants 60 days and younger at low risk for serious bacterial infections. *JAMA Pediatr.* 2019;173(4):342-351.

Levine D, et al. Risk of serious bacterial infection in young febrile infants with respiratory syncytial virus infections. *Pediatrics.* 2004;113(6):1728-1734.

Pantell RH, et al. Management and outcomes of care of fever in early infancy. *JAMA.* 2004;29(10):1203-1212.

154

Fever 2 Months Old and Beyond

Anne Whitehead, MD, FAAEM

Very little strikes as much fear into the heart of a parent as a high fever in their child. They rush out of bed in the wee hours of the morning worried that the fever will melt their little brains. Yet, the vast majority of these children are subsequently discharged from the emergency department (ED) with little more than acetaminophen and parental re-assurance. Fever is a symptom, but not a problem by itself. It is important not only to know when a fever requires a more extensive work-up, but also to reduce fever phobia in families and in your ED.

Unlike hyperthermia, which can lead to brain damage and death from an environmental cause, fever is an adaptive responsive mediated by the hypothalamus. There is no evidence that a true fever itself can cause serious problems. The harms of fever are typically mild and include discomfort, decreased oral intake, and febrile seizures, which are scary to parents but benign. Only rarely, in very ill children with conditions like sepsis or congenital heart disease, the increased metabolic demand associated with fever can have a deleterious effect.

The medical literature generally defines the minimum temperature to qualify for fever between 38°C (100.4°F) and 38.4°C (101.1°F). Invariably though, the question on parents' minds is "how high is *too* high?" It is best not to answer this question with a number but rather to encourage parents to focus on how the child is doing rather than what the thermometer says. Are they lethargic? Are they able to hydrate? It is more worrisome if a child with a 38.1°C fever is lethargic and not drinking, than if a child who is running around the room with a 39.5°C fever.

Who Needs a Work-Up?

Brief fever, well-appearing child: In healthy children ≥2 months old, a brief fever most often requires no more than a history and physical. Often these fevers are the result of a self-limited viral process, otitis media, or another infection that can be identified on examination. Children <2 years old without a clear source of fever may have a urinary tract infection (UTI). Girls <2 years and boys <12 months (<6 months if circumcised) are at higher risk for UTI.

Immunocompromised child: Well-appearing immunocompromised children, including children with sickle cell disease, should get at least a complete blood count, blood cultures, and a dose of empiric antibiotics (typically ceftriaxone). Depending on the underlying condition, often they can be discharged with close follow-up. While unvaccinated children or children <4 months are not necessarily "immunocompromised," they are at higher risk for occult bacteremia and other serious infections. They likely resemble the children of the prevaccine era, who had rates of occult bacteremia as high as 3%-5% with fever. Have a low threshold to initiate this more comprehensive work-up on any unvaccinated or undervaccinated child, especially under age 3.

Fever >5 days, >7 days, and beyond: Be explicit in determining if the patient was truly febrile and truly sustained for consecutive days. Caregivers will often include temperatures <100.4°F or <38.0°C or confuse back to back illnesses with one prolonged illness.

After 5 days of fever, Kawasaki disease must be considered. Often this can be ruled out by diagnostic criteria alone. Once a child has 7 days of fever without a clear source, the fever is then classified as "fever of unknown origin" (FUO). The differential for FUO includes occult infection, malignancy, and collagen vascular disease. The recommended work-up includes bloodwork and urine testing, as well as any other testing indicated by history and examination.

Do

Treat the patient, not the number! The goal of antipyretics should be to increase patient comfort and oral intake. Antipyretics can also help determine if significant tachycardia is simply due to fever as the heart rate should improve as patients defervesce. Children with fever may have blankets, despite what parents (or medical providers) may have heard to the contrary.

Do Not

Do not use aspirin in children, which can put them at risk for Reye syndrome. Do not insist that a child's fever resolve before they leave the ED. This gives parents the false impression that they must keep the patient afebrile at home. Discourage alcohol baths as there is a risk for systemic absorption. Lukewarm water baths are not dangerous, but should only be used if they help the patient feel better.

KEY POINTS

- Treat the child, not the number! Do not worry about the number on the thermometer as much as the condition of the child.
- Be aware of things that make parents worry about height of fever.
- The goal of antipyretics should be comfort, normalizing heart rate, and improved oral intake, all of which can help reassure you that there is not a more serious underlying illness.
- At 5 days, think about Kawasaki disease. After 7 days, work to identify a source.
- Age <2 years? Think about UTI.

Suggested Readings

Antoon JW, et al. Pediatric fever of unknown origin. *Pediatr Rev*. 2015;36(9):380-391.

Mace SE, et al. Clinical policy for well-appearing infants and children younger than 2 years of age presenting to the emergency department with fever. *Ann Emerg Med*. 2016;67(5):625-639.

Sullivan JE, Farrar HC. Fever and antipyretic use in children. *Pediatrics*. 2011;127(3):580-587.

Hot to the Touch: Differentiate Between Fever Without a Source and Fever of Unknown Origin

Courtney Jacobs, MD

Fever, defined as temperature $\geq 100.4°F$ or $38°C$, is one of the most common pediatric presentations in the emergency department (ED). Most pediatric fever is the result of viral illnesses and only requires symptomatic treatment. Other sources of fevers have a significant potential for morbidity and mortality. A thorough history eliciting the exact temperature of the patient, if and how it was measured, time course of fever, additional symptoms, recent travel, past medical history, and a comprehensive physical examination should, in most cases, reveal the cause of the fever. Depending on the age of the patient and clinical features (or lack thereof), some fevers may need additional workup.

Fever Without a Source

Fever without a source (FWS) is a fever <7 days duration without an apparent cause after a history and physical examination. Management strategies for febrile children without a source depend on the age of the patient, vaccination status, and well vs ill appearance on examination. Identification of serious bacterial infections (SBI) such as meningitis, urinary tract infections, pneumonia, and occult bacteremia is the goal. This does not require a full panel of tests necessarily; it can often be accomplished simply with a clinical assessment and risk stratification. Management of fever <90 days will be discussed in another chapter.

Previously healthy, vaccinated, well-appearing infants older than 90 days presenting with FWS have a very low risk for SBI. Infants and children who are toxic appearing or who have abnormal vital signs require a more thorough evaluation including blood work, urine studies, and potentially a lumbar puncture to evaluate for possible SBI. These children may require admission pending culture results with empiric antibiotics to treat the most likely pathogen depending on their age group. Unimmunized patients with FWS may also require more through testing as they are at higher risk than immunized patients. Well-appearing children FWS can typically be discharged home with recommendations for supportive care. They should be instructed to have follow-up care within 24-48 hours if fevers persist.

Fever of Unknown Origin

FWS becomes fever of unknown origin (FUO) if the fever lasts >7 days without a clear cause for the fever. FUO can be further categorized into presumed infectious (ie, viral, bacterial, atypical infections, and other) vs noninfectious (oncological, vascular, autoimmune, or other) etiologies. The majority of pediatric FUO are caused by occult infection, followed by collagen vascular disease process and malignancy.

The evaluation of FUO depends on the history and physical, previous testing, and well vs ill appearance on examination. Pseudo-FUO defined as "successive episodes of benign, self-limited infections with fever that parents perceive as one prolonged fever episode" (aka overlapping or abutting infections) must also be considered. Instruct parents to keep a fever diary with actual recorded temperatures to help distinguish pseudo-FUO from FUO. The fever pattern (sustained, relapsing/remitting, intermittent), a history of previous infections or neutropenia, the patient's race, ethnicity, family history, and geographical location including recent travel and exposures (especially to animals) can help rule-in or rule-out certain conditions.

Laboratory testing for FUO may include complete blood count with differential, complete metabolic panel, blood and urine cultures, acute phase reactants such as C-reactive protein, erythrocyte sedimentation rate, and ferritin, and potential cerebrospinal fluid studies if neurological symptoms are present. Imaging such as chest x-ray may be performed, but studies have found limited utility in more advanced modalities without a specific diagnosis in mind. Stopping all nonessential medication to exclude drug fever is the first step in management. In well-appearing pediatric patients, empiric antibiotics are not recommended unless a diagnosis is highly suspected. Furthermore, steroids should not empirically be used unless there is high suspicion of serious autoimmune disease. Fortunately, progression from FWS to FUO in children tends to have better outcomes than in adults. Referral to a tertiary care center or specialist may help further identify the causes of FUO.

<hr>

KEY POINTS

- Fever is the most common presenting symptom in the pediatric ED and most likely is caused by a viral illness.
- FWS is any fever (temperature >38°C or 100.4°F) without an apparent cause after a history and physical examination.
- FUO is any fever >7 days that persists without an apparent source.
- FWS and FUO often require laboratory testing and/or imaging depending on factors such as age of the patient, well vs ill appearing, other comorbidities, additional presenting symptoms, and vaccine status.

Suggested Readings

Antoon JW, Potisek NM, Lohr J. A pediatric fever of unknown origin. *Pediatr Rev.* 2015;36(9):380-390.
Chow A, Robinson JL. Fever of unknown origin in children: a systematic review. *World J Pediatr.* 2011;7(1):5-10.

It Is a Small World After All: Know the Differential for Fever, Diarrhea, and Rash in the Traveling Child

Nicholas Sausen, MD and Stephen Mac, MD

More children than ever are traveling, resulting in more children with unexpected infectious souvenirs. Compared to adults, children get less pretravel screening and fewer region-specific vaccinations and are thus are more susceptible to infection. They tend to present earlier after travel and require more hospitalizations. The most common complaints are fever, diarrhea, and dermatologic infections. Most travel infections will be the same "bugs" acquired at home. The "zebra" illnesses are rare. Diagnosis requires a systematic approach.

Consider all travel destinations from the previous 12 months, asking specifically about dates and purpose of travel, pretravel screening, appropriate vaccinations, and prophylactic medications. Risk factors include children visiting friends and relatives, extended travel periods, living in local populations or remote settings, eating local foods, exposure to wild animals, and freshwater exposure through drinking or recreation. The basic workup will include complete blood counts, complete metabolic profile, thick and thin blood smears, chest x-ray, stool studies, and antigen tests or PCR based on symptoms and geography. Use universal precautions or isolation if concerned for communicable disease. In complex cases, obtain early guidance from infectious disease specialists.

Fever

Fever is worrisome due to the breadth of possible diseases. Narrow the differential diagnoses by pairing location with syndromic patterns.

- Nonspecific symptoms—malaria, dengue, leptospirosis
- Nervous system involvement—meningitis, encephalitis, trypanosomiasis
- Respiratory symptoms—influenza, tuberculosis, pneumonia
- Diarrhea—gastroenteritis, giardiasis, amebiasis
- Rash—measles, chikungunya, rickettsia

Fever with hemorrhage, neurologic impairment, or respiratory distress are of emergent concern for the patient and public health. Consider malaria or dengue in anyone returning from endemic areas. Malaria can have a highly varied symptomatology with respiratory, gastrointestinal, or neurologic symptoms. Treat with artesunate upon diagnosis, high suspicion, or severe symptoms. Dengue is the most common cause of fever in travelers after travel to Asia or Latin America. Treatment is supportive. Admit any suspicious fevers for monitoring, further diagnostic evaluation, and treatment.

Diarrhea

Traveler's diarrhea is the most frequent travel-related illness that children will acquire. Children often have a more severe and longer course when compared to adolescents or adults. Food and water exposure are main risks for acquisition of diarrhea. Typical presentation is cramping abdominal pain with loose, nonbloody stool. Dehydration is the greatest threat. Traveler's diarrhea is more likely to be bacterial, protozoal, or helminthic. Evaluate stool ova and parasite studies, perform antigen testing, and consider PCR. Azithromycin is the drug of choice for children. Ciprofloxacin is an alternative in children older than 12 months, but avoid in return from Asia due to high resistance. Probiotics have been shown to reduce duration of diarrhea. Avoid antidiarrheal agents due to risk of toxic megacolon.

Skin and Soft Tissue Infections

Nearly one-third of posttravel evaluation is for skin problems. If rash is accompanied by fever or arthralgias, systemic disease is likely; consider dengue, chikungunya, and enteric fever. The most common diagnoses are insect bites, cutaneous larva migrans, and bacterial infections. Cutaneous larva migrans is the extremely pruritic, serpiginous rash of larval hookworm. Treat with antihelminthics. Fungal infections such as tinea versicolor and tinea corporis can present with scaling, macular lesions. Treat with topical or systemic antifungals. Tungiasis and myiasis are caused by the larva of sand fleas, botfly, or tumbu fly. Treat by occlusive dressing and extraction of asphyxiated larva. *Staphylococcus aureus* and *Streptococcus pyogenes* are the most common bacteria. In the tropics they have increased antibiotic resistance.

KEY POINTS

- The most common pathologies of the returning pediatric traveler are fever, diarrhea, and rash.
- Most children have globally common illnesses, not "zebras."
- Suspect malaria or dengue in any febrile child returning from endemic areas.
- The treatment of choice for traveler's diarrhea in children is azithromycin.
- Fever with hemorrhage, neurologic impairment, or respiratory distress requires emergent management, may have public health implications, and necessitates isolation.

Suggested Readings

Brunette GW. *CDC Yellow Book 2018: Health Information for International Travel.* New York, NY: Oxford University Press; 2017.

Flores MS, et al. A "syndromic" approach for diagnosing and managing travel-related infectious diseases in children. *Curr Prob Pediatr Adolesc Health Care.* 2015;45(8):231-243.

Fox TG, Manaloor JJ, Christenson JC. Travel-related infections in children. *Pediatr Clin.* 2013;60(2):507-527.

Halbert J, Shingadia D, Zuckerman JN. Fever in the returning child traveller: approach to diagnosis and management. *Arch Dis Child.* 2014;99(10):938-943.

Swanson SJ, John CC. Health advice for children traveling internationally. In: Kliegman RM, et al. *Nelson Textbook of Pediatrics.* Elsevier Health Sciences; 2015:1268-1277.

Diagnose Outpatient Pediatric Pneumonia Clinically and Avoid the X-Ray

Devan Pandya, MD and Tommy Y. Kim, MD

Community acquired pneumonia (CAP) is the most common cause of mortality in children worldwide with the majority of deaths occurring in developing countries. The pathogen associated with CAP varies with age. Neonates are particularly susceptible to bacterial pathogens acquired through the birthing process, including Group B *Streptococcus* and *Escherichia coli.* Viruses such as respiratory syncytial virus, parainfluenza, influenza, and adenovirus are the most common during the toddler years. The incidence of viral pathogens decreases with as children get older with *Streptococcus pneumoniae,* nontypeable *Haemophilus influenzae, Mycoplasma pneumoniae,* and *Staphylococcus aureus* being more common in school-aged children and adolescents. *S. pneumonia* remains the most common bacterial cause of CAP across all age groups beyond the neonatal period.

Presentation can differ significantly with age or pathogen. Symptoms of fever, cough, and some degree of respiratory distress are common to all age groups. Neonates and infants can present with nonspecific symptoms of poor feeding, lethargy, irritability, or temperature instability. Older children can present with atypical symptoms such as abdominal pain. Viral CAP often presents with fever, runny nose, congestion, myalgia, and/or bilateral lung findings on auscultation. In contrast, bacterial pathogens usually present with higher fevers, localized findings on auscultation, or a more toxic appearance. Complications such as sepsis, effusion, and empyema are often associated with streptococcal or staphylococcal infections. Patients with atypical CAP such as mycoplasma gradually develop symptoms of fever, malaise, or cough over several days. Unfortunately, there is no single diagnostic examination finding for pneumonia, but the combination of examination findings such as fever, cough, and tachypnea or prolonged symptoms of fever and cough increase the likelihood.

The diagnosis of CAP is usually based on clinical findings. With the exception of neonates, laboratory and radiographic studies are not routinely recommended for mild uncomplicated pneumonia as they do not distinguish bacterial from viral causes and rarely alter management. However, it should be considered in patients with moderate to severe illness requiring hospitalization. When available, clinicians should consider bedside lung ultrasound (US) instead of chest radiographs as lung US is inexpensive, radiation free, and performs similarly, if not better, than chest radiographs. Common findings on lung US include a change in lung echogenicity over the area of consolidation, increased B-lines arising from the area of consolidation, and dynamic air bronchograms. Additionally, complications such as effusion and empyema are more accurately diagnosed with US compared to chest radiographs.

Treatment is divided into outpatient and inpatient therapy and is largely dependent on the age of the patient and the severity of illness. Indications for hospitalization include neonates with pneumonia, inability to tolerate oral medications, hypoxemia, moderate to severe respiratory distress, toxic appearance, or failed outpatient therapy. Admission to an intensive care unit should be considered for the patient with respiratory failure, impending respiratory failure, or sepsis. Antibiotic treatment choices should be informed by local antibiograms. Inpatient antibiotics targeting *S. pneumoniae* include ampicillin or a third-generation cephalosporin for patients who are penicillin allergic, toxic, underimmunized, or infants. Macrolides can be added for coverage of atypical pathogens. Vancomycin or clindamycin should be considered for CAP complicated with sepsis, effusion, or empyema. Oseltamivir should be considered for CAP from influenza based on regional recommendations.

Empiric first-line therapy for the outpatient treatment of mild uncomplicated CAP is high-dose (90 mg/kg/d) amoxicillin targeting *S. pneumoniae*. In fact, high-dose amoxicillin has greater activity against pneumococcal strains than oral cephalosporins or clindamycin. Macrolide antibiotics can be considered for atypical CAP although it cannot be used for empiric coverage as *S. pneumoniae* has significant macrolide resistance.

KEY POINTS

- The presentation of pneumonia in children can differ significantly depending on the age of the patient and the acquired pathogen.
- Laboratory and radiographic tests are not recommended in outpatient management of uncomplicated pneumonia.
- Consider the use of bedside lung US instead of chest radiographs in the diagnosis of CAP.
- Treatment is divided into outpatient and inpatient therapy and is largely dependent on the age of the patient and the severity of illness.

Suggested Readings

Bradley JS, Byington CL, Shah SS, et al. The management of community-acquired pneumonia in infants and children older than 3 months of age: clinical practice guidelines by the Pediatric Infectious Diseases Society and the Infectious Diseases Society of America. *Clin Infect Dis*. 2011;53(7):e25-e76.

Harris M, Clark J, Coote N, et al. British Thoracic Society guidelines for the management of community acquired pneumonia in children: update 2011. *Thorax.* 2011;66:ii1-ii23.

Leroux DM, Zar HJ. Community-acquired pneumonia in children—a changing spectrum of disease. *Pediatr Radiol.* 2017;47(11):1392-1398.

I Thought It Was Just a Cold: Do Not Forget to Consider Sepsis

Danielle Dardis, MD and Jennifer Plitt, MD

Pediatric sepsis is potentially life threatening and must be identified and treated as quickly as possible. Few would argue that it is abnormal for a 15-month-old to lay listlessly sprawled out on the bed, oblivious to the nurses and doctors around them trying to poke them with needles. More difficult is identifying these patients before they get to this point. How can you tell if the tachycardic, febrile child with a cough has the common cold or is critically ill?

First, let us start with some definitions. Sepsis is systemic inflammatory response syndrome (SIRS) secondary to suspected or proven infection. Most commonly, it presents with fever or hypothermia, tachypnea, tachycardia, leukocytosis or leukopenia, thrombocytopenia, or altered mental status. Severe sepsis is sepsis with either cardiovascular dysfunction, acute respiratory distress syndrome, or two or more signs of organ dysfunction. Finally, septic shock is sepsis with cardiovascular dysfunction.

Your first indication of sepsis should be the child's vital signs and/or mental status. A somnolent child is a sick child until proven otherwise. It is even more important in these children to pay attention to vital signs. If something is abnormal, you have to ask, "Why?" Children often compensate for shock by increasing their heart rate long before they become hypotensive. However, agitation, fever, dehydration, and compensated shock are all possible explanations for tachycardia. It is easy for a child with compensated shock to get lost in the pool of the far more numerous children presenting to the ED with fever and subsequent tachycardia without sepsis. Repeating vital signs and close monitoring are important. Persistently abnormal vital signs should catch your attention. Capillary refill is another easy, noninvasive way to assess for shock. Poor perfusion should prompt immediate intervention.

Some hospitals have started using an electronic sepsis alert system, which looks for abnormal vital signs in association with clinical signs (such as delayed capillary refill or altered mental status) and physician evaluation to increase identification of sepsis in its earlier phases. Once you have identified a child at risk, obtaining labs showing a leukocytosis or elevated lactate can further support your concerns. Initiating treatment for early sepsis could prevent progression and decrease overall hospital stays.

If the child presents initially in severe sepsis or septic shock, or happens to progress to this stage while in the ED, early goal-directed therapy should be initiated. Many hospitals have order sets based on accepted pediatric sepsis guidelines to hasten treatment. However, placing orders does not mean things get done in a timely manner. In a busy ED, it is easy to assume things are happening and move on to evaluate the next patient. One of the biggest areas for delay in treatment is communication. It is important to discuss your concerns and plan of care with staff who may or may not recognize the severity of the patient's condition. A septic patient takes up more time and resources and they will need to plan accordingly. It is also important for staff to communicate any delays to physicians so this can be addressed quickly.

There is conflicting information regarding how much fluid should be given and which vasopressors are best. There is no argument that timing is important; use what you can get quickly and tailor your treatment to the patient. For fluid resuscitation, do not focus on a specific volume goal. Start with a 20-mL/kg isotonic bolus and reevaluate for improvement or volume overload. In a shocky patient, this should be pushed manually or given via pressure bag, rather than over a pump. Re-bolus until clinical improvement, and stop when there are signs of volume overload (hepatomegaly, rales) or improvement has occurred. Some children will need 40-60 mL/kg or more of fluids, ideally within the first hour along with broad-spectrum antibiotics. If the child is still shocky after fluid resuscitation, begin vasopressors. Do not delay pressor infusion for placement of a central line. Begin using the best IV (or IO) available, and work on central access after. Most infants and small children present with a "cold shock" picture and epinephrine is a good choice, however, consider using what you have immediately available in the ED and changing it later as clinically indicated.

KEY POINTS

- Have a reference for pediatric vital signs and do not ignore them when they are abnormal.
- Repeat vitals and reevaluate often for clinical improvement or worsening.
- Begin early goal-directed therapy with fluids and antibiotics as soon as sepsis suspected.
- Make sure everyone involved understands the importance of acting quickly.

Suggested Readings

Alder MN, et al. Fuhrman & Zimmerman's pediatric critical care. In: Fuhrman BP, et al., eds. *Fuhrman & Zimmerman's Pediatric Critical Care.* 5th ed. Amsterdam: Elsevier; 2017:1520-1540.

Balamuth L. Interventions for pediatric sepsis and their impact on outcomes: a brief review. *Healthcare (Basel).* 2018;7(1).

Balamuth F, et al. Improving recognition of pediatric severe sepsis in the emergency department: contributions of a vital sign based electronic alert and bedside clinician identification. *Ann Emerg Med.* 2017;70(6):759-768.

Scott W, Pomerantz W. Septic shock in children: rapid recognition and initial resuscitation (first hour). *UpToDate.* July 30, 2018; www.uptodate.com/contents/septic-shock-in-children-rapid-recognition-and-initial-resuscitation-first-hour#H9034264.

Woods J. PEM Pearls: Pediatric Sepsis Management—Understanding the Basics. ALiEM; 2017 March 2019.

Meningitis—Do Not Delay the Lumbar Puncture in Patients With High Suspicion for Bacterial Meningitis

Amanda Dupont, MD, Ayush Gupta, MD and Whitney Minnock, MD

Bacterial meningitis carries a mortality of up to 4% in children and up to 30% in neonates. The most common pathogen varies with age. Group B *Streptococcus* (GBS) and *Escherichia coli* are the most common etiologies in neonates with GBS being most common between 1 and 3 months. *Streptococcus pneumoniae* and *Neisseria meningitidis* are seen in children 3 months to 10 years with *N. meningitidis* being most common between 10 and 19 years.

Prior to vaccines, *Haemophilus influenza* type b (HIB) was the main cause of bacterial meningitis in children <5 years. *S. pneumoniae* then replaced HIB as the leading cause of bacterial meningitis after HIB vaccination was widely administered. Pneumococcal vaccination, intrapartum prophylaxis against GBS, and herd immunity have decreased the overall rate of bacterial meningitis. Underimmunized children <2 years have remained the highest risk group.

Presentation and Physical Examination

The presentation of bacterial meningitis differs with age. Infants can present with temperature instability, apnea, a full fontanelle, irritability, rash, or seizures. In young children, the chief complaint may be fever, vomiting, or altered mental status. In older children, headache, neck pain/nuchal rigidity, or photophobia are the predominant symptoms. The absence of fever on presentation may reduce the likelihood of bacterial meningitis but does not rule out the disease, particularly in the young infant.

Examination findings of a child with potential bacterial meningitis focus on abnormal vital signs and neurological examination. Irritability or lethargy, a full fontanelle, or decreased muscle tone should raise concern. Toddlers should have motor skills consistent with their developmental stage. Older children can be lethargic or irritable. Nuchal rigidity is more often seen in older children than in infants. Any child with suspected meningitis should be given a meningitic dose of antibiotics immediately. This should be simultaneous with or immediately followed by a lumbar puncture (LP).

Laboratory Tests

While lab tests have been used in the past to help guide the decision of whether to perform a LP, they should not be used in place of a LP for diagnosis. White blood cell count (WBC), blood culture (BC), procalcitonin (PCT), C-reactive protein (CRP), and urinalysis (UA) should all be obtained. In neonates, meningitis is more likely with a positive BC though you should not wait for a BC to result before treating. The WBC has little value in the diagnosis of neonatal meningitis. PCT is more sensitive and specific than CRP for distinguishing bacterial infections and may have diagnostic utility. The percentage of concurrent bacterial meningitis in infants with febrile urinary tract infections (UTI) is 0.2%.

Prediction Rule

There is a low threshold to perform a LP on infants 28-60 days due to a high mortality rate and severe neurological sequelae. Kuppermann et al. derived and validated a clinical decision instrument to identify febrile infants ≤60 days who are at low risk for serious bacterial infections (SBIs) including meningitis. This rule used a negative UA, an ANC of <4091/μL, and serum PCT of 1.71 ng/mL or less with a high sensitivity and negative predictive value in the validation cohort. This study successfully identified infants ≤60 days who are at low risk for SBIs using the above lab values. Clinical application of the rule has potential to reduce health care costs, unnecessary LPs, and hospital admission rates.

Contraindications to the LP

Contraindications include but are not limited to cerebral herniation, focal neurological signs, hemodynamic instability, underlying coagulopathies, and spinal epidural abscess. Signs and symptoms of herniation occur in 4%-6% of children with bacterial meningitis, accounting for 30% of deaths from bacterial meningitis. This complication of bacterial meningitis can occur even when a LP has not been done. A head computed tomography (CT) should be performed on any patient with suspected increased intracranial pressure, papilledema, prolonged seizures, altered mental status, or focal neurologic findings. Death secondary to herniation can still occur even with a normal CT, thus obtaining a CT is not always helpful. If CT head is indicated, then obtain BC and administer antibiotics first.

KEY POINTS

- Obtain a LP when there is suspicion of bacterial meningitis as early diagnosis decreases mortality and risk of neurological sequela.
- Labs and prediction rules can help guide your medical decision-making, but they do not replace the gold standard of the LP to diagnose bacterial meningitis.
- If clinical suspicion is high, do not delay giving antibiotics.
- If LP is contraindicated, obtain a BC and promptly start antibiotics.

Suggested Readings

Bedetti L, Marrozzini L, Baraldi A, et al. Pitfalls in the diagnosis of meningitis in neonates and young infants: the role of lumbar puncture. *J Matern Fetal Neonatal Med*. 2019;32(23):4029-4035.

Kuppermann N, Dayan PS, Levine DA, et al. A clinical prediction rule to identify febrile infants 60 days and younger at low risk for serious bacterial infections. *JAMA Pediatr*. 2019;173(4):342-351.

Posadas E, Fisher J. Pediatric bacterial meningitis: an update on early identification and management. *Pediatr Emerg Med Pract*. 2018;15(11):1-20.

Riordan FA, Cant AJ. When to do a lumbar puncture. *Arch Dis Child*. 2002;87(3):235-237.

Pertussis Infection in Infants and Children: Do Not Miss the Early Signs

Suzanne E. Seo, MD and Derya Caglar, MD

Pertussis, or whooping cough, is a respiratory infection caused by *Bordetella pertussis* characterized by paroxysmal coughing followed by an inspiratory "whoop." It can be associated with cyanosis, post-tussive emesis, or apnea, particularly in young infants. It affects 24.1 million children under 5 years of age and causes 160 700 deaths annually. Infants <1 year make up the most vulnerable population, comprising 53% of deaths each year. Fortunately, mortality from pertussis has declined significantly due to vaccines, though the disease has yet to be eradicated.

Pertussis infection is defined by three phases: the catarrhal phase, the paroxysmal phase, and the convalescent phase. The catarrhal phase consists of 1-2 weeks of nonspecific upper respiratory infection symptoms such as mild cough, coryza, and rhinorrhea. Low-grade fever may also be present during the catarrhal phase, but often, children are afebrile. Though patients have mild symptoms during this stage, they are highly contagious.

The paroxysmal phase occurs next lasting between 2 and 4 weeks. This phase is characterized by bursts of staccato coughs followed by the inspiratory "whoop," though not all children will present classically. During this phase, young infants may develop cyanosis and/or apnea. Importantly, many children with pertussis may not have tachypnea or increased work of breathing between coughing episodes. This is important to note, as children with persistent respiratory distress may have alternative diagnoses such as bronchiolitis or pneumonia.

Finally, the illness progresses to the convalescent phase during which the cough becomes less severe and the patient makes a gradual recovery with occasional exacerbations. This phase can persist for weeks to months. For this reason, in addition to being called "whooping cough," pertussis has been called the "100-day cough."

Children are most likely to be diagnosed during the paroxysmal phase when the cough is severe and cyanosis, apnea, gagging, or post-tussive emesis are present. Children with severe disease are at risk for serious complications during this stage such as pneumonia, seizure, anoxic brain injury, and respiratory failure requiring mechanical ventilation. Diagnosis is ideally made during the catarrhal stage. To do so, the clinician should ask about potential exposures and the immunization status of the patient and close contacts, particularly in infants <4 months.

Laboratory testing can also help with early diagnosis, ideally before the whooping starts. Consider testing for pertussis in young infants with cough, in unimmunized patients with cough, and in patients presenting with cough and apnea or cyanosis. A respiratory viral PCR or culture from a nasopharyngeal swab or serology is used for testing. Patients may also have leukocytosis with lymphocytic predominance on a complete blood count. Chest radiographs are often normal but may also show nonspecific signs of infection such as perihilar infiltrates, enlarged lymph nodes, and atelectasis.

Pertussis can be treated with macrolide antibiotics, such as azithromycin, clarithromycin, or erythromycin, to decrease disease severity and duration. Azithromycin is the antibiotic of choice in infants <1 month as erythromycin is associated with increased risk for hypertrophic pyloric stenosis in this age group. Chemoprophylaxis with macrolides should also be considered for close contacts of those with known pertussis infection. Treatment with antibiotics is most effective when initiated in the first

21 days of illness, when signs and symptoms are often nonspecific, making the diagnosis challenging. Even with antibiotic treatment, many infants with severe disease require admission for IV fluids and observation given their risk for apnea and cyanosis with coughing episodes. Some infants and children will require escalation of respiratory support in the setting of severe disease.

The best treatment, however, is prevention. The pertussis vaccine, usually given in the form of acellular pertussis as part of the DTaP vaccine, is part of the primary immunization series, which starts at 2 months and continues through 18 months. Following the completion of the primary series, 98% of children are protected against pertussis for 1 year and 71% are protected for 5 years after completion of the series. Because of waning immunity, it is essential to continue booster immunizations in adolescence and throughout adulthood. Infants <2 months cannot get the vaccine, so the CDC recommends that pregnant women receive the Tdap immunization in the second or third trimester to confer passive immunity to infants.

KEY POINTS

- Pertussis can lead to apnea, cyanosis, and death in infants.
- Early diagnosis of pertussis infection is important as antibiotics can reduce disease severity and duration if started during the first 21 days of illness.
- The clinician should ideally diagnose pertussis before severe signs of illness start. Ask about immunization status and pertussis exposures in at-risk patients.
- A CBC may show leukocytosis with a lymphocytic predominance and the diagnosis can be confirmed with culture, bacterial PCR, or serology.

Suggested Readings

Cherry JD. Pertussis in young infants throughout the world. *Clin Infect Dis.* 2016;63(suppl 4):S119-S122.

Koenig KL, Farah J, McDonald EC, et al. Pertussis: the identify, isolate, inform tool applied to a re-emerging respiratory illness. *West J Emerg Med.* 2019;20(2):191-197.

Yeung KHT, Duclos P, Nelson EA, et al. An update of the global burden of pertussis in children younger than 5 years: a modelling study. *Lancet Infect Dis.* 2017;17(9):974-980.

Bronchiolitis: Value Aggressive Airway Clearance Over Nebulizers, X-Rays, and Steroids in Bronchiolitis

Sarah Becker, DO, FAAP

Bronchiolitis Basics

Managing bronchiolitis with evidence-based practice means not getting caught up in the ineffective treatment patterns. By recalling the pathophysiology of bronchiolitis, we can target treatments proven to work. Bronchiolitis is the result of a viral infection of the epithelial cells lining the small airways of the lungs. The cascade of inflammation, edema, and mucus production causes small airway obstruction, leading to cough, tachypnea, and increased work of breathing. Painting this picture for parents (and for ourselves), we can help set expectations for what will and will not help their child.

Bronchiolitis Pitfalls

Albuterol is commonly trialed for acute bronchiolitis in the emergency department (ED). However, the 2014 American Academy of Pediatrics (AAP) guidelines recommends *against* bronchodilator use in bronchiolitis. In general, airway obstruction in bronchiolitis is *not* a result of bronchospasm but rather from secretions. Several meta-analyses and systematic reviews have shown that bronchodilators may improve clinical symptom scores but do not affect disease resolution, need for hospitalization, or length of stay. Steroids have also not shown efficacy. It is reasonable to assume steroids would decrease inflammation, but studies have found no difference in outcomes with steroid use in moderate to severe bronchiolitis. Parents often expect a chest x-ray for children with respiratory symptoms. However, research has shown little clinical utility for chest x-rays in bronchiolitis. Though some may argue that imaging is needed to confirm the diagnosis, always remember that bronchiolitis is a *clinical* diagnosis.

Despite evidence and guidelines, we often ask ourselves "what is the harm in trying?" As enticing as it might be, these therapies are not benign. In addition to their side effects, we subject ourselves to confirmation bias, influencing reassessment and sending patients down a potentially unnecessary treatment pathway. Parents incur unnecessary cost for medications that will not work and may ignore supportive care or delay a return visit for reevaluation.

Evidence-Based Bronchiolitis Management

There are really only three reliable interventions in managing bronchiolitis: airway clearance/respiratory support, supplemental oxygen, and hydration. Often saline drops combined with a bulb suction or other suction device will improve the work of breathing. It should be done gently to prevent direct trauma and edema. By removing secretions from the nasopharynx, we can relieve the upper airway obstruction from these often obligate nose breathers, thus ameliorating much of their work of breathing. Sometimes admission for more frequent suctioning is necessary.

It is a difficult paradigm shift to accept lower oxygen saturations. However, instead of reflexively starting supplemental oxygen, consider suctioning first. If a patient still has saturations lower than a level you are comfortable with, look at the work of breathing. If it is normal or mildly increased, consider eliminating oxygen level from your disposition decision-making equation. Additionally, consider spot-checking oxygen saturations instead of continuous pulse oximetry, and using the AAP recommendation of an oxygen saturation <90% to prompt intervention. On the other hand, if the patient is unable to feed or develops significant hypoxia while feeding, admission for IV hydration may be warranted.

If there is significant work of breathing despite all our best efforts, then high-flow nasal cannula (HFNC) therapy, noninvasive positive pressure ventilation, or intubation with mechanical ventilation may be indicated. Depending on acuity, consider titrating up from least invasive to most invasive as HFNC therapy may prevent intubation.

In deciding the disposition for your patient, consider high-risk features (eg, prematurity, chronic lung disease, congenital heart disease, etc.), ability to maintain adequate hydration, the projected disease course (symptoms tend to peak on day 3-5), the caregiver's comfort, and ability to follow-up.

KEY POINTS

- Bronchodilators, systemic steroids, and x-rays are not recommended routinely.
- Airway clearance, respiratory support, hydration, and oxygen are the mainstay of treatment.
- HFNC, noninvasive positive pressure ventilation, and mechanical ventilation should be based largely on patient's work of breathing and mental status.

Suggested Readings

Fernandes RM, Bialy LM, Vandermeer B, et al. Glucocorticoids for acute viral bronchiolitis in infants and young children. *Cochrane Database Syst Rev.* 2013;6:CD004878.

Gadomski AM, Scribani MD. Bronchodilators for bronchiolitis. *Cochrane Database Syst Rev.* 2014;6:CD001266.

Ralston SL, Lieberthal AS, Meissner HC, et al. Clinical practice guideline: the diagnosis, management, and prevention of bronchiolitis. *Pediatrics.* 2014;134(5):e1474-e1502.

Schuh S, et al. Evaluation of the utility of radiography in acute bronchiolitis. *J Pediatr.* 2007;150:429-433.

Zorc JJ, Hall CB. Bronchiolitis: recent evidence on diagnosis and management. *Pediatrics.* 2010;125(2):342-349.

Bad to the Bones—Do Not Let a Child Limp Out of the ED Without Considering Septic Joint

Seth Ball, MD and Getachew Teshome, MD, MPH

Background

The three most common causes of limp in children <10 years are transient synovitis, septic arthritis, and osteomyelitis. Transient synovitis is a benign, self-limited postinfectious inflammatory response. The exact cause is poorly understood but often preceded by viral infection. Septic arthritis is caused by hematogenous spread, local spread, or direct inoculation, most commonly seen in the hip, knee, and elbow. The most common pathogens are *Staphylococcus aureus* and streptococcal species, though *Streptococcus pneumoniae* and *Kingella kingae* are also seen. Group B *Streptococcus* and *Escherichia coli* are more likely in neonates, and *Neisseria gonorrhoeae* should be considered in adolescents. Osteomyelitis is similarly caused by hematogenous or local spread or vascular insufficiency, most commonly affecting the femur or tibia. Bacterial pathogens are similar to those found in septic arthritis and a concurrent septic joint can be found in about 50% of neonates.

Presentation and Examination

Most children will present with some combination of pain, fever, and refusal to use an extremity or bear weight. Patients with septic arthritis and osteomyelitis more often are ill appearing and febrile. The child might hold the affected extremity in a position of comfort and resist passive range of motion. The affected area may be warm, swollen, erythematous, or tender. Transient synovitis is more difficult to differentiate from early infection and thus is a diagnosis of exclusion. These patients may be more well appearing, afebrile, and tolerant of passive range of motion. Refusal to bear weight may be the only symptom so fracture should also be considered.

Evaluation

When presented with the undifferentiated limping child, it is reasonable to start with nonsteroidal anti-inflammatory drugs (NSAIDs) for pain control and radiographs of the affected joint or limb. In transient synovitis, the radiograph will look normal or will show mild widening/effusion. In septic arthritis, radiographs often show soft tissue swelling, joint space widening, and displacement of the fat pads. These changes can be subtle, and a contralateral image can be helpful. Osteomyelitis may have no radiographic findings if early in the disease process; late radiographic findings include periosteal elevation and bony destruction. If the joint examination is worrisome or joint space widening is seen on plain film, an ultrasound (US) may reveal an effusion, though 70% of patients with transient synovitis will also have an effusion.

The Kocher criteria may be helpful in guiding your suspicion for septic arthritis. Risk factors include non–weight bearing, temperature >38.5°C, ESR >40 mm/h, and WBC count >12 000 cells/mm³. The more risk factors present, the higher the probability of septic joint as follows: 1 risk factor: 3%, 2: 40%, 3: 93%, and 4: 99%. Inflammatory markers will be elevated with septic arthritis and osteomyelitis but not with transient synovitis. However, they are often normal in neonates and in children with sickle cell disease. Blood cultures should be drawn but will be positive in only a third of septic arthritis cases and half of those with osteomyelitis. Lyme serology may be warranted if the child lives in or has traveled to a Lyme-endemic area.

If concern for septic arthritis is high, synovial fluid should be sent for cell count, protein, glucose, Gram stain, and culture. Findings suggestive of septic arthritis include a cell count >50 000 with

>80% neutrophils, positive Gram stain, and glucose <30% of serum. The synovial fluid will be positive in 50%-75% of septic arthritis cases but sterile in transient synovitis. If the evaluation is inconclusive, a bone scan or magnetic resonance imaging may be considered.

Management

Patients who are afebrile and well appearing, with low risk of septic joint and clinical improvement after minimal pain control, can be sent home with a likely diagnosis of transient synovitis. Treatment includes NSAIDs, supportive care, and close outpatient follow-up.

Definitive management of septic arthritis includes parenteral antibiotics and surgical drainage. The surgical team should be involved as early as possible. Ideally, antibiotics would be administered after arthrocentesis so the culture results can help narrow antibiotic therapy. However, antibiotics should never be delayed in a septic patient. Empiric antibiotics for septic include gram-positive coverage such as nafcillin/oxacillin, clindamycin, or cephalexin. Adding gram-negative coverage for neonates and ceftriaxone for adolescents is recommended. Initial management of osteomyelitis is similar with special considerations to include vancomycin for methicillin-resistant *S. aureus* concerns, *Salmonella* coverage with ceftriaxone for children with sickle cell disease, and pseudomonal coverage with piperacillin-tazobactam, meropenem, or ceftazidime for those with osteomyelitis after stepping on a nail.

KEY POINTS

- Osteomyelitis and septic arthritis commonly affect the proximal lower extremities.
- Septic arthritis and osteomyelitis require early, aggressive antibiotic therapy.
- Transient synovitis is a diagnosis of exclusion.
- A child who cannot walk out of the ED needs further investigation, even if x-rays are normal.

Suggested Readings

Conrad D. Acute hematogenous osteomyelitis. *Pediatr Rev.* 2010;31(11):464-447.
Dodwell E. Osteomyelitis and septic arthritis in children: current concepts. *Curr Opin Pediatr.* 2013;25(1):58-63.
Harowitz R. Pediatric orthopedic emergencies. In: Adams J, ed. *Emergency Medicine Clinical Essentials.* Philadelphia, PA: Elsevier Saunders; 2013:204-208.
John J, Chandran L. Arthritis in children and adolescents. *Pediatr Rev.* 2011;32(11):470-448.

HEMATOLOGY/ONCOLOGY

Tumor Lysis Syndrome

Mahnoosh Nik-Ahd, MD, MPH

When your patient's "Results" section has more red than black and the electrolytes are all deranged, think of tumor lysis syndrome (TLS), whether they have a known malignancy or not (everything has to start somehow!).

Overview

Tumor lysis syndrome (TLS) is caused by the rapid lysis of malignant cells—especially after initiation of therapy—most commonly from non-Hodgkin lymphoma, acute myeloid leukemia, and acute lymphoblastic leukemia. It is defined by metabolic abnormalities such as hyperkalemia, hyperphosphatemia, hypocalcemia, and hyperuricemia. These abnormalities can lead to complications such as renal failure, seizures, and cardiac arrest, making TLS a true oncologic emergency. While TLS is most likely in patients with a known malignancy, less commonly a previously undiagnosed malignancy may present with TLS; please see the "New-Onset Cancer" chapter for more information on ED evaluation for suspected pediatric cancer.

Laboratory TLS is defined by at least two of the following abnormalities: hyperuricemia, hyperkalemia, hyperphosphatemia, or hypocalcemia. Clinical TLS is defined by the presence of Laboratory TLS along with at least one of the following: renal insufficiency, seizures, arrhythmias, or sudden death.

Treatment

Treatment of TLS includes aggressive fluid management, allopurinol, and rasburicase. TLS patients should have labs every 6 hours and careful monitoring of fluid balance until resolution. Urgent consultation with a pediatric nephrologist is recommended, as these patients may require dialysis. When TLS is suspected, patients should be transferred to a facility with pediatric critical care, nephrology, and hematology/oncology.

Fluid Management

With the exception of patients with renal insufficiency/failure or decreased cardiac function, aggressive hydration is the mainstay of treatment of TLS. For children who are 30 days old or less, give 1.5-2 times maintenance IVF (mIVF) of 5% dextrose/half normal saline. For children over 30 days old, give 1.5-2 times mIVF using 5% dextrose/normal saline. For obvious reasons, fluids should not contain additional electrolytes. Close monitoring of urine output is necessary, with a goal urine output of 4-6 mL/kg/h for patients ≤10 kg and goal of at least 2-4 mL/kg/h for patients >10 kg. For patients without hypovolemia or acute obstructive uropathy, diuretics can be used to maintain goal urine output.

Allopurinol

Allopurinol decreases the formation of uric acid through the inhibition of xanthine oxidase, an enzyme critical for the catabolism of purines to uric acid. By slowing uric acid formation, high levels can be suppressed, thus preventing its precipitation and renal injury. However, because allopurinol cannot decrease existing hyperuricemia, patients with a uric acid level of ≥7.5 mg/dL should be treated with rasburicase instead of allopurinol.

Rasburicase

Rasburicase is recommended in patients with a uric acid level of ≥ 7.5 mg/dL. As opposed to allopurinol, which prevents production of uric acid, rasburicase (recombinant urate oxidase) works to break down uric acid to a degradation product (allantoin) that is more readily excreted by the kidney. Rasburicase is contraindicated in patients with G6PD deficiency and pregnant or breast-feeding females. Uric acid levels should be checked 4 hours after administration of rasburicase, and then every 6 hours. Uric acid samples must be sent to the lab on ice, as rasburicase causes degradation of uric acid at room temperature. Additionally, allopurinol should not be added when patients are receiving rasburicase, as allopurinol can decrease rasburicase effectiveness. Additionally, allopurinol is not benign, as it can ultimately lead to precipitation of xanthine crystals in the kidney, which can lead to acute obstructive uropathy.

Electrolyte Management

Hyperkalemia, hypocalcemia, and hypo/hyperphosphatemia caused by TLS are managed in the same manner as electrolyte derangements from other etiologies.

KEY POINTS

- Suspect TLS in a patient with malignancy who presents with hyperkalemia, hyperphosphatemia, hypocalcemia, hyperuricemia, and/or renal failure.
- Hyperhydrate to goal urine output. Use allopurinol or rasburicase to lower uric acid levels.
- Check labs at least every 6 hours.
- Early discussion with pediatric nephrology, hematology/oncology, and ICU is vital.

Suggested Readings

Cairo MS, Coiffier B, Reiter A, et al. Recommendations for the evaluation of risk and prophylaxis of tumour lysis syndrome (TLS) in adults and children with malignant diseases: an expert TLS panel consensus. *Br J Haematol.* 2010;149(4):578-586.

Coiffier B, Altman A, Ching-Hon P, et al. Guidelines for the management of pediatric and adult tumor lysis syndrome: an evidence-based review. *J Clin Oncol.* 2008;26(16):2767-2778.

Howard SC, Jones DP, Ching-Hon P. The tumor lysis syndrome. *N Engl J Med.* 2011;365(17):1844-1854.

Jones GL, Will A, Jackson GH, et al. Guidelines for the management of tumour lysis syndrome in adults and children with haematological malignancies on behalf of the British Committee for Standards in haematology. *Br J Haematol.* 2015;169(5):661-671.

164

Do Not Get Caught Unaware: Recognizing NEW-ONSET CANCER

Alexander Werne, MD, Saharsh Patel, MD and Efrat Rosenthal, MD

Though rare, childhood malignancies can imitate common pediatric illnesses. Judicious evaluation and early diagnosis is critical; this chapter reviews key "red flag" findings, as well as initial ED management.

Initial Presentation

In contrast to adults, leukemia is by far the most common childhood malignancy, and, along with lymphomas, can present with a constellation of vague symptoms. It is therefore vital to keep both on the differential, especially if the vague symptoms are persistent. Most pediatric patients with a new diagnosis of leukemia present with at least one of the following:

- *Palpable liver or spleen* (most common, approximately two-thirds of patients)
- *Fever* (secondary to disease process itself or due recurrent infections)
- *Pallor/fatigue, bruising, or petechiae/purpura*
- *Lymphadenopathy* (typically any node that is >10 mm; an enlarged, nontender posterior auricular, lower cervical, or epitrochlear node is most concerning)
- *Musculoskeletal pain, limp, or refusal to bear weight*

Less commonly, patients can present with respiratory symptoms secondary to a mediastinal mass, headaches from increased intracranial pressure, gingival hypertrophy, and, very rarely, unilateral, painless testicular enlargement (more common with relapsed acute lymphoblastic leukemia than in initial presentation).

A careful physical examination, including examinations of the skin (undress the child completely!), mucous membranes, abdomen, lymph nodes, and genitals, is critical in patients with persistent, undifferentiated complaints.

Less common cancers may also present with vague symptoms, including the following:

- *Brain tumor*—in children, unlike adults, more likely to occur in the lower brain (cerebellum or brain stem) with associated symptoms such as ataxia, headaches, vomiting, cranial nerve palsies (double vision), or seizures
- *Neuroblastoma*—abdominal mass, pain, constipation, back pain with no history of trauma, "raccoon eyes," ipsilateral Horner syndrome, and opsoclonus myoclonus ("dancing eyes and dancing feet")
- *Wilms tumor*—abdominal mass, pain, and/or gross hematuria
- *Retinoblastoma*—white pupil may be noticed by parents from a camera flash

Diagnosis

With a hematologic cancer high on the differential, send a CBC with manual differential, comprehensive metabolic panel, LDH, uric acid, coagulation studies, and type and screen, as well as a blood culture if fevers are present. A chest x-ray can evaluate for a mediastinal mass. For solid malignancies, consider further imaging, such as ultrasound or CT of the chest, abdomen, and/or pelvis.

Early Management in ED

Initial management includes assessment and stabilization of airway, breathing, and circulation. This is followed by early identification and management of life-threatening conditions, including the following:

- *Severe blood count abnormalities*: Seen mostly in the setting of hematologic malignancies.
  - *Anemia*—transfuse patients with hemoglobin <7 g/dL or symptomatic anemia. If severely anemic, transfuse slowly to avoid volume overload.
  - *Thrombocytopenia*—spontaneous bleeding, including intracranial hemorrhage, may occur at platelets <20 000/μL.
  - *Neutropenia*—blood culture and broad-spectrum antibiotics should be initiated in the setting of fever (high risk for sepsis).
- *Severe electrolyte abnormalities*: Tumor lysis syndrome in leukemia/lymphoma, or SIADH or DI from brain tumors.
- *Intravascular leukostasis*: End organ damage due to sludging effects from hyperleukocytosis (WBC > 100 000), with high risk for respiratory distress and neurological abnormalities. Prompt initiation of chemotherapy, rather than leukapheresis, is the most effective approach to treatment.
- *Superior vena cava syndrome*: Mediastinal leukemia/lymphoma infiltration or neuroblastoma invasion of posterior mediastinum causing chest pain, swelling, respiratory compromise, and/or dysphagia from recurrent laryngeal nerve involvement. Emergent steroids may be indicated.

- *Cord compression:* may be from neuroblastoma infiltration of spinal canal, a spinal cord tumor, or chloroma (mass of leukemic blasts).
- *Elevated intracranial pressure:* dexamethasone is indicated in the setting of brain tumors.

Once treatment of emergent complications has been initiated, the hematology-oncology team should be consulted immediately for admission and further management of the patient. Almost all patients will need to be admitted to a pediatric cancer center, though level of care (PICU vs floor) will depend on associated complications.

KEY POINTS

- The incidence of childhood malignancies is low; however, a high index of suspicion should be present with persistent vague complaints.
- Hematologic malignancies are the most common malignancy of childhood and require blood work to assess for severe blood count or electrolyte abnormalities.
- Following initial stabilization and treatment of emergent complications, consultation with hematology-oncology and/or transfer to a pediatric cancer center is essential.

Suggested Readings

Dorshow JH, Kastan MB, Tepper JE, eds. *Abeloff's Clinical Oncology.* 5th ed. Philadelphia, PA: Elsevier; 2013:1849-1872.
Hunger SP, Mullighan CG. Acute lymphoblastic leukemia in children. *N Engl J Med.* 2015;373:1541.
Hutter JJ. Childhood leukemia. *Pediatr Rev.* 2010;31:234-240.
Jefferson MR, Fuh B, Perkin RM. Pediatric oncologic emergencies. *Pediatr Emerg Med Rep.* 2011;16:57-67.

Sickle Cell Disease Is Not Just Anemia: Be Prepared for Complications Affecting All Organ Systems

Gregory Hall, MD, MHA, FACEP and Evan Verplancken, MD

Sickle cell disease (SCD) is a common disorder seen in the emergency department, and SCD and its complications manifest clinically with a wide array of presentations. Early identification is essential in providing appropriate care for pediatric patients.

Mechanism of Disease

SCD is a genetic disorder that results from a single point mutation causing an altered form of hemoglobin (Hb S) that precipitates intracellularly with resultant cell deformity (sickling). This is the basis for the two main mechanisms of disease, vasoocclusion and hemolysis.

Vasoocclusive Complications

Vasoocclusive Pain Crisis

The most common presentation related to sickle cell disease is vasoocclusive pain crisis. Typically, patients present with pain in the long bones but frequently have pain in the back, chest, and abdomen as well. Patients may have precipitating factors including physiologic or emotional stress, extremes of temperature, dehydration, hypoxia, or anemia to name a few. Dactylitis, a painful inflammation of an entire digit, is particularly common in children <5 years old with SCD. Treatment includes early analgesic medications, beginning with NSAIDs and advancing to opioid medications, supplemental oxygen, and hydration. Rapid initiation of patient-directed pain medication is important both to treat pain and potentially avoid admission. Incentive spirometry should also be initiated early to help prevent respiratory complications.

Splenic Vasoocclusion

Splenic vasoocclusion may lead to splenic sequestration, or pooling of erythrocytes in splenic tissue, and subsequent precipitous drop in hemoglobin on laboratory testing. This should be suspected with splenomegaly on physical examination and is most common in infants with HbSS disease as older children have typically already infarcted their spleen. Early identification and transfusion of pRBC is of utmost importance, and definitive splenectomy is often required.

Priapism

Priapism is also seen frequently in SCD patients due to sickling in penile sinusoids, blocking appropriate venous drainage. This is an emergent situation and requires prompt treatment of pain, hydration, and possibly urology consultation if conservative measures fail. For prolonged priapism lasting >4 hours, aspiration of the corpus cavernosum along with irrigation is the preferred treatment. Injections of phenylephrine into the corpus cavernosum can then be used for full detumescence.

Stroke

Sudden onset of neurological deficits should raise suspicion for acute ischemic stroke secondary to occlusion, with definitive diagnosis often requiring MRI. After prompt recognition, treatment is exchange transfusion.

Acute Chest Syndrome

Acute chest syndrome (ACS) is a particularly concerning SCD complication due to its high morbidity and mortality, particularly in the pediatric population. ACS is most commonly caused by infection; however, it may be secondary to infarction or fat embolus. Symptoms and signs of ACS include cough, chest pain, dyspnea, fever, and hypoxia. Patients should be evaluated with chest x-ray while initiating treatment with oxygen, antibiotics (third-generation cephalosporin), pain management, and possibly blood transfusion. IV fluids should be used judiciously to maintain hydration without fluid overload.

Hemolytic Complications

Both intravascular and extravascular hemolysis is seen with SCD. This results in a chronic hemolytic state that is prone to acute or chronic decompensation. Complications of this include aplastic crisis and splenic or hepatic sequestration. Treatment of acute symptomatic anemia is with transfusion of packed red blood cells.

Infectious Complications

Functional asplenia predisposes patients to infection from encapsulated organisms, including *Haemophilus influenzae*, *Neisseria meningitidis*, and *Streptococcus pneumoniae*. Increasing vaccination rates have reduced rates of bacterial infection. However, any fever >38.5°C in a child with SCD warrants evaluation with a thorough infectious workup including blood cultures and antibiotic therapy, typically with a third-generation cephalosporin.

KEY POINTS

- Treatment of vasoocclusive pain crises require adequate pain control; opioid medications should be used if needed.
- Manage ACS with supplemental oxygen, pain control, maintenance fluids, and antibiotics.
- Sudden onset of neurological symptoms warrants advanced imaging to evaluate for stroke and consideration of exchange transfusion.
- Suspect splenic sequestration with enlarged spleen and drop in hemoglobin and treat with blood transfusion.
- Fever in SCD patients should prompt evaluation with complete blood count and blood cultures and treatment with parenteral antibiotics.

Suggested Readings

Azar S, Wong TE. Sickle cell disease: a brief update. *Med Clin North Am.* 2017;101(2):375-393.

Marshall J. Sickle cell disease in children. In: Tintinalli JE, Stapczynski J, Ma O, Yealy DM, Meckler GD, Cline DM. eds. *Tintinalli's Emergency Medicine: A Comprehensive Study Guide.* 8th ed. New York, NY: McGraw-Hill; 2016.

Shilpa J, Bakshi N, Krishnamurti L. Acute chest syndrome in children with sickle cell disease. *Pediatr Allergy Immunol Pulmonol.* 2017;30(4):191-201.

Ware RE, de Montalembert M, Tshilolo L, Abboud MR. Sickle cell disease. *Lancet.* 2017;390(10091):311-323.

Hemolytic Anemia: Think Before You Transfuse

Yongtian Tina Tan, MD, MBA, Rosy Hao, MD, and Carol C. Chen, MD, MPH, FAAP

Hemolytic anemia can stem from a variety of causes, and some causes can worsen anemia with blood transfusions. It is important to determine the cause to appropriately initiate therapy. Figure 166.1 shows a decision tree to help in this determination.

Sickle Cell Disease and Thalassemia

Sickle cell disease (SCD) patients in particular can have vaso-occlusive crises, which can present as pain, acute chest syndrome, and splenic sequestration. Diagnosis and management of acute chest syndrome is similar to that of adults, including obtaining a chest radiograph to look for new pulmonary infiltrate(s), oxygen as needed, antibiotics, and analgesia.

Splenic sequestration results from splenic pooling of RBCs. Pediatric patients typically present with tender splenomegaly, a hemoglobin drop ≥2 points, thrombocytopenia, and/or reticulocytosis. Giving isotonic fluid to maintain euvolemia is crucial to management. Transfusion is considered only if the patient has symptomatic anemia, as it may precipitate hyperviscosity and increase the risk of sickling.

SCD and thalassemia patients are functionally asplenic, so infection can be deadly. Infection can also trigger hemolytic crisis in SCD patients. When these patients present with fever, they need a blood culture, complete blood count, reticulocyte count, and empiric ceftriaxone.

Hereditary Spherocytosis and Glucose-6-phosphate Dehydrogenase Deficiency

Hereditary spherocytosis (HS) patients may have mild chronic anemia, whereas in glucose-6-phosphate dehydrogenase (G6PD) this is often absent. In both conditions, patients are asymptomatic unless

Approach to the Child with Hemolytic Anemia in the Emergency Department

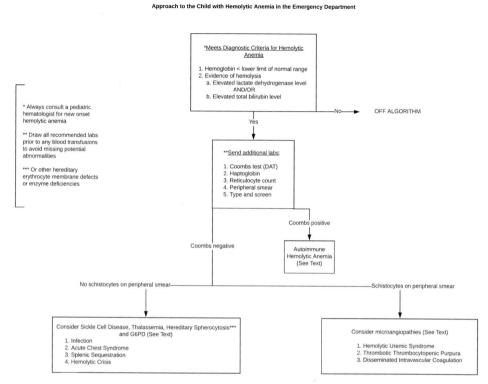

Figure 166.1 Approach to the child with hemolytic anemia in the emergency department.

they are triggered into hemolytic crisis. The most common trigger is infection; for G6PD patients other triggers include certain foods and/or medications. Management includes treating/removing the offending agent, intravenous hydration, and protecting kidney function. Transfusion for symptomatic patients can be helpful and will not precipitate further hemolysis.

Autoimmune Hemolytic Anemia

In autoimmune hemolytic anemia (AIHA), autoantibodies bind to RBCs, leading to premature destruction. It can be caused by "warm" (more common) or "cold" antibodies, both with a positive Coombs test. Management is generally the same; in "cold" type, keeping the patient warm and avoiding cold fluids can prevent further hemolysis.

Patients with AIHA generally warrant hospitalization for close observation and treatment. RBC transfusions in AIHA can lead to additional hemolysis and should only be considered in children with severe anemia and signs of hypoxemia or cardiac failure. When transfusions are necessary, infuse 5 mL/kg over 10-15 minutes; if signs of acute hemolysis develop, stop and administer normal saline until a new unit can be prepared. In severely anemic patients, an immediate trial of either corticosteroid therapy or intravenous immunoglobulin (IVIG) may reduce the need for RBC transfusion.

Microangiopathies

Schistocytes with negative Coombs test suggest a microangiopathic process, such as hemolytic uremic syndrome (HUS) or thrombotic thrombocytopenic purpura (TTP).

HUS is the simultaneous occurrence of microangiopathy, thrombocytopenia, and acute kidney injury, and is most commonly caused by Shiga toxin in *Escherichia coli*. The hemolysis is the result of small vessel disease in the kidney, and thus treatment is targeted at supportive care and preventing renal failure. This may include RBC and platelet transfusions, fluid/electrolyte management, and initiating dialysis.

Consider TTP with fever, hemolysis, neurologic and renal abnormalities, and thrombocytopenia. Prompt institution of plasma exchange in TTP can be lifesaving. Untreated, TTP has a mortality rate as high as 90%, largely due to delayed recognition and treatment. Consider RBC transfusion only when the anemia is symptomatic.

KEY POINTS

- Children with new-onset hemolytic anemia need subspecialty consultation and a baseline laboratory workup prior to blood transfusion.
- Do not transfuse patients with splenic sequestration unless they have severe symptomatic anemia, as the transfusion can worsen vaso-occlusion.
- AIHA warrants close observation, but RBC transfusions can cause additional hemolysis and should only be considered in children with severe anemia and hypoxemia.
- Prompt recognition and treatment of TTP with plasma exchange can be lifesaving.

Suggested Readings

Barros MM, Langhi Jr DM, Bordin JO. Autoimmune hemolytic anemia: transfusion challenges and solutions. *Int J Clin Transfus Med*. 2016;5:9-18.

Joly B, Coppo C, Veyradier A. Thrombotic thrombocytopenic purpura. American Society of Hematology. *Blood*. 2017;129:2836-2846.

Sieff CA, Kesselheim JC. Hematologic emergencies. In: Fleisher GF, Ludwig SL, eds. *Textbook of Pediatric Emergency Medicine*. 6th ed. Philadelphia, PA: Lippincott Williams & Wilkins; 2010:862-886.

Vachinsky E. Overview of the clinical manifestations of sickle cell disease. *UpToDate*. 2019.

Feeling Blue Despite O₂?: Consider Methemoglobinemia

Morgan J. Sims, MD, FAAP and Benjamin F. Jackson, MD, FAAP, FACEP

When confronted with a case of cyanosis in the absence of known respiratory or cardiac disease, clinicians should maintain a high index of suspicion and an open differential diagnosis. Methemoglobinemia is an uncommon but not infrequent etiology that must be kept in mind to initiate appropriate and timely treatment.

In patients with methemoglobinemia, cyanosis will persist despite use of supplemental oxygen. Despite low oxygen saturation and refractory cyanosis, these patients have a normal PaO_2. Another hallmark of methemoglobinemia is abnormally colored blood, often described as chocolate brown. Normally, iron in hemoglobin is in the ferrous state (Fe^{2+}), which allows it to effectively deliver oxygen; about 1% is ferric (Fe^{3+}) in typical, healthy individuals. However, under oxidative stress, more iron is pushed to the ferric state, which renders it incapable of reversibly binding oxygen. Oxygen cannot be released to the tissues, which causes end-organ dysfunction.

A methemoglobin level of 15% produces visible cyanosis. As levels rise, patients may start to experience anxiety, headache, dizziness, fatigue, confusion, tachycardia, and tachypnea. Methemoglobin >30% is considered life threatening as complications like seizures and arrhythmias may occur. Methemoglobin levels of 70% or greater are fatal. Symptomatic thresholds may be lower in an anemic individual, as there is less normally functioning hemoglobin available prior to onset of methemoglobinemia.

Methemoglobinemia may be congenital or acquired. Congenital methemoglobinemia is most commonly caused by cytochrome b5 reductase deficiency, which is the enzyme predominately responsible for converting methemoglobin back to hemoglobin. Patients are usually asymptomatic despite high levels of methemoglobin. Acquired methemoglobinemia can come from a wide variety of environmental insults including various foods, chemicals, and medications. Common etiologies include benzocaine teething gels, dapsone, nitrates, and sulfa-containing antibiotics. Ingested products high in nitrates such as well water have also been known to cause methemoglobinemia. If ingestion is suspected, consider involving toxicology or poison control. Finally, methemoglobinemia may occur as part of another disease process, most notably severe gastroenteritis causing acidosis and sepsis.

In all cases of methemoglobinemia, the offending oxidative agent should be identified and removed. If patients are only mildly symptomatic or have a methemoglobin level <20%, medical therapy is not required as patients will convert methemoglobin back to hemoglobin within hours. However, treatment should be considered when methemoglobin levels exceed 20% or when patients have significant symptoms. Preferred treatment is methylene blue 1-2 mg/kg IV. If symptoms persist, or if methemoglobin levels exceed 30%, after 60 minutes, a dose may be repeated. Be cautious—at high levels, methylene blue is an oxidant that can potentiate methemoglobinemia. Total dose of methylene blue should not exceed 7 mg/kg.

Methylene blue should not be used in patients with known or suspected glucose-6-phosphate dehydrogenase (G6PD) deficiency. In such children, it can precipitate a hemolytic crisis. In cases where methylene blue is unable to be used or when it is unavailable, ascorbic acid (vitamin C) may also be used as treatment. Current evidence for ascorbic acid in methemoglobinemia is limited but suggests it may be beneficial and is a reasonable treatment option. While methylene blue works quickly, ascorbic acid is a more gradual process that takes days to significantly lower methemoglobin levels. For cases that are refractory to methylene blue or in patients with G6PD deficiency who need acute treatment, consider exchange transfusion.

Children with methemoglobinemia should be admitted to the hospital after receiving treatment, whether that be for observation or further intervention. Certain agents may cause rebound methemoglobinemia, requiring subsequent treatment.

KEY POINTS

- Patients with a methemoglobin level of ~15% will have cyanosis; as levels rise, this will progress to cardiorespiratory abnormalities and altered mental status.
- Treat cases with a methemoglobin level exceeding 20% or a severely symptomatic patient.
- Treatment is with methylene blue 1-2 mg/kg IV, but this should not be used in patients with G6PD deficiency.
- In cases where methylene blue cannot be used or is not available, consider ascorbic acid or exchange transfusion.

Suggested Readings

Cash C, Arnold DH. Extreme methemoglobinemia after topical benzocaine: recognition by pulse oximetry. *J Pediatr.* 2017;181:319.

Cortazzo JA, Lichtman AD. Methemoglobinemia: a review and recommendations for management. *J Cardiothorac Vasc Anesth.* 2014;28:1043-1047.

Croteau SE, Fleegler EW, Brett-Fleegler M. Hematologic emergencies. In: Shaw KN, Bachur RG, ed. *Fleischer & Ludwig's Textbook of Pediatric Emergency Medicine.* 7th ed. Philadelphia, PA: Wolters Kluwer; 2016:804-837.

DeBaun MR, Frei-Jones M, Vichinsky E. Hereditary methemoglobinemia. In: Kleigman RM, ed. *Nelson Textbook of Pediatrics.* 19th ed. Philadelphia, PA: Elsevier Saunders; 2011:1672-1673.

Rehman HU. Methemoglobinemia. *West J Med.* 2001;175:193-196.

168

Pediatric Neutropenia: Worth a Pause, but Not Always Panic

Cortlyn Brown, MD and Heidi Werner, MD, MSHPEd

The lab calls and says that the ANC for your well-appearing 3-year-old is 640. Sound the alarm? Or not so much…? Pediatric neutropenia is more common than you may think, and should give us pause, though not necessarily panic, as we will soon see.

Neutropenia is an absolute neutrophil count (ANC) <1500/µL, with severe neutropenia being an ANC < 500/µL. In children, neutropenia may be acquired or congenital, with infections, medications, and immune disorders as the most common acquired causes. Many pediatric patients will present with asymptomatic neutropenia, found incidentally on laboratory testing, and those patients often do not require ED workup; however, febrile neutropenia requires special consideration.

Febrile Neutropenia

Early identification of febrile neutropenic patients is critical, especially those who are ill appearing and require immediate evaluation and resuscitation. While some data suggest that neutropenia in well-appearing, immunocompetent, febrile patients is frequently an outcome of viral illness, prompt identification of neutropenia and underlying risk factors remains imperative. Ill-appearing patients and those with underlying diseases require broad-spectrum antibiotics to be administered without delay. ED providers should assess for a history of prior infections, as well as height of fever and current constitutional symptoms, focusing on possible sources, including oral, mucosal, pulmonary, GI, urinary, and CNS locations. A thorough medication history should assess for immunosuppressive medications such as chemotherapy. A family history of early infant deaths, neutropenia, or recurrent infections could point to congenital causes of neutropenia. A focused physical examination may yield an infectious source keeping in mind that the absence of neutrophils may diminish visible inflammation. The examination should also look for adenopathy and organomegaly (most notably splenomegaly).

The most common cause of mild-to-moderate neutropenia is viral bone marrow suppression; some examples include varicella, measles, rubella, hepatitis A and B, influenza, cytomegalovirus (CMV), ebstein barr virus (EBV), parvovirus b19, adenovirus, and coxsackievirus. Bacterial endotoxin suppression, most notably with gram-positive cocci and gram-negative bacilli, can also cause neutropenia.

Febrile neutropenic patients require a CBC and blood culture. Testing, including chest x-ray, urinalysis/urine culture, viral PCR, or abdominal imaging, should be tailored to the patient's symptoms and risk factors. When evaluating the CBC, also evaluate for thrombocytopenia and anemia, because these in addition to neutropenia suggest a generalized marrow process such as aplastic anemia or leukemia. Initial regimens for well-appearing febrile neutropenic patients includes ceftriaxone or other monotherapy with broad coverage. Ill-appearing patients should receive double or triple coverage (eg, cefepime, vancomycin, and metronidazole).

Afebrile Neutropenia

Chronic benign neutropenia is the most common cause of afebrile neutropenia in children younger than 4 who do not have an infection. Certain medications, most notably analgesics/anti-inflammatories (ibuprofen, indomethacin), antibiotics (sulfonamides, penicillins, chloramphenicol), anticonvulsants (phenytoin, carbamazepine), antithyroid agents propylthiouracil (PTU), and cardiovascular drugs (hydralazine, procainamide), can cause neutropenia. There are also autoimmune causes, such as primary autoimmune neutropenia, which is typically seen in girls younger than 2 who have mild skin and upper respiratory infections. This neutropenia spontaneously resolves and is associated with a good prognosis. Lastly, there are inherited causes of neutropenia, such as IgA deficiency, and hereditary causes, such as Kostmann syndrome, familial benign, Shwachman-Diamond syndrome, and Fanconi anemia.

Disposition

Disposition depends on the patient's underlying marrow function and appearance more than the ANC. Well-appearing children with normal marrow function may be managed outpatient with follow-up labs to ensure resolution. Ill-appearing children or those with poor marrow function require inpatient monitoring and IV antibiotics. If discharged, families should be instructed to monitor for continued fever, signs or symptoms of new infectious sources, or change in baseline level of functioning. Close follow-up with the primary subspecialist or primary care physician is imperative.

KEY POINTS

- Neutropenia is an absolute neutrophil count (ANC) of <1500/μL, with severe neutropenia <500/μL.
- Febrile neutropenia in the ill-appearing child is an emergency, and requires evaluation with CBC and blood culture, as well as identification of the underlying source of infection.
- Ill-appearing children or those with marrow suppression and febrile neutropenia require prompt administration of broad-spectrum antibiotics.

Suggested Readings

Approach to the patient with neutropenia in childhood. https://pedemmorsels.com/neutropenic-fever/

Klastersky J, de Naurois J, Rolston K, et al.; ESMO Guidelines Committee. Management of febrile neutropaenia: ESMO clinical practice guidelines. *Ann Oncol.* 2016;27(suppl 5):v111-v118.

Meckler G, Lindemulder S. Fever and neutropenia in pediatric patients with cancer. *Emerg Med Clin North Am.* 2009;27(3):525-544.

Pascual C, Trenchs V, Hernández-Bou S, Català A, Valls AF, Luaces C. Outcomes and infectious etiologies of febrile neutropenia in non-immunocompromised children who present in an emergency department. *Eur J Clin Microbiol Infect Dis.* 2016;35(10):1667-16672.

Fever and Neutropenia: Be Prepared When That Oncology Patient Arrives

Ian Kane, MD

Background

Fever and neutropenia remains a feared complication among children treated with chemotherapy for cancer. Neutropenia is formally diagnosed at levels below 1500 cells/μL; however, the risk of complications due to neutropenia increases as the absolute neutrophil count (ANC) drops below 500 cells/μL, and this limit has been widely adopted as the definition of neutropenia among this patient population. Fever is defined among these children as one temperature >38.3°C (101°F) or two temperature readings >38.0°C (100.4°F) separated by at least 1 hour. Children with fever and neutropenia are at risk for severe infectious complications due to their weakened immune system.

Prearrival Preparation

Emergency department management of these children must be accomplished quickly and efficiently, as studies have documented that delays in antibiotic administration beyond 60 minutes are associated with increased morbidity and mortality. This is most often accomplished through the use of an institution-specific clinical practice guideline that has been developed in concert with the Pediatric Oncology department. Current guidelines in use highlight the importance of communication between the ED and the Oncology department prior to a patient's arrival. Prior communication allows for neutropenic or potentially neutropenic patients to be triaged and evaluated urgently so that the appropriate laboratory studies and antibiotics can be ordered without delay.

Initial Evaluation

Triage vital signs should be reviewed to assess for signs of severe sepsis and shock, which would necessitate immediate resuscitative measures. A thorough history and physical examination is required to assess for any potential infectious source. Particular attention should be paid to all indwelling devices such as a central venous line (CVL), the mouth to assess for mucositis, and the abdomen to check for tenderness and distention as would be seen with neutropenic enterocolitis. Blood cultures from every lumen of the CVL and a CBC with differential should be obtained on all patients. Bacteremia is the most common severe infection among children with fever and neutropenia, occurring in up to 25% of all cases. The routine acquisition of a peripheral culture is controversial and institution specific as the management of CVL-related and peripheral bacteremia is managed similarly in these patients. Other investigations such as urinalysis, urine culture, viral testing, and chest radiography are not routinely obtained unless specifically suggested by the child's clinical presentation. Importantly, invasive testing such as urinary catheterization or rectal temperature measurement should be avoided in all neutropenic patients.

Antibiotic Selection

Antibiotics are vital for any child with suspected or confirmed neutropenia and should be initiated as soon as possible. Empiric antibiotic choices for typical chemotherapy-induced fever and neutropenia should provide broad gram-positive, gram-negative, and pseudomonal coverage and options include piperacillin-tazobactam, cefepime, or meropenem. Monotherapy with any one of these agents has been shown to be similar to combination therapy with an improved side effect profile. Vancomycin should only be added in cases where a gram-positive infection is suspected; for example among children with hypotension, pneumonia, signs of a soft tissue infection, or those who were recently treated with high-dose cytarabine.

Disposition

At most institutions, all children meeting criteria for fever and neutropenia are admitted for continued IV antibiotics as the cultures are followed. However, some smaller studies have suggested that certain low-risk populations of children with fever and neutropenia may be discharged with oral antibiotics and close Oncology follow-up.

KEY POINTS

- Having an institutional algorithm in place is essential for the prompt evaluation and treatment of children with fever and neutropenia.
- Among children with fever and neutropenia, a delay in antibiotics beyond 60 minutes is associated with worse outcomes.
- For most children, empiric treatment with piperacillin-tazobactam, cefepime, or meropenem is sufficient.
- The addition of empiric vancomycin should be reserved for those children with hypotension or those with signs of a gram-positive infection such as a localized skin or soft tissue infection.

Suggested Readings

Henry M, Sung L. Supportive care in pediatric oncology: oncologic emergencies and management of fever and neutropenia. *Pediatr Clin North Am.* 2015;62:27-46.

Ku BC, Bailey C, Balamuth F. Neutropenia and the febrile child. *Pediatr Emerg Care.* 2016;32:329-336.

Yoshida H, Leger KJ, Xu M, et al. Improving time to antibiotics for pediatric oncology patients with suspected infections. *Pediatr Emerg Care.* 2018;34:47-52.

170

Hemophilia—Do Not Undertreat the Bad Bleeds

William White, MD, MA, Jessica L. Chow, MD, MPH and Dina Wallin, MD

A huge thigh hematoma after vaccinations. Bleeding gums with teething. The circ that will not stop oozing. Top of the differential? Hemophilia!

Hemophilia is X-linked and leads to a deficiency of clotting factors; hemophilia A is a deficiency in factor VIII, while hemophilia B is a factor IX deficiency. Clinical manifestations are seen mostly in males, and although hemophilia is commonly inherited, up to one-third of diagnosed children have de novo mutations.

Baseline plasma factor VIII and IX activity levels correlate with clinical severity and bleeding risk, with severe hemophilia defined as factor levels <1% of normal, moderate as 1%-5%, and mild as 5%-40%. Hemophilia B tends to be milder and may not be diagnosed until later in life.

Historical factors suggesting hemophilia in children include easy bruising, spontaneous bleeding, and persistent or severe bleeding after trauma, surgery, or procedures such as heel sticks, venipuncture, vaccinations, and circumcision. However, the differential also includes platelet disorders, vasculitides, coagulopathies, and nonaccidental trauma.

Bleeding Presentations

Joint and Soft Tissue Bleeds

The hallmark of hemophilia is joint bleeding (hemarthrosis). Patients may present only with pain, without examination ination findings; often, the first sign is tingling, followed by pain, swelling, and reduced range of motion. Factor treatment is advised—untreated hemarthrosis can lead to chronic arthropathy. Avoid nonsteroidal anti-inflammatories (increased bleeding risk) and intramuscular injections. Arthrocentesis is not required unless evaluating for infection or for pain control (replace factor *pre*procedure). The joint may require splinting and non–weight bearing. Most hemarthroses are managed as an outpatient; indications for hospitalization include disruption of a major joint, initial delay in treatment, failure of outpatient therapy, and poor pain control.

Other common clinical manifestations include oral mucosal bleeding and intramuscular hematomas. Bleeding from a tooth eruption may be an initial sign of hemophilia. Muscle hematomas may vaguely present as pain or swelling, often after trauma or injections. Factor replacement is recommended for muscle hematomas to decrease the risk of compartment syndrome, nerve damage, and muscle atrophy.

Treatment

Do Not Delay: Treat First and Evaluate Second

The main goal is to increase deficient circulating factor levels as soon as possible. In suspected acute life-threatening bleeds (eg, intracranial hemorrhage or bleeding of the airway, abdomen, or gastrointestinal tract) do *not* wait for lab or imaging results to initiate emergent replacement.

Dose to target to specific factor activity percentages. Life-threatening bleeds need 100% activity, and minor/moderate bleeds target lower percentages (30%-80%).

Hemophilia A

Each unit/kg of factor VIII concentrate increases plasma levels by 2%; infuse 25 IU/kg for minor bleeds or 50 IU/kg for major bleeds. Cryoprecipitate or tranexamic acid (TXA) may be used if factor VIII concentrate is unavailable. Desmopressin has been shown to increase endogenous factor VIII levels in some patients.

Hemophilia B

Each unit/kg of factor IX concentrate increases plasma levels by 1%; infuse 40 IU/kg for minor bleeds or 100 IU/kg for major bleeds. Fresh frozen plasma (FFP) or TXA may be used if factor IX concentrate is unavailable.

Some patients may present to the emergency department with their own doses of recombinant factor. In the setting of life-threatening bleeding, use patient-provided factor for replacement to significantly expedite the process of factor replacement.

Additional Considerations

Ask the patient if he or she has known factor inhibitors. If the patients know they have inhibitors OR if the factor infusion does not raise their activity to desired percentages, then they may need activated prothrombin complex concentrate (such as FEIBA [factor eight inhibitor bypassing activity]) or recombinant activated factor VII.

More recently, a new therapeutic option, treatment with the monoclonal antibody emicizumab, has become available for patients with hemophilia A. This monoclonal antibody to factors IXa and X has been shown to decrease the incidence of bleeding in patients with and without factor VIII inhibitors. Managing bleeding in patients on emicizumab is treated as above.

KEY POINTS

- Patients with hemophilia may present with easy bruising or spontaneous or persistent bleeds in early childhood, even without family history.
- Do not delay factor replacement treatment for life-threatening bleeds!
- Treat first and evaluate (diagnostics, consultations) second, with a goal to raise factor activity levels to 100% for severe bleeds. For hemophilia A: 50 units (per kg) to raise to 100%. For hemophilia B: 100 units (per kg) to raise to 100%.

Suggested Readings

Kulkarni R, Soucie JM. Pediatric hemophilia: a review. *Semin Thromb Hemost.* 2011;37(7):737-744.

Morgan LM, Kissoon N, de Vebber BL. Experience with the hemophiliac child in a pediatric emergency department. *J Emerg Med.* 1993;11:519-524.

World Federation of Hemophilia. Guidelines for the management of hemophilia. *Haemophilia.* 2012. https://www.wfh.org/en/resources/wfh-treatment-guidelines. Accessed on February 10, 2019.

171

How Much Is Too Much: Spotting Abnormal Bleeding Disorders

Gabriel Paul Devlin, MD/CM and Tatyana Vayngortin, MD

Children often present to the emergency department (ED) for bleeding, whether after a fall from the monkey bars or nose-picking. While usually nothing of concern, bleeding may be a harbinger of an underlying coagulopathy. Be aware of the warning signs and know when to pursue a more comprehensive evaluation.

History and Physical Examination

To no clinician's surprise, the first step is a good history. Providers should ask about the severity and duration of the current episode of bleeding, as well as any significant prior episodes. In children, this includes hematomas after minimal or no trauma as well as any prolonged bleeding after routine procedures such as vaccinations, heel pricks, circumcision, dental extractions, tonsillectomies, and other surgeries.

About one-fourth of patients presenting to the ED with epistaxis or abnormal uterine bleeding (AUB) have an underlying bleeding disorder. Red flags for epistaxis include age <2 years old, absence of provoking factors, occurrence more than twice per week, duration longer than 30 minutes, or bleeding that requires cauterization or packing. Red flags in AUB include heavy bleeding since menarche, duration longer than 7 days, soaking one pad or tampon every hour, passing clots larger than the size of a quarter, and soaking through clothing or onto bedding.

Clinicians should always ask basic questions about past medical history, medications, review of systems, and family history. In addition to aspirin and NSAIDs, certain herbal supplements (eg, ginger, feverfew, ginkgo biloba) can also cause bleeding. The review of systems should evaluate for malignancy, liver dysfunction, and infection. A negative family history is useful but does not rule out an inherited bleeding disorder (one-third of patients with hemophilia have no known family history!).

Certain situations should always prompt an evaluation for a bleeding disorder. These include spontaneous hemarthrosis (especially in a newly mobile child), bleeding gums, bleeding from multiple organs, or frequent health care visits for bleeding. Furthermore, any infant presenting with significant bleeding requires special attention, as ~50% of patients with severe inherited coagulopathy are diagnosed within the first month of life.

The physical examination should survey all skin, joints, and mucocutaneous areas. While small bruises (<1 cm) on the forehead, chin, anterior knees, and shins are common in older children due to falls, bruises in premobile infants (typically <9 months old) are highly concerning for nonaccidental trauma or coagulopathy. Larger bruises or bruises located on the arms, abdomen, back, and thighs are more concerning, but these can be seen in healthy ambulatory children as well. Diffuse petechiae or any purpura merit laboratory evaluation.

Laboratory Evaluation and Management

Laboratory screening for coagulopathy includes a complete blood count (CBC), blood smear, prothrombin time (PT), and activated partial thromboplastin time (aPTT). Additional evaluation can include liver function enzymes and aspirin/acetaminophen levels as indicated. Patients younger than 6 months have lower levels of coagulation factors, so clinicians should ensure their institution's laboratory reference ranges are appropriately adjusted for age. Many disorders such as von Willebrand disease, mild hemophilia, factor XIII deficiency, and platelet function disorders will have normal screening labs. Some institutions offer lab test panels (such as a von Willebrand's panel or bleeding panel) that can provide useful information for the family in follow-up. Nevertheless, clinicians should always refer any patient with features suspicious for a bleeding disorder to a pediatric hematologist for further evaluation, regardless of lab results.

KEY POINTS

- Red flags for a bleeding disorder include significant bruising/bleeding in infancy, two or more sources of bleeding, diffuse petechiae, purpura, mucocutaneous bleeding, spontaneous hematomas, hemarthrosis, or multiple ED visits for bleeding.
- Consider the patient's age and developmental milestones when evaluating whether bruising is normal.
- Basic screening tests for a bleeding disorder include CBC, blood smear, PT, and aPTT. However, normal screening labs do not rule out a bleeding disorder. If there is sufficient concern, refer to pediatric hematology.

Suggested Readings

Collins PW, Hamilton M, Dunstan FD, et al. Patterns of bruising in preschool children with inherited bleeding disorders: a longitudinal study. *Arch Dis Child*. 2017;102:1110-1117.

Khair K, Liesner R. Bruising and bleeding in infants and children—a practical approach. *Br J Haematol*. 2006;133(3):221-231.

Revel-Vilk S, Rand ML, Israels SJ. An approach to the bleeding child. In: Blanchette VS, Breakey VR, Revel-Vilk S, eds. *Sick Kids Handbook of Pediatric Thrombosis and Hemostasis*. Basel: Karger; 2013:14-22.

GENETICS/METABOLISM

172

Recognition and Management of Inborn Errors of Metabolism—The Needle in the Haystack

James (Jim) Homme, MD

Inborn errors of metabolism (IEM) present with a spectrum of signs of symptoms, the majority of which overlap significantly with other disease conditions. Newborn screening has improved early detection; however, patients may present prior to the results of the newborn screen and many conditions remain that evade detection under currently offered screening methods. It is important to have a basic understanding of how to recognize and manage these disorders.

The clinical manifestations of IEM are typically the result of either an interruption in energy production or accumulation of toxic metabolites. Glucose is the primary energy source for most cellular activities with the ultimate result of metabolism ending in oxidative phosphorylation and energy production. Cells also utilize ketone bodies from the breakdown of fatty acids to feed into the system when glucose is not available. Interruptions in metabolic pathways either decrease substrates for utilization or block pathways for production. In addition, accumulation of metabolites can either have direct toxic effects or disrupt metabolism. General knowledge of the subtle and overt manifestations of IEM as well as a few key laboratory tests are all clinicians need to be able to identify and address this heterogeneous group of disorders.

Recognition of the subtle and overt signs and symptoms of an IEM (Table 172.1) is the critical first step. Key initial laboratory studies to obtain in suspected IEM are listed in Table 172.2. It is vital to obtain samples during the acute illness as treatment may erase key evidence of the disorder delaying diagnosis. Saving extra serum and urine for future testing is recommended.

Table 172.1 ■ Potential Signs and Symptoms of an IFM	
Subtle	Overt
Poor feeding/feeding refusal	Persistent hypoglycemia
Vomiting	Acidosis
Somnolence	Lethargy/coma
Irritability	Seizure
Tachypnea	Arrhythmia
Abnormal tone	Apnea
Prostration with mild illness	Cardiomyopathy
Tachycardia	Sudden unexplained death
Poor weight gain	
Bleeding and cytopenias	

Table 172.2 ■ Laboratory Investigations for Potential IEM	
Primary Evaluation	Secondary Evaluation
Blood	**Blood**
Glucose[a]	Primary evaluation laboratory tests *plus*
Electrolytes (Na$^+$, K$^+$, Cl$^-$, HCO$_3^{-a}$, anion gap[a])	Plasma carnitine, acylcarnitine profile
CBC with differential	Amino acid profile (quantitative)
Venous blood gas	± Biotinidase
Ammonia[a]	
Lactate[a] & pyruvate	
Hepatic transaminases, ± bilirubin	
± Coagulation studies, ± Creatinine Kinase	
Urine	**Urine**
Ketones[a]	Primary evaluation laboratory tests *plus*
Reducing substances	Organic acids, orotic acids, and amino acids
pH	Acylglycines

[a]Key labs to guide initial management.

Laboratory indicators in the acute care setting suggestive of an inborn error of metabolism include:

- Profound hypoglycemia → Disorders of carbohydrate metabolism
- Hypoketotic hypoglycemia → Fatty acid oxidation (FAO) defect
- Hyperammonemia without acidosis → Urea cycle defect
- Hyperammonemia with acidosis → Secondary effect on urea cycle from other IEM like organic acidemia, FAO, etc.
- Respiratory alkalosis + tachypnea (and seizures or altered mental status) → Hyperammonemia
- Lactic acidosis without sepsis, poor perfusion, or hypoxia → Mitochondrial disorder
- Profound acidosis → Organic acidemia
- Neonate with ketosis → Organic acidemia

Some IEM, such as many of the aminoacidopathies (eg, phenylketonuria [PKU]) and lysosomal storage diseases (eg, mucopolysaccharidosis) can only be diagnosed by specific tests with symptoms manifesting as a result of cumulative exposure. Of special note, disorders of branched chain amino acid metabolism (eg, Maple Syrup Urine Disease [MSUD]) can be rapidly fatal and should be suspected and ruled out in neonates presenting with subtle symptoms of poor feeding, irritability, and lethargy followed by spasticity, seizures, and coma.

Initial management of any patient suspected of an IEM focuses on *stopping catabolism* by providing an alternative energy source. This is typically done with infusion of D10 ½NS or D10NS at 1½ maintenance rate after correction of initial hypoglycemia with boluses. Some patients require concomitant insulin or intralipid infusions. In addition, correction of metabolic acidosis may require boluses/infusions of bicarbonate. Removal of toxic metabolites through cessation of feeding as well as administration of scavenger agents or replacing depleted cofactors is also important. Ammonia is a potent neurotoxin, and patients with elevated ammonia and altered mental status *should* be rapidly transferred to a facility that can provide dialysis. All patients receive supportive care and treatment of potential infections. Early consultation with a specialist in genetics is strongly recommended.

KEY POINTS

- Presentation of an IEM can be subtle or overt with significant overlap with other more common disorders.
- Utilization of some simple tests (glucose, electrolytes with anion gap, lactate, pyruvate, ammonia, pH, and ketones) can help raise suspicion for IEMs.
- Initial treatment of IEMs focuses on *stopping catabolism* and *removal of toxic metabolites*.
- Obtain samples for expanded diagnostic testing early in presentation to avoid erasing evidence of the disorder with treatment.

Suggested Readings

MacNeil EC, Walker CP. Inborn errors of metabolism in the emergency department (undiagnosed and management of known). *Emerg Med Clin North Am.* 2018;36(2):369-385.
Rice GM, Steiner RD. Inborn errors of metabolism (metabolic disorders). *Pediatr Rev.* 2016;37(1):3-15.

Have No Fear; an Inborn Error of Metabolism Is Here! Managing Patients With Known Inborn Errors of Metabolism

James (Jim) Homme, MD

Patients with known underlying inborn errors of metabolism (IEM) can be intimidating due to the notion that these conditions are vast and unknowable without specialized training. Memories of complex metabolic pathways quickly memorized and more rapidly forgotten generate a sense of helplessness even in experienced providers. However, a basic understanding of the main parts of metabolism coupled with detailed emergency care plans and the "phone a metabolic specialist" friend option allows any practitioner to efficiently and confidently manage this heterogeneous group of patients.

The very first thing any provider should ask when a patient with an IEM presents for care is "Does the patient have an established emergency care plan or emergency information form (EIF) and where can I access it?" These documents typically summarize the underlying condition, outline the situations that may result in metabolic decompensation, and provide guidance on initiation of appropriate labs and treatment. In addition, key subspecialist contact information is often included. Care providers are instructed to bring these documents with them but may not present them for fear of seeming too pushy or demanding. Alternatively, they may have forgotten the document exists especially if the child has experienced an extended period of health. It is critical to engage the care providers immediately when determining a plan of care for the patient. They have the perspective of the child's baseline, propensity for decompensation along with established goals of care.

A basic understanding of the "buckets" into which the majority of IEMs fall help clinicians understand the rationale for recommended evaluation and therapies. The four major classes are disorders of carbohydrate, lipid, and protein metabolism as well as defects in primary energy production. Carbohydrate metabolism disorders affect the availability of glucose through interruption of glycogenolysis (glycogen breakdown), gluconeogenesis (glucose production), or glycolysis (metabolism of glucose into Acetyl-CoA to be fed into the Krebs cycle). Pyruvate is a key intermediary in this process. Hepatic-based glycogen storage diseases (GSD) lead to hypoglycemia in the fasting state whereas muscle-based

GSD lead to muscle breakdown with preserved blood glucose levels. Other carbohydrate disorders include galactosemia and hereditary fructose intolerance. Clinical manifestations of these disorders result from the toxic effects of buildup of galactose or fructose-1 phosphate.

Individuals with fatty acid oxidation disorders develop a hypoketotic hypoglycemia during fasting or increased metabolic demand. Examples include medium chain, long chain, and very long chain acyl CoA dehydrogenase enzymes or disorders of carnitine metabolism. Clinical manifestations result from the hypoglycemia, hypoketonemia, and buildup of toxic metabolites.

Aminoacidopathies develop when the initial step of amino acid metabolism, deamination (removal of the amine group), is interrupted. They are typically clinically silent in their presentation with dysfunction occurring over prolonged exposures. Organic acidemias result from defects in enzyme metabolism of the remaining keto acid. These disorders result in severe acidosis and secondary hyperammonemia. Urea cycle defects produce profound hyperammonemia without acidosis due to the inability to properly metabolize ammonia into urea. Neurologic morbidity and overall mortality are directly related to magnitude and duration of hyperammonemia.

Disorders of energy production, often referred to as mitochondrial disorders, are a heterogenous group of conditions that result in decrease in ATP production (arguably an oversimplification). The highest energy–utilizing tissues (brain, muscles, heart and lungs) are most affected. Manifestations include encephalopathy, neuromuscular diseases, seizures, strokes, and developmental delay. Typically, multiple organ systems are involved in these disorders.

Management of all IEMs rely on halting the catabolic process, providing alternative substrate (typically dextrose) for energy production, repletion of diminished cofactors, and removal of toxic metabolites through hydration, scavenging agents, or dialysis. One very important cofactor is carnitine. It plays a critical role in the transportation of fatty acids across the mitochondrial membrane for oxidation into energy and in the generation and stabilization of acetyl-CoA. It also binds to excess organic acids and free fatty acids permitting excretion, which can lead to a secondary carnitine deficiency during metabolic decompensation. Thus, carnitine is commonly utilized in the treatment of many IEMs. Dosing of medications and monitoring response to treatment may be tailored to the individual patient and his or her current metabolic state. Therefore, it is exceptionally important to engage subspecialty input early in care.

KEY POINTS

- Determine immediately if a patient with a known IEM has an emergency care plan.
- Early communication with the geneticist or primary provider for a patient with a known IEM is critical—do not try and manage them on your own.
- Despite a well appearance, patients with known IEM can decompensate quickly—do not deviate from the care plan or discount caregiver concerns.

Suggested Readings

MacNeil EC, Walker CP. Inborn errors of metabolism in the emergency department (undiagnosed and management of known). *Emerg Med Clin North Am.* 2018;36:369-385.

Rice GM, Steiner RD. Inborn errors of metabolism (metabolic disorders). *Pediatr Rev.* 2016;37(1):3-15.

Be Aware of Abnormal Newborn Screens

Cree Kachelski, MD, FAAP and Jason (Jay) Homme, MD, FAAP

Universal newborn screening aims at early detection of multiple genetic diseases, hearing loss, and critical congenital heart disease (CCHD). Front-line providers will have to deal with both true and false positives as well as recognition of the disorders that may present prior to state newborn screening results. With the rise of alternative birthing options, more newborns are not undergoing routine screening. There are some important presentations all emergency department providers need to recognize and treat emergently in order to decrease morbidity and mortality. Providers should also know the resources to use if a child with a known abnormal newborn screen has been sent to the emergency department for care. The best resource to utilize quickly is the American College of Medical Genetics and Genomics Newborn Screening ACT sheets and algorithms all located online.

Not to Miss Presentations

The lethargic newborn presenting to the emergency department can be from multiple causes. Inborn errors of metabolism (IEM) are one such cause. These should be suspected in newborns that are hypotonic, have poor weight gain, persistent poor feeding, unusual jaundice, and laboratory evidence including acidosis, ketosis, elevated ammonia, or hypoglycemia. The neonate with galactosemia may present with sepsis as they are prone to *Escherichia coli* infections.

Another condition to not miss in a hypotonic, poorly feeding newborn is congenital hypothyroidism. This condition is twice as likely in female infants and more prevalent in Down syndrome. These patients may also have abdominal distension, constipation, and prolonged jaundice.

CCHD is a leading cause of infant mortality. Not all infants are diagnosed in the neonatal period despite screening and prenatal ultrasounds. If a newborn presents with cyanosis, tachypnea (without lung problems), hypoxemia, tiring quickly with feedings, or hypotension; CCHD should be considered.

Emergency Care

In all lethargic newborns, a point-of-care glucose should be obtained immediately. Correction of hypoglycemia is urgent in the newborn aiming for a sugar >45. Other laboratory studies to obtain include a CBC, lactate, blood gas, electrolyte panel, hepatic function panel, and ammonia. An IEM should be considered in the infant with unexplained hypoglycemia or hyperammonemia. Administer IV fluids and dextrose to correct hypoglycemia. Emergent treatment of hyperammonemia includes scavenging agents and may require dialysis so prompt consultation with metabolic genetics, critical care, and nephrology is imperative. Feedings should be discontinued and replaced by infusion of D10 0.45 normal saline at 1.5 maintenance rate to stop catabolism as protein intake can worsen some IEMs.

If there is concern for congenital hypothyroidism, obtain TSH and free T4 levels and start levothyroxine before testing comes back. Initiation of therapy within the newborn's first 2 weeks of life can preserve cognitive development. The risks of early treatment are minimal and outweighed by the potential harms of waiting for test results.

For the newborn you are concerned could have CCHD, a chest x-ray can be helpful to look for heart size and pulmonary vascular markings. A heart murmur may or may not be present on your examination. An echo is diagnostic, but if not readily available, an EKG can be helpful. If you believe that the presentation of this infant is due to a ductal dependent lesion (eg, rapid decline in clinical status with cyanosis and/or cardiovascular collapse), early prostaglandin infusion is necessary to save the infant's life in consultation with pediatric cardiology. Be prepared to support the respiratory status as apnea is a known side effect of prostaglandin treatment.

KEY POINTS

- Newborns that are lethargic with hypoglycemia, ketosis, or hyperammonemia have an inborn error of metabolism until proven otherwise. Make them NPO and give IV fluids with dextrose. Hyperammonemia requires an emergent multispecialty approach.
- If you suspect congenital hypothyroidism, check TSH and free T4 and start empiric levothyroxine.
- Newborns with CCHD may present with cyanosis and unexplained hypoxia. An echo is diagnostic; however, chest x-ray and EKG can be helpful. For suspected ductal dependent lesions, start prostaglandin and monitor closely for apnea.
- Consult your state health department for full screening panels and treatment guidelines.

Suggested Readings

Chakrapani, A, Cleary MA, Wraith JE. Detection of inborn errors of metabolism in the newborn. *Arch Dis Child Fetal Neonatal Ed*. 2001;(84):205-210.

Rose S, Brown R; American Thyroid Association; American Academy of Pediatrics. Update of newborn screening and therapy for congenital hypothyroidism. *Pediatrics*. 2006;117(6):2290-2303. doi: 10.1542/peds.2006-0915.

Yun SW. Congenital heart disease in the newborn requiring early intervention. *Korean J Pediatr*. 2011;54(5): 183-191.

175

Umbilical Care: Do Not Confuse the Normal Granulation With the Purulence of Omphalitis

Robert Peterson, MD

The umbilical cord is the fetal lifeline for oxygen and nutrition before birth. Once severed from mom, it becomes a potential site for infectious spread and a site of much consternation for both parents and doctors. The adage "less is more" regarding umbilical cord care is true as is the adage "all hands-on deck" for umbilical infections. Here we will discuss umbilical anatomy, cord care, basic cord complications, and the "not to miss" infection omphalitis with associated abdominal wall necrotizing fasciitis.

The Umbilicus

The umbilicus is the last reminder of our direct biologic connection to our mothers. Normally composed of one vein and two arteries, the umbilical cord carries oxygenated blood and nutrients to the newborn from mom and can serve as a site for emergent vascular access if needed.

In general, following delivery the umbilical vessels will thrombose and detach by the end of the first week of life. Dry cord care, leaving the cord outside the diaper, only wiping it down when the cord is soiled is what both the American Academy of Pediatrics and World Health Organization advocate in high resource settings. An initial cleaning with chlorhexidine is recommended in developing countries and suggested for out-of-hospital births. Of note, delayed cord clamping of 30-60 seconds when safe for both mother and baby is recommended by the American College of Obstetricians and Gynecologists. Finally, the use of sterile instruments when cutting the cord helps prevent neonatal infections arising from the umbilical cord stump, including tetanus neonatorum.

Umbilical Cord Stump Complications

Once cut, the umbilical cord transitions from a lifeline into a potential for systemic infection for the neonate. Fortunately, most often umbilical cord stump concerns are about serosanguinous drainage with or without a small area of granulation tissue. Appearing like a small pyogenic area in the stump, this granulation tissue can be cauterized as needed with a silver nitrate stick.

However, not all serosanguinous drainage is physiologic. It might be pathologic if it is secondary to a patent urachus. The urachus, a connection from the fetal bladder to the umbilicus, usually closes and obliterates during the first trimester. A patent urachus can lead to urine leaking from the umbilicus requiring surgical consultation. Partial obliteration of this track may lead to a urachal cyst, which can serve as potential space for infection.

This leads us to the not to miss infection of the umbilical stump, omphalitis. Often the first sign and presenting complaint is purulent discharge from the umbilicus. This purulence often develops in a urachal remnant and can be expressed with inferior, midline pressure below the umbilicus. Untreated this can develop into surrounding cellulitis and progress rapidly into abscesses, septicemia, or necrotizing fasciitis. It is important to note that purulent discharge, while common, is not required to make the diagnosis of omphalitis.

Progression of omphalitis is a leading cause of necrotizing fasciitis in children, which carries a high mortality risk. Physicians must carefully evaluate erythema and induration around the umbilical cord stump and manage accordingly. Unfortunately, there are no clear clinical criteria or definitive lab tests to assist the physician in making the diagnosis of omphalitis.

In general, suspected omphalitis should be managed aggressively. Even in the absence of fever, clinicians should obtain cultures and start antibiotics. Empiric antibiotic coverage must be directed at both aerobic and anaerobic bacteria as omphalitis is a polymicrobial infection. In these cases, ultrasound should be performed to evaluate the depth and extension of the infection, helping to determine the need for immediate surgical intervention.

In general, medical treatment of omphalitis should always be in conjunction with surgical consultation. In most cases, this will require transfer to center with both pediatric surgeons and a pediatric intensive care unit. If not deemed an emergent surgical case, disposition should be discussed with the intensive care unit as the neonate will require close monitoring for the development of either septicemia or necrotizing fasciitis. These complications make omphalitis the not to miss complication of the umbilical stump.

KEY POINTS

- The umbilical vein may be the easiest site for intravenous access in the newborn.
- The WHO and AAP advocate the use of dry umbilical cord care in high-resource settings.
- Fever is not required to make the diagnosis of omphalitis and lack of fever should not delay obtaining cultures and starting antibiotics.
- For omphalitis, surgical consultation is required as omphalitis can rapidly progress to necrotizing fasciitis of the abdominal wall.

Suggested Readings

Fraser N, Davies B, Cusack J. Neonatal omphalitis: a review of its serious complications. *Acta Paediatr*. 2006;95:519-522.

Stewart D, Benitz W. Umbilical cord care of the newborn infant. Committee on Fetus and Newborn. *Pediatrics*. 2016;138(3):e20162149 doi: 10.1542/peds.2016-Open Access.

Video of emergent umbilical vein catheterization. https://vimeo.com/35337127

Zundel S, Lemaréchal A, Kaiser P, Szavay P. Diagnosis and treatment of pediatric necrotizing fasciitis: a systematic review of the literature. *Eur J Pediatr Surg*. 2017;27(2):127-137. doi: 10.1055/s-0036-1584531.

176

I Am So Hungry! Know the Right Questions to Ask About Feeding Difficulty in the Neonate

Katina M. Summerford, MD and Rachel E. M. Cramton, MD

Overview

The importance of adequate nutrition in the first 30 days of life cannot be understated. Infants are at risk of rapid dehydration or hypoglycemia with poor feeding or emesis. Poor feeding indicates an anatomical defect or indolent illness or a more benign issue. Poor feeding can lead to failure to thrive, a life-threatening complication of chronic malnutrition and/or poor feeding. Parental concerns regarding neonatal feeding are common in the emergency department (ED), and providers must differentiate normal feeding from "cannot miss" pathology.

What Is Normal?

The basics of feeding for neonates revolve around adequate feeding time, feeding volume, and emesis volumes. Infants may transiently lose up to 10% of their birth weight but should regain birth weight by 14 days of life. Exclusively breast-fed infants typically lose more weight compared to those who are formula fed. Newborns should feed on-demand, typically every 1-3 hours. Neonates are at risk for hypoglycemia and should never go >3 hours without feeding. Breast-fed infants should feed for ≥15 minutes, and bottle-fed infants should take ≥3-4 oz per feed. However, these are merely guidelines as adequate weight gain is the best measure.

Feeding Problems

Ask how often the infant feeds and how much they take per feed (or how long feeding lasts, if breast-fed). Always ask how formula is being mixed as improper mixing can result in improper caloric intake as well as serious electrolyte abnormalities such as hyper-/hyponatremia. If emesis/spit-up is the predominant complaint, estimate the volume, frequency, and color.

GER is one of the most common causes of spit-up or emesis in infants. Often parents will report vomiting occurring after feeds or that the baby is gassy and fussy with grimacing or back arching. Vomiting with every feed or an infant who is not gaining weight is concerning for pathologic reflux. To the parent who has had to change their clothes hourly, it is hard to quantify volume. Squirt a 10-mL syringe of water onto a paper towel for comparison, and the parent may realize that their child is not actually "vomiting everything." Easy remedies for GER include upright positioning for a minimum of 30 minutes after a feed and adequate burping. In cases of chronic or severe GER, a trial of ranitidine may be appropriate; however, the decision to start this is best left to the PCP. Formula changes should not be made in the ED. Formula should be changed in stepwise fashion after >2 weeks before switching. If parents have formula concerns, recommend follow-up with a PCP who can devote adequate time to this nonemergent problem.

Signs of a more concerning etiology of emesis and poor feeding include bilious vomiting, GI bleeding, consistently forceful ("projectile") vomiting, and severe abdominal tenderness or distension. Tracheoesophageal fistula (TEF), duodenal atresia or web, hiatal hernia, diaphragmatic hernia, intestinal malrotation, and hypertrophic pyloric stenosis are known to cause neonatal feeding problems, particularly emesis. TEF patients typically have a prolonged history of mild respiratory distress associated with feeding and/or recurrent episodes of pneumonia. Any of these more concerning historical or physical examination findings should warrant further workup including imaging and/or labs.

Finally, children with non-GI illnesses may present with feeding difficulty. A baby who is sweating with feeds may have heart disease. Listen for a murmur, ensure all pulses are equal and adequate, and ask about cyanotic episodes. An infant that is not waking for feeds or is refusing feeds may be ill, as neonates have very few ways of telling us they are sick. Lethargy, irritability, or refusal to feed may indicate systemic illness, such as sepsis or simply hypoglycemia. If the infant repeatedly has milk dribbling from nares, check for any palpable or visible palate defects. Infants with poorly coordinated suck/swallow/breath function may have an underlying neurologic cause, but most often are simply uncoordinated, requiring appropriate positioning and pauses during feeds. These patients would benefit from lactation consultation as an outpatient.

KEY POINTS

- Weight loss up to 10% is common, but they should regain birth weight by 14 days of life.
- Newborns should feed on demand about every 1-3 hours, but never >3-4 hours.
- Reflux is one of the most common causes of spit-up and emesis in infants and is usually benign. Formula changes should not be made in an ED setting.
- Sweating, disinterest, bilious emesis, GI bleeding, abdominal distension, or fatigue with feeding are concerning signs of underlying pathology.
- Long-term, poor feeding can lead to failure to thrive requiring admission.

Suggested Readings

Anonymous. Bright futures—nutrition issues and concerns. In: *AAP Bright Futures Guidelines*. American Academy of Pediatrics. brightfutures.aap.org/

Fortunato JE, Tarbell SE. Vomiting and nausea in the pediatric patient. *Nausea Vomit*. New York, NY: Springer International Publishing; 2016;175–190.

Lightdale JR, Gremse DA. Gastroesophageal reflux: management guidance for the pediatrician. *Pediatrics*. 2013;131(5):e1684–e1695.

Mccollough M, Sharieff GQ. Abdominal surgical emergencies in infants and young children. *Emerg Med Clin North Am*. 2003;21(4):909–935.

Rosen R, et al. Pediatric gastroesophageal reflux clinical practice guidelines. *J Pediatr Gastroenterol Nutr*. 2018;66(3):516–554.

Is It Supposed to Look That Way?: Know What Is Normal Postcircumcision So You Can Reassure Parents

Alyssa Bernardi, DO and Rachel E. M. Cramton, MD

It is common for worried parents to show up to the emergency department (ED) late at night with questions about what is normal and abnormal after a circumcision. In this chapter, we will examine techniques used to circumcise male infants, review basic postoperative care, and describe worrisome complications that need prompt attention from the ED provider.

Circumcision Techniques

To understand normal and abnormal, there must be a familiarity with the circumcision procedure. Analgesia is usually achieved with dorsal penile nerve block and oral sucrose. The procedure typically takes <15 minutes. There are three techniques that can be used to remove the penile foreskin. Two of the three circumcision techniques use a metal or plastic piece to protect the glans penis as the foreskin is removed. The Gomco clamp technique fits a metal bell over the glans and under the foreskin. The clamp is then fitted over the foreskin and left in place for 5 minutes to achieve tissue hemostasis. The foreskin is then circumferentially excised using a scalpel. A similar technique is used with the Plastibell; a plastic ring slides over the glans and the foreskin is tied off with a string. The string and plastic part are left on the infant's penis for up to a week; eventually the foreskin becomes necrotic and sloughs as a result of the ligature cutting off blood supply to the tissue. If the Plastibell device has not fallen off after a week, or has migrated proximally, it can be removed using a ring cutter. The last technique uses the Mogen clamp, in which the foreskin is spread flat and slid through a linear clamp before being excised.

Postoperative Instructions for Parents

Many parents are distracted or worried before and after their infant's circumcision so discharge instructions are not always remembered or followed. The most important message to convey to parents is to keep the glans covered. A barrier emollient, such as petroleum jelly, can be applied liberally to the glans penis immediately after circumcision. Apply a nonadhesive dressing over the glans or apply a barrier ointment to the diaper itself to prevent the skin from adhering to the diaper. Parents should reapply with every diaper change for up to 5 days postcircumcision in order to prevent meatal stenosis and adhesions. Unless the glans area is completely covered in stool, there is no need to wipe down the entire penis during diaper changes. Note that the glans penis is highly vascularized and will appear very erythematous and slightly edematous after circumcision. This is normal and there is no need to worry unless the meatal opening is occluded or the infant has not urinated for 6-8 hours following circumcision.

Circumcision Complications

Bleeding and local infection in a newly circumcised patient are the most likely complications an ED provider will treat. That being said, an international meta-analysis in 2015 reported that the median frequency of all complications postcircumcision was only 1.5%.

Most postcircumcision bleeding is limited and self-resolves or resolves with pressure. Techniques for treatment of bleeding in the ED include application of small amount of silver nitrate (use only if bleeding is limited to several small spots), application of oxidized cellulose polymer (Surgicel), or several small sutures using fine absorbable suture. Never use cautery to stop bleeding in newly circumcised patients, as this may lead to tissue necrosis and affect penile function and cosmetic appearance. If bleeding is severe or recalcitrant to silver nitrate, ask about hemophilia or bleeding in family history and consider bloodwork for coagulopathy evaluation. Consult urology or pediatric surgery for surgical exploration if bleeding is severe or persistent.

Infection in a postcircumcision patient is usually local and can be treated with a dressing change. If the infection appears mild, or you are worried about a developing infection, be sure to reiterate the importance of barrier ointment and frequent diaper changes to the parents (ie, do not let the infant sit in a wet diaper for prolonged periods of time). A local infection can be treated with bacitracin or similar topical antibiotic ointment. Consider systemic infection (*and full septic work up*) if the infant is demonstrating lethargy, poor feeding, or fever. Remember, a fever in a newly circumcised neonate is always concerning and should be worked up accordingly.

KEY POINTS

- If the Plastibell device has not fallen off after a week, or has migrated proximally, it can be removed using a ring cutter.
- Keep the glans covered with petroleum jelly. There is no need to wipe down the diaper area between every diaper change.
- Never use cautery to stop bleeding in newly circumcised patients.
- A localized infection can be treated with bacitracin or similar topical antibiotic ointment.
- Fever in the circumcised neonate should be evaluated with the same concern as the uncircumcised neonate with a focus toward a septic workup.

Suggested Readings

Cancian MJ, Caldamome AA. Special considerations in the pediatric patient. In: Taneja SS, Shah O, eds. *Complications of Urologic Surgery*. 4th ed. Edinburgh, UK: Elsevier; 2010:581-590.

Smith AW, Hebra A, Mansfield JM, et al. Management of Plastibell circumcision ring migration and glans penis incarceration. *J Pediatr Surg Case Rep*. 2013;7:186-188.

Srinivasan M, Hamvas C, Coplen D. Rates of complications after newborn circumcision in a well-baby nursery, special care nursery, and neonatal intensive care unit. *Clin Pediatr*. 2015;12:1185-1191.

178

Skin and Bones, or Normal Growth: Identifying Failure to Thrive

Marci Macaraeg, MD and Rachel E. M. Cramton, MD

Failure to thrive (FTT) is difficult to define acutely as the true diagnosis is made over time. However, it can be suspected acutely by history, exam, or numbers. The patient may be brought in due to nutritional concerns from the pediatrician or guardians. The patient may look or act malnourished on exam. The patient's growth chart may demonstrate <5% or a drop in weight of ≥2 percentiles over 3-6 months. Term infants <2 years should be measured on World Health Organization growth charts, while older children should be measured on Center for Disease Control growth charts. There are also special growth charts for special kids, including premature infants, trisomy 21, Prader-Willi, and many others that are readily available online.

Fortunately, it is pretty rare for children with FTT to present with life-threatening conditions. Dehydration and hypoglycemia are the most common serious conditions warranting ED treatment. In an infant, signs of dehydration include tachycardia for their age, capillary refill >2 seconds, lack of tear production with crying, a sunken fontanelle, or lethargy. Ask the guardians if the baby has had a normal amount of wet diapers that day. Children and adolescents will have more typical signs of dehydration, such as tachycardia, decreased capillary refill, dry mucous membranes, and decreased urine output. For all of these patients, rehydration is key. The typical bolus in pediatrics is 10-20 mL/kg of isotonic fluid with reassessment.

Some life-threatening conditions that can present as FTT and cannot be missed include intermittent malrotation with or without volvulus, congenital adrenal hyperplasia, congenital heart disease, inborn errors of metabolism, and acute infection or sepsis. Much of FTT is social, so neglect or abuse should always be considered. Most FTT patients, including neonates, can be managed in the outpatient setting. If the history and physical exam are not significant for any abnormalities except for a child who is small for his or her age and who is otherwise strong, vigorous, and eating, then the patient should be discharged with good outpatient follow-up.

Initiating a workup for a child with FTT will depend on the history and exam because the differential diagnosis is exceedingly broad. If anything is concerning in the history or physical exam, pursue the appropriate tests for the abnormal findings. A complete blood count and complete metabolic panel should be collected to evaluate for anemia, iron deficiency, and renal and hepatic function. If there is a heart murmur, consider a chest x-ray and echocardiogram. Thyroid studies, glucose, and lactate and ammonia levels may indicate an inborn error of metabolism. For the most part, FTT is due to inadequate caloric intake and should be managed in the outpatient setting with parental education and guidance. The child should be admitted if the child is ill, the child will not feed in the ED, or there is concern that the child's family cannot guarantee reliable follow-up or a safe home.

Refeeding syndrome occurs when nutrition is aggressively reintroduced to a severely malnourished child. The adolescent with long-standing anorexia nervosa is the prototypical example. Clinical manifestations of refeeding syndrome include vomiting, diarrhea, and fluid imbalances. Laboratory findings include hypophosphatemia, hypokalemia, hypomagnesemia, and glucose imbalance. Fluid imbalances can lead to edema, hypotension, and shock. This, in addition to the electrolyte abnormalities, can be fatal, usually via arrhythmias or cardiac failure. Management of refeeding syndrome includes aggressive correction of electrolyte abnormalities, particularly of phosphorus, potassium, and magnesium. These patients should be placed on cardiac monitoring with telemetry and should receive more frequent checks of both vital signs and electrolytes.

KEY POINTS

- FTT is defined as a child who is <5% on the appropriate growth chart, or a child who has fallen >2 percentiles in 3-6 months.
- The majority of FTT cases, from neonates to adolescents, can and should be discharged and managed in the outpatient setting.
- Always consider dehydration, abuse/neglect, and life-threatening causes of FTT.
- Much of FTT is social requiring parental counseling and guidance. Work up and admit only when there is clinical concern for disease.
- Beware of refeeding syndrome in severely malnourished children.

Suggested Readings

Ammoury RF. Malabsorptive disorders of childhood. *Pediatr Rev*. 2010;31(10):407-415.

Growth Charts. Washington State Academy of Nutrition and Dietetics. https://www.eatrightwashington.org/pnpg/page/growth-charts

Jaffe AC. Failure to thrive: current clinical concepts. *Pediatr Rev*. 2011;32(3):100-107.

Mehler PS, Winkelman AB, Andersen DM, Gaudiani JL. Nutritional rehabilitation: practical guidelines for refeeding the anorectic patient. *J Nutr Metab*. 2010;2010.

Motil K. Poor weight gain in children younger than two years: etiology and evaluation. In: Drutz J, Jenson C, eds. *UpToDate*, Accessed January 14, 2010 from https://www.uptodate.com/contents/poor-weight-gain-in-children-younger-than-two-years-in-resource-rich-countries-etiology-and-evaluation?search=Poor%20weight%20gain%20in%20children%20younger%20than%20two%20years:%20etiology%20and%20evaluation&source=search_result&selectedTitle=1~150&usage_type=default&display_rank=1

179

Anaphylaxis: It May Come as a Shock, but It Does Not Have to End in Tragedy...

Lindsey Retterath, MD and Melissa E. Zukowski, MD, MPH, FACEP,FAAP

Anaphylaxis has to be one of the most well-known medical emergencies among children of the 90s. If you have not seen the movie *My Girl*—spoiler alert—it ends with a tragic death of Macaulay Culkin's character due to a swarm of bees. However, with appropriate early recognition, management, and anticipatory guidance about anaphylaxis in high-risk children, this admittedly scary medical emergency does not have to end in tragedy. This begs a question: how do we prepare pediatric patients and their caregivers for management of anaphylaxis before they arrive in the emergency department (ED)?

Anaphylaxis

Any allergic reaction involving two or more systems constitutes anaphylaxis. These may include the cardiovascular system, the respiratory system, skin, eyes, and the GI tract. Although a patient with hives and vomiting may more readily trigger concern for anaphylaxis, it is even more critical to consider anaphylaxis as an etiology for hemodynamic compromise and respiratory distress. Be on the lookout for subtle signs/symptoms of end-organ malperfusion. Mortality from anaphylaxis most commonly occurs as asphyxia or bronchospasm, usually correlating with a concomitant asthma history and/or delayed epinephrine administration.

For anaphylaxis, give IM epinephrine 1:1000 (1 mg/mL). Just give it, and give it quickly. For anaphylaxis, epinephrine is the only evidence-based pharmacologic intervention. Furthermore, most cases with high morbidity or mortality involve delayed administration. Do not rely on antihistamines or glucocorticoids as these second-line medications are not lifesaving in the emergent condition. Auto-injectors come in three sizes. Use the "infant" (0.1 mg) size for <1 year, "pediatric" (0.15 mg) for >1 year and under 30 kg, and the "adult" (0.3 mg) dose for children >30 kg. Weight-based dosing is 0.01 mg/kg or 0.1 mL/kg. The typical max dose is 0.3 mg/dose; however, up to 0.5 mg/dose can be given per dose as long as the dose is not >0.01 mg/kg.

Patients with a history of anaphylaxis often have already used an autoinjector or otherwise received epinephrine prior to arrival. Confirm prehospital dosing and strongly consider redosing if prehospital dosing was inadequate or unknown. In addition to asthma/atopy/eczema histories, ask about fevers, possible foreign bodies, environmental exposures, respiratory history, and cardiovascular history. If a patient requires more than one IM epinephrine dose, consider starting an epinephrine infusion and admitting to the ICU. Usual starting dose would be 0.05 mcg/kg/min, but titrate up as needed until perfusion and/or breathing improves. Fortunately, the majority of these patients are discharged home. Anticipatory guidance for recurrence is crucial as biphasic anaphylaxis occurs in up to 15% of children.

Anticipatory Guidance

Allergic exposures are rarely planned, making ready access to an autoinjector critical. Whenever possible, educate all caretakers, not just the caretaker present in the ED. Consider discharging with an "Allergy and Anaphylaxis Emergency Plan," which includes a list of the patient's likely allergies, dosages and indications for medications, and comorbid conditions. Instructions should include when to seek help, when to self-treat with an autoinjector, and the importance of removing the offending agent. The patient's pediatrician and/or allergy specialist should update the plan at least annually, keeping copies at home and at school. Advise parents and patients to obtain a medical alert bracelet for severe allergies. This allows for prompt recognition and treatment in the instance that the patient is too ill to communicate their medical history.

Children can generally recognize anaphylaxis by age 9 and reliably self-administer IM epinephrine by age 12. Caretakers, in turn, must be instructed on recognition of anaphylaxis as well as administration of autoinjectors.

Anticipatory guidance is most critical in kids with severe allergies or anaphylaxis and a history of asthma. Children with asthma are the most likely to have life-threatening respiratory symptoms during an allergic reaction. Early epinephrine is the only intervention shown to change morbidity and mortality. Good guidance for appropriate prehospital administration of epi autoinjectors may be truly lifesaving.

KEY POINTS

- Epinephrine—give it fast, give it early!
- Be on the lookout for subtle signs of end-organ malperfusion: Respect it!
- Biphasic anaphylaxis—may occur in up to 15% of your pediatric patients.
- Anticipatory guidance—although not as exciting as anaphylaxis treatment in the ED, arguably just as CRITICAL for your patients and their families.

Suggested Readings

Alquarashi W, Stiell I, Chan K, et al. Epidemiology and clinical predictors of biphasic reactions in children with anaphylaxis. *Ann Allergy Asthma Immunol.* 2015;115:217.

Bock SA, et al. Further fatalities caused by anaphylactic reactions to food, 2001-2006. *J Allergy Clin Immunol.* 2007;119(4):1016-1018.

Simons E, Sicharer SH, Weiss C, Simons FE. Caregivers' perspectives on timing the transfer of responsibilities for anaphylaxis recognition and treatment from adults to children and teenagers. *J Allergy Clin Immunol Pract.* 2013;1(3):309-311.

Turner PJ, Gowland MH, Sharma V, et al. Increase in anaphylaxis-related hospitalizations but no increase in fatalities: an analysis of UK national anaphylaxis data, 1992-2012. *J Allergy Clin Immunol.* 2015;135(4):956-963.

Wang J, Sicherer SH; Section on Allergy and Immunology. Guidance on Completing a Written Allergy and Anaphylaxis Emergency Plan. *Pediatrics.* 2017;139(3):e20164005. doi: 10.1542/peds.2016-4005.

Primary Immunodeficiency: Know What to Expect When Cell Lines Go Awry

Monica Hajirawala, MD and Julia Schweizer, MD, FAAP

Common Clinical Features of Immunodeficiency

A patient with recurrent upper respiratory tract infections, pneumonias, ear infections, abscesses, serious sinus infections, bronchitis, fungal infections, or diarrhea may have had a run of bad luck or they may have signs of an immunodeficiency. Be suspicious if a patient has had intermittent fevers, failure to thrive, an infection with unusual organisms, severe bacterial infections, a family history of immunodeficiency, a severe clinical course from common infections, or infections that persist with partial response or no response to therapy. When parts of the immune system fail, the pattern of infections can help identify the problem.

Patients with innate immunity defects such as natural killer cell deficiencies or chronic granulomatous disease present with impaired wound healing, pyogenic infections, and rapid progression of infection. Since the innate system is responsible for creating an inflammatory response, these patients may not present with a fever, may not have associated pain, and may have normal inflammatory markers in the setting of an infection. Unfortunately, their lack of symptoms could delay diagnosis and worsen the outcome so be cautious in a patient with a known innate deficiency.

B-cell defects such as IgA deficiency, common variable immune deficiency, and X-linked agammaglobulinemia most commonly cause recurrent sinus, ear, and pulmonary infections, especially with encapsulated organisms due to issues with antibody production or function. These occur more frequently after maternal immunoglobulins fade around age 6 months. They often have autoimmune diseases, malignancy, cytopenias, and sensorineural hearing loss as well. T-cell disorders are functionally similar to AIDS with a similar pattern of opportunistic infections such as *Candida* and *Mycobacterium*. Consequentially, HIV infection should be considered in the differential for these patients.

Screening Tests for Immunodeficiency

The best initial screening tests for any child with recurrent infections are a complete blood count with manual differential and an erythrocyte sedimentation rate (ESR). Pay close attention to the absolute lymphocyte count (ALC) (which varies by age), absolute neutrophil count (ANC), and platelet count. A low ANC could indicate a leukocyte adhesion defect, congenital neutropenia, or acquired neutropenia. Keep in mind a low ANC is very common in children after a viral infection or secondary to drug exposure. A low ALC can indicate a T-cell deficiency. Platelet abnormalities along with immune issues can point to Wiskott-Aldrich syndrome. Chronic bacterial and fungal infections are less likely if the ESR is normal. Refer the patient to a pediatric immunologist for a thorough evaluation if there is any concern for an immunodeficiency.

A thorough history, physical, and complete metabolic profile would also help evaluate for secondary immunodeficiencies such as malignancy, HIV, immunosuppressive medications, sickle cell disease, asplenia, diabetes mellitus, severe liver disease, liver failure, and protein loss.

Management of Immunodeficiency in the Emergency Department (ED)

Any patient with a primary or secondary immunodeficiency should receive a thorough infectious workup in the ED setting if they are having concerning symptoms, fever, or vital signs. Immunocompromised patients of any etiology are at high risk for bacterial infections, occult bacteremia, and severe illnesses, thus a thorough history and physical can guide infectious workup. Inserted medical devices should be considered as potential infectious sources. If the patient is ill appearing, hospitalization and empiric antibiotics are strongly recommended. Even if physical examination, vital signs, and lab results are reassuring, a blood culture should still be considered due to the high risk of bacteremia. Also consider consultation with the specialty involved (eg, oncology, nephrology) and empiric antibiotics. If the patient is deemed stable for discharge, they will need frequent follow-up over the first week to reevaluate their clinical status.

KEY POINTS

- Suspect an immunodeficiency for patients with recurrent infections, serious infections from common bacteria, unusual infections, opportunistic infection, family history of immunodeficiency, diarrhea, or failure to thrive.
- Obtain CBC with manual differential and ESR as initial screening tests.

Suggested Readings

Alkhater SA. Approach to the child with recurrent infections. *J Fam Community Med*. 2009;16(3):77-82.

Kliegman RM, et al. *Nelson Textbook of Pediatrics, vols. 1 and 2*. 20th ed. Elsevier; 2016.

O'Keefe AW, et al. Primary immunodeficiency for the primary care provider. *Paediatr Child Health*. 2016;21(2): e10-e14.

Reust CE. Evaluation of primary immunodeficiency disease in children. *Am Fam Physician*. 2013;87(11):773-778.

181

Do Not Forget to Look for the Five W's of Cutaneous Injuries

Caroline Wang, MD and Julia N. Magana, MD

Bruises are the most common visible clue to child physical abuse, but unfortunately clinicians often downplay its significance. Some skin injuries should not be overlooked as they may be an indicator of child abuse or a signal of internal injury. Often, mobile children present with bruises overlying bony surfaces such as the shins, knees, elbows, and forehead—these are a normal and an expected part of childhood. So what cutaneous lesions should we be worried about? Consider bruises in the context of the five W's:

Who: The nonmobile child rarely bruises. To bruise oneself accidentally, one must be able to generate enough momentum to crush tissue. Studies have repeatedly shown "those who do not cruise rarely bruise." Any bruise without a clear trauma history on a nonmobile infant should trigger an additional evaluation for child abuse. Injuries on older children who are nonmobile due to developmental delay should trigger the provider to ask more questions.

What: Patterned injuries and large quantities of bruises are concerning. If an object is used to inflict trauma, it can leave an outline or a pattern of the object, such as belt and belt-buckle marks or looped-cord marks from whipping. A large number of bruises should also raise the suspicion for abuse.

Where: Protected areas of the body are bruised less frequently. An easy way to remember this is with the mnemonic TEN-4 FACES: bruises on the torso, ears, neck, frenulum, angle of the jaw, cheek, eyelid, or sclera of a child <4 years old without a public, confirmed accident or any bruise on an infant <4 months old.

When: If an infant presents to the ED with a medical chief complaint and the concerning bruise is found incidentally.

Why: If no there is no "why" or a trauma history that explains a bruise in a nonmobile infant or a confirmable story that makes sense developmentally in an older child, take a moment to think about abuse.

The principles of the five W's can be applied to burns as well. Inflicted burns are more severe than accidental ones. Immersion scald burns without associated splash marks, dip burns in a stocking-glove distribution, or symmetrically burned buttocks/genitals are red flags for abuse. Inflicted contact burns or branding injuries are usually well-demarcated, deep, and leave a clear imprint of the object used—for example, from a cigarette or hot iron.

What should be done with concerning bruises or cutaneous injuries? A skeletal survey should be done in children <2 years with any obvious or suspicious injury. The lesions should be photographed with a measuring instrument. If any injuries are on the face or head, there should be a low threshold to obtain a CT scan of the head in children 12 months of age or less. Remember that imaging decision rules such as the PECARN head injury guidelines do not apply to abuse. Labs should also be considered to screen for occult injuries including a CBC, BMP, AST/ALT, and a UA. Proper documentation and thorough history should be taken. Medical providers also have a legal responsibility to report abuse when suspected.

KEY POINTS

- Who: Those who do not cruise rarely bruise.
- What: Patterned injuries and a large number of bruises are concerning.
- Where: Worry about TEN-4 FACES bruises. They are on the torso, ears, neck, the frenulum, angle of the jaw, cheek, eyelid, or sclera of a child <4 years old.
- When: If a young infant presents with a bruise without a trauma chief complaint that is concerning.
- Why: There should be a "why" for weird bruises in young children.

Suggested Readings

Christian CW; Committee on Child Abuse and Neglect, American Academy of Pediatrics. The evaluation of suspected child physical abuse. *Pediatrics.* 2015;135(5):e1337-e1354.

Pierce MC, Kaczor K, Aldridge S, et al. Bruising characteristics discriminating physical child abuse from accidental trauma. *Pediatrics.* 2010;125(1):67-74.

Sheets LK, Leach ME, Koszewski IJ, et al. Sentinel injuries in infants evaluated for child physical abuse. *Pediatrics.* 2013;131(4):701-707.

Do Not Miss Abusive Head Trauma!

Leah Sitler, MD and Julia N. Magana, MD

Children with abusive head trauma (AHT) can present with a variety of symptoms, some of which can be subtle. It is therefore critical to maintain a high degree of suspicion as AHT is the most common cause of fatal abuse, yet providers often miss it. When missed, AHT can results in significant clinical and social impact including long-term physical and mental health impacts on patients and can potentially be fatal.

AHT has historically been called shaken baby syndrome because the most well-known mechanism of AHT is when a caregiver shakes the child. This whiplash-like motion causes shearing forces that can tear the bridging veins, which leads to intracranial hemorrhages such as subdural hemorrhages. Diffuse anoxic injury frequently results from rapid acceleration/deceleration forces complicated by bleeding, swelling, axonal shearing, and decreased cerebral perfusion. Forceful shaking can also cause retinal hemorrhages. AHT involves many findings such as intracranial/spinal injury, rib and other fractures, and complex retinal hemorrhages inconsistent with the mechanism provided. There is no single diagnostic test and the diagnosis is made after thorough consideration. Because the mechanism for AHT is multi-part the best term is AHT as suggested by the American Academy of Pediatrics.

When Should I Suspect AHT?

Providers miss AHT because the signs of AHT appear similar to infections, accidental trauma, or even an ostensibly normal infant. Signs and symptoms can include vomiting, seizure, change in cry, change in activity level, decreased interest in feeding, apnea, color change, and more. Patients can present with a trauma history that, on the surface, may seem plausible or they may have no history of trauma. It is incumbent on the provider to differentiate between a benign etiology and abuse. The history should focus on the trauma mechanism if provided, parental response, subsequent symptoms, patient's developmental capability, and the social history.

Infants should have a full head to toe skin exam with the child completely undressed. Bruises, scleral hemorrhages, or a torn frenulum in a nonmobile infant should raise a red flag, especially in conjunction with the previously mentioned signs and symptoms of AHT. Palpate the entire body for bony tenderness, scalp injury, and abdominal tenderness or distention. The infant should be observed in the ED drinking and interacting with family for any subtle neurological abnormalities.

What Do I Do When I Have AHT on My Differential?

Providers miss AHT when they do not obtain a head CT because they attribute the symptoms of AHT to more benign causes, do not think of AHT, or utilize the PECARN TBI rules to reduce radiation. The PECARN traumatic brain injury (TBI) rules cannot be applied to AHT because they rely on an accurate patient history, which is notoriously inaccurate in abuse. Also, the PECARN rules are looking clinically important TBI, whereas diagnosing even a subtle AHT can drastically change a child's life.

If symptoms, injuries, or stories do not add up, get a noncontrast CT. Consider AHT in any intracranial hemorrhage without a clear cause. Transfer the patient to a pediatric trauma center for further evaluation with subspecialists.

The diagnosis of AHT carries enormous implications for the child and the family, and many physicians hesitate to make the diagnosis. However, our job is not to apportion blame, but rather to provide the best possible care and medical workup for that child. Providers should file a report with the proper authorities (ie, child protective services or law enforcement) with any reasonable suspicion for abuse.

KEY POINTS

- Always consider the possibility of AHT! Sometimes the only symptom can be vomiting.
- Take cutaneous wounds seriously, especially in the context of possible AHT symptoms.
- Decision rules do not apply! If you suspect AHT, get a head CT.
- If you suspect abuse, be sure to report to the proper authorities.

Suggested Readings

Choudhary AK, Servaes S, Slovis TL, et al. Consensus statement on abusive head trauma in infants and young children. *Pediatr Radiol.* 2018;48(8):1048-1065.

Christian C, Block R; Committee on Child Abuse and Neglect, American Academy of Pediatrics. Abusive head trauma in infants and children. *Pediatrics.* 2009;123(5):1409-1411.

Magana J, Kuppermann N. The PECARN TBI rules do not apply to abusive head trauma. *Acad Emerg Med.* 2017;24(3):382-384.

Broken Bones in Broken Homes: When to Get a Skeletal Survey

Lily Anne Jewett, MD and Julia N. Magana, MD

Clinicians who care for patients where there is a suspicion of possible child abuse must decide how to pursue the diagnosis. Emergency medicine providers use radiographs to screen for occult fractures. But in an attempt to avoid radiation, they can order inappropriate radiographs that either falsely reassure or inappropriately expose a child to unnecessary tests. A skeletal survey is a crucial tool in the evaluation of suspected abuse, and clinicians must know what it involves and when to obtain one.

A skeletal survey as defined by the American College of Radiology is a series of 20 x-rays and is primarily used to assess for occult fractures in children with concern for abuse. The American College of Radiology skeletal survey recommendations include AP and lateral views of the skull, lateral views of the cervical spine and thoracolumbar spine, and single AP views of the long bones, hands, feet, chest and abdomen and obliques of the ribs. Among infants with concern for abuse, 11%-20% will have an unsuspected fracture detected by the skeletal survey. The highest rates of positive results have been found in children <6 months, and children with a history of BRUE/ALTE or seizure.

While a skeletal survey is an appropriate test for many children at risk for abuse, it exposes a child to the equivalent of 1-2 months of background radiation (~0.2 mSv). For comparison, a computed tomography scan of the head is equivalent to ~12-18 months of background radiation (1.5-1.9 mSv). Other downsides include cost, length of stay, and need for an expert to read the films. The skeletal survey requires a radiology technician and radiologist familiar with the series and may therefore not be available at every institution. Thus, the patient may need close follow-up at an appropriate facility or transfer to a center capable of obtaining and reading these films. It is sometimes tempting to order a "babygram" (single film of an entire infant) instead of a skeletal survey in an attempt to reduce radiation, but this is not an adequate substitute. Babygrams are not sufficiently sensitive for occult fractures and are liable to miss evidence of abuse.

The primary purpose of the skeletal survey is to detect occult fractures in children at risk for abuse who are nonverbal, unable to provide a reliable history, or otherwise unable to indicate a history of trauma. For this reason, providers should order a skeletal survey when they suspect abuse in children <2 years old and in children >2 years old and the patient cannot verbalize areas of injury or pain during the exam. If the older child can identify areas of injury or lack thereof, imaging can focus on the areas of clinical concern.

The 2015 American Academy of Pediatrics Clinical Report on Abuse recommends a skeletal survey in all children <2 years old with (1) obvious abusive injuries or (2) any suspicious injuries including

- Oral injuries, bruises, or other skin injuries in nonambulatory infants
- Injuries not consistent with the history provided
- Infants with unexplained, unexpected sudden death (discuss with coroner)
- Infants and young toddlers with unexplained intracranial injuries
- Infants and siblings <2 years old and with household contacts of an abused child

Also, a fracture in a nonambulatory infant should trigger concern for abuse, especially those without a clear history of trauma and without a known medical condition that predisposes them to bone fragility. The appropriate use of the skeletal survey as a screening tool for children at risk for abuse has the potential to make a lifetime of difference for a child.

KEY POINTS

- A skeletal survey is used to detect occult trauma in young suspected victims of physical abuse that are unable to give a reliable history.
- A skeletal survey consists of MANY films that capture all extremities in specific views; a "babygram" cannot substitute for a skeletal survey.
- Get a skeletal survey when there are obvious or suspected abusive injuries such as bruises, fractures, or oral injuries in nonambulatory children.

Suggested Readings

Borg K, Hodes D. Guidelines for skeletal survey in young children with fractures. *Arch Dis Child Educ Pract Ed.* 2015;100(5):253-256.

Christian CW; Committee on Child Abuse and Neglect, American Academy of Pediatrics. The evaluation of suspected child physical abuse. *Pediatrics.* 2015;135(5):e1337-e1354.

Expert Panel on Pediatric Imaging; Wootton-Gorges SL, Soares BP, et al. ACR Appropriateness Criteria® suspected physical abuse-child. *J Am Coll Radiol.* 2017;14(5S):S338-S349.

Wood JN, Fakeye O, Mondestin V, et al. Development of hospital-based guidelines for skeletal survey in young children with bruises. *Pediatrics.* 2015;135(2):e312-e320.

184

Sentinel Moments, Sentinel Injuries: Know How to Recognize the Signs of Abuse

Leslie Palmerlee, MD, MPH

Approximately 20%-30% of children who die from abuse are seen in the emergency department (ED) for injuries before the child's death. Victims of abuse can present to the ED with apparently minor injuries or confounding symptoms. Each of these visits is a potential missed opportunity to intervene and save a life. ED clinicians can miss the subtle signs of abuse and therefore miss the opportunity to prevent further abuse and even death.

Certain children are at higher risk for abuse. It can be useful to think of risk factors in three categories: factors relating to the child, to the caregiver, and to the environment. Children <4 years old, particularly infants <12 months, as well as those with special needs (including those with disabilities and mental illness) are at higher risk for abuse. Caregivers with a history of mental illness, substance abuse, or were themselves the victims of violence are at higher risk to abuse their children. Finally, children growing up in areas with high rates of poverty, high unemployment, and with poor social connections are at higher risk for abuse. While the presence of risk factors can help point a provider to the possibility of abuse, the opposite cannot be said of their absence. Providers should never be reassured by the lack of traditional risk factors. Children without obvious risk factors for abuse are more likely to be missed than those with known risk factors, and clinicians need to be cautious to avoid bias in abuse evaluations. These risk factors can be elicited by the social worker or by the provider with gentle, normalizing language (Pierce et al., 2014).

One simple way to screen for abuse is to perform a thorough skin examination on all young children in the ED for any reason. All young children should be exposed and examined from head to toe with an eye for sentinel injuries. Sentinel injuries are injuries that may be overlooked as inconsequential but could be a red flag for abuse because they are not developmentally capable of the injury, or the explanation is implausible. Sentinel injuries in children <12 months old include subconjunctival hemorrhages, frenulum injuries, unusual bruising, burns, bites, and fractures that are not age or developmentally appropriate. When a clinician finds one of these injuries, the first step is to obtain a more thorough history. It is essential to find out more about the mechanism of injury such as how it happened, when the injury occurred, who was present, and the circumstances surrounding the event. If there was a fall, find out the mechanics of the fall, the surface the child landed on, the height of the fall, and how they landed. If there are significant inconsistencies in the story, or the story does not match the developmental capabilities of the child, obtain further workup and consultation. Obtain a skeletal survey in all children <6 months with any bruising and in those <24 months with concerning bruising. Have a low threshold to obtain a head CT in children with any face/head injuries and those with subtle signs of head injury such as fussiness, lethargy, vomiting, or poor feeding. In all cases of suspected abuse, consult social work or child protective services. Consider transfer or hospital admission if a full workup cannot be obtained or there is concern about a safe discharge.

KEY POINTS

- Know the risk factors for abuse, but in their absence, forget about them.
- Always have abuse in the differential diagnosis when treating children.
- Do a full skin examination on high risk and young children.
- Be aware of sentinel injuries and take them as seriously a sentinel bleed of a subarachnoid hemorrhage.

Suggested Readings

Lindberg DM, Beaty B, Juarez-Colunga E, et al. Testing for abuse in children with sentinel injuries. *Pediatrics.* 2015;136:831-838.

Maguire-Jack K, Font SA. Community and individual risk factors for physical child abuse and child neglect: variations by poverty status. *Child Maltreat.* 2017;22(3):215-226.

Pierce MC, Kaczor K, Thompson R. Bringing back the social history. *Pediatr Clin North Am.* 2014;61(5):889-905.

Thorpe EL, Zuckerbraun NS, Wolford JE, et al. Missed opportunities to diagnose child physical abuse. *Pediatr Emerg Care.* 2014;30:771-776.

Wood J, Fakeye O, Mondestin V, et al. Development of hospital-based guidelines for skeletal survey in young children with bruises. *Pediatrics.* 2015;135:312-320.

Cannot Miss: Adolescent Sexual Assault

Molly Hallweaver, MD and Angela Jarman, MD, MPH

Sexual assault is an unfortunate reality, and one in three female rape victims was first assaulted between 11 and 17 years of age. Sexual assault has profound consequences on the short- and long-term physical, mental, and reproductive health of survivors. We define adolescent as between 11 and 18 years of age and sexual assault as an all-encompassing term for any nonconsensual sexual act between minors or illegal sex acts between an adolescent and an adult as defined by local laws. Emergency clinicians must be prepared to identify, treat, and refer victims of sexual assault in the ED.

Who to Screen

No single risk factor is sufficient to identify victims, and a high index of suspicion is mandatory in the pediatric setting. While there are differences between victims of sexual assault and commercial sexual exploitation, practically for most clinicians these populations should be considered together. If a patient has any of the red flag characteristics shown in Table 185.1, screen the patient for sexual assault.

How to Screen

When speaking to adolescent victims of assault, use nonjudgmental language to create a safe space and avoid retraumatization. It is important to use a trauma-informed approach. This treatment approach is patient centered and acknowledges the multiple and complex factors that can lead to trauma and that these traumatic experiences can influence all aspects of how our patients function including how they think, behave, and interact with others.

- Reiterate confidentiality while also being sure to explain mandatory reporting obligations.
- Speak to the patient one-on-one in a private space.
- Always use a hospital translator if the patient does not speak fluent English. Do not use family/ friends.
- Be direct with adolescents, and ask questions like "Has anyone forced you to have sexual contact against your will?" or "Have you ever had to exchange sex for money, food, drugs, shelter, or other favors?"
- Be explicit about what constitutes sexual activity as not all patients may recognize what is sexual assault.

Table 185.1 ■ Red Flags for Patients at High Risk of Sexual Assault

Red Flags
- Discrepancy between history and physical/clinical presentation
- High-risk chief complaint (pelvic pain, vaginal/penile discharge, pelvic/genital pain, request for STI testing, request for pregnancy testing, intoxication/ingestion, suicide attempt/ideation, homicidal ideation, acute sexual assault, traumatic assault, behavioral complaints)
- Signs of physical abuse
- Vulnerable population (homeless/runaway, LGBTQI, concurrent substance use disorder, mental health disorder, developmental delay)

Clinical Implications

When a patient shares that she/he has been assaulted, it is important to test and treat for physical complications of sexual assault. As mandated reporters of assault in children, law enforcement should be notified per local policies.

- Evidentiary exams are conducted by specially trained providers, which may require transfer to a different facility.
- Adolescents must consent to the forensic exam, though the age at which a patient has the ability to legally consent varies from state to state.
- Female patients should always be screened for pregnancy.
- The patient should also be screened for HIV, STIs, and other communicable diseases. Prophylactic treatments such as Plan B for pregnancy prevention, antibiotics for chlamydia/gonorrhea, and HIV prophylaxis should also be offered when appropriate.

Report the history with verbatim quotes and describe objective physical exam findings. Avoid statements like "*consistent with* assault" in your documentation. Physical injury to the anogenital area can be from both consensual and nonconsensual sexual activity. Likewise, many confirmed victims of sexual assault have normal physical exams.

Survivors of sexual assault are at high risk of a number of downstream sequelae including chronic pain, mood symptoms, and adverse life events; ensuring proper follow-up and continuity of care is important for the patients' long-term physical and mental health.

KEY POINTS

- The majority of sexual assault victims are seen in acute care settings. Be aware of the warning signs and screen high-risk patients.
- Identifying sexual assault victims can impact the patient's acute care and has profound consequences for their long-term mental and physical health.
- Use a nonjudgmental, trauma-informed approach in caring for these patients. Enlist a multidisciplinary team when possible (social work, primary care, psychiatry, etc.).
- Familiarize yourself with local legal protocols for mandatory reporting and handling of sexual and physical assault in your state.

Suggested Readings

Crawford-Jakubiak JE, Alderman EM, Leventhal JM. Care of the adolescent after an acute sexual assault. *Pediatrics*. 2017;139(3). doi:10.1542/peds.2016-4243.
https://www.nctsn.org/trauma-informed-care
https://www.cdc.gov/std/tg2015/sexual-assault.htm
https://www.freelists.org/archives/hilac/02-2014/pdftRo8tw89mb.pdf=

It Is Normal to Be Normal: Understand Unique Aspects of the Prepubescent Sexual Assault Examination

Samantha Kerns, MD and Mary Bing, MD, MPH

Frightened parents often come to the emergency department (ED) when they are worried their child has been sexually abused. Clinicians often feel ill prepared to recognize and care for potential victims because the principles of adult sexual assault do not translate easily to child sexual abuse. To provide compassionate and appropriate care in the ED, it is critical for providers to understand the unique aspects of pediatric sexual abuse.

Medical History

A child who has experienced sexual abuse might present to the ED with a concern for sexual abuse or with nonspecific symptoms like headaches, abdominal pain, behavioral changes, encopresis, or enuresis. During a busy shift, it is easy to speed through the history, expecting examination findings or lab results to make the diagnosis of child sex abuse. But the history is the most critical aspect of the evaluation, as most examinations of sexually abused children demonstrate no abnormalities.

The adult should be interviewed separately to not influence the child's account. Because prepubescent children are susceptible to suggestion, they should be interviewed by trained practitioners. Early coordination with a multidisciplinary team will help avoid repeated interviews that can both create trauma for the child and put potential evidence at risk. The provider should document verbatim anything the child discloses. Important questions for the caregiver include who the suspect is, when was last contact with the suspect, where did the potential abuse occur (important for legal jurisdiction), and does the suspect have continued contact with the child.

Physical Examination

While adult sexual assault often leaves physical findings, even in legally confirmed cases of sexual abuse, the majority of children do not have clinically apparent injuries or infections. It is normal to be normal, even in an abused child. Injuries are rare despite a history of penetration because the common types of abuse (touching, oral-genital contact, genital-genital contact without penetration) rarely leave marks and minor genital injuries heal rapidly. Clinicians should perform a medical clearance examination to ensure there are no injuries that require emergent care. For the evidentiary examination, the clinician should refer to local protocols, which determine who approves and performs the examination and in what timeframe. Unlike adult sexual assault, evidence in children deteriorates rapidly, and evidentiary examinations are rarely authorized after 72 hours. For medical clearance, an external examination of the genitalia should suffice and is usually performed in the frog-leg or prone knee-to-chest position. Providers who rarely perform prepubescent evidentiary examinations have a tendency to conclude that unexpected or nonspecific findings such as erythema, anal, and/or hymenal dilation are a result of abuse. Nonspecific findings should be documented and communicated but not considered evidence of abuse, especially if there is no reported history of abuse. Photographic documentation can be used to supplement (but not substitute for) physical examination findings.

Workup and Treatment

Sexually transmitted infections (STIs) are rare in children, but when found are highly concerning for abuse. Local protocols should guide testing. Strongly consider testing for STIs in symptomatic children or if the perpetrator possesses high-risk features. The preferred way to screen for Chlamydia and Gonorrhea is with a dirty urine nucleic acid amplification test (NAAT). Treat STIs if results are positive, not prophylactically. Regardless of examination findings, a concerning history of abuse must be reported.

KEY POINTS

- The history is key, but get it from the guardian. Let trained professionals interview prepubescent children about anything other than medical aspects.
- Document child's responses in quotes.
- It is normal to be normal. Most sexual abuse victims will have no physical findings of injury. Leave nonspecific findings such as erythema, anal/hymenal dilation to the experts to determine the cause.
- Report when suspicious for sexual abuse, even if the examination is normal.

Suggested Readings

Adams JA. Understanding medical findings in child sexual abuse: an update for 2018. *Acad Forensic Pathol.* 2018;8(4):924-937.

Adams JA, Harper K, Knudson S, Revilla J. Examination findings in legally confirmed child sexual abuse: it's normal to be normal. *Pediatrics.* 1994;94(3):310-317.

Adams JA, Kellogg ND, Farst KJ, et al. Updated guidelines for the medical assessment and care of children who may have been sexually abused. *J Pediatr Adolesc Gynecol.* 2016;29(2):81-87.

Jenny C, Crawford-Jakubiak JE; Committee on Child Abuse and Neglect; American Academy of Pediatrics. The evaluation of children in the primary care setting when sexual abuse is suspected. *Pediatrics.* 2013;132(2): e558-e567.

Center for Disease Control. 2015 Sexually Transmitted Disease Treatment Guidelines. https://www.cdc.gov/std/tg2015/default.htm. Accessed April 29, 2019.

187

Treat the Patient, Not the Poison

Michelle Odette, MD and Daniel K. Colby, MD

The rates of substance use and substance use disorder (SUD) by young people around the world are high. While teens are commonly understood to be an at-risk population, clinicians are nonetheless often caught off guard in the emergency department (ED) by the young age of these patients, the severity of drug toxicity, and variety of substances used.

General Tips on Substance Use

The most common error regarding substance use in the ED is not asking about it or asking in front of caregivers. For teens, it is important to ask parents to step out of the room and ask sensitive questions about alcohol and drugs. Drug testing is often not necessary, as patients often provide the answers themselves. In patients with severe drug intoxication, a focused examination is typically the best source of information, as many present with classic toxidromes. Recalling toxidrome patterns can point to the diagnosis even with a suboptimal history.

Unfortunately, not every intoxicated patient reads the textbook on toxidromes or the history conflicts with the examination, and the exact substance itself is frequently never identified. As a result, when you treat acute drug toxicity, make sure to *treat the patient, not the poison*. Antidotes are often not necessary, especially when they distract from the supportive care most of these patients require. Once stabilized, the substance can be further identified if necessary.

A test often used in the ED as a quick way to screen for common drugs of abuse is the urine drug screen (UDS). However, the UDS is a remarkably flawed tool. Labs have different UDS panels with wildly varying levels of sensitivity and specificity and many cross-reactions that can create a false positive. For example, a ubiquitous medication like ibuprofen use can cause false-positive results for barbiturates, phencyclidine (PCP), and tetrahydrocannabinol (TCH). The most egregious example is the amphetamine screen, which has nearly a dozen agents that provide a false-positive result. Moreover, the false-negative rate is profound as there are many drugs not detected, including the increasingly commonly abused drug fentanyl. Due to these limitations, the utility of the UDS is limited as it rarely changes acute management. A thorough history and examination by a clinician familiar with toxidromes are more valuable than any drug testing.

Commonly Used Substances

Alcohol

- Make sure to include alcohol on your differential for pediatric patients who present with altered mental status. Alcohol ingestion can cause hypoglycemia and seizures in children.

Caffeine

- While most caffeine toxic patients present with mild symptoms of nausea and palpitations, severe caffeine toxicity can occur even accidentally in patients who use multiple sources of caffeine, such as energy drinks and caffeine pills.
- Patients with severe caffeine toxicity can present with symptoms similar to a sympathomimetic toxidrome, including hyperthermia, tachycardia, irritability, and even drowsiness. Severe metabolic derangement can occur, such as hypokalemia. Rhabdomyolysis is also common.

Marijuana

- Marijuana toxicity does not present with only one classic toxidrome. The symptoms can be variable.
- Young children and youth can get into marijuana in the house, and edibles are very appealing to children. The marijuana of today is significantly more potent than then marijuana of our parents. Consider ingestion of this ubiquitous drug in any child with altered mental status. Caregivers are more likely to disclose marijuana in the house with nonjudgmental language.
- For teens presenting with recurrent nausea and abdominal pain, make sure to enquire about marijuana, as chronic use is associated with cannabis hyperemesis syndrome. Symptoms typically resolve with cessation of marijuana, although complete resolution can take weeks to months as marijuana is stored in fat long after exposure ends.

Dextromethorphan

- Intentional use of dextromethorphan, also known as "robotripping," results in a dissociative state with a "zombie-like" altered mental status and nystagmus.
- Patients will often ingest over-the-counter cough/cold preparations for the dextromethorphan. However, these preparations often contain additional ingredients, such as acetaminophen, guaifenesin, antihistamines, and/or pseudoephedrine. As a result, for patients possibly "robotripping," also consider toxicity from concomitant exposures.

KEY POINTS

- Treat the patient, not the poison.
- The UDS is significantly flawed and rarely changes management.
- Look for toxidrome patterns to make the diagnosis instead of relying on the UDS.

Suggested Readings

Algren DA, Christian MR. Buyer beware: pitfalls in toxicology laboratory testing. *Mo Med.* 2015;112(3):206-210.
Levy S. Youth and the opioid epidemic. *Pediatrics.* 2019;143(2):e20182752.
Nanda S, Konnur N. Adolescent drug & alcohol use in the 21st century. *Pediatr Ann.* 2006;35(3):193-199.

188

The Minefield of Minor Consent: Be Sure That You Are Following Your State's Legal Statutes

Rachel J. Heidt, MD and Kendra Grether-Jones, MD

What do you do when an unaccompanied minor shows up in the ED? See them! Federal law under the Emergency Medical Treatment and Active Labor Act (EMTALA) mandates a medical screening examination to determine the existence of an emergency medical condition (EMC). An EMC is any threat to the patient's life or health.

An attempt should be made to contact the patient's parent/legal guardian to seek consent without delaying stabilization of the patient. If an EMC is *not* identified, the EMTALA regulations no longer apply and state laws determine the minor's authority to consent based on conditions for which the minor seeks care and the status of the child.

Emancipation, Mature Minor Doctrine, and Condition-Specific Exceptions

Emancipation: Most states recognize minors as emancipated if they are married, economically self-supporting and not living at home, or active-duty status in the military. In some states, a minor who is a parent or who is pregnant is considered emancipated. Some states require a court to declare emancipation.

Mature Minor Exception: Many states also recognize the consent rights of a mature minor, usually 12 years or older, who is determined to have the ability to understand and appreciate the benefits, risks, and alternatives of the proposed treatment. State laws vary in whether a physician can make this determination, and in states without this law, parent/guardian consent for nonemergent treatment is required.

Condition-Specific Exceptions: Many states allow a minor to consent for evaluation/treatment for mental health services, drug and alcohol addiction, pregnancy-related care, contraceptive services, and testing/treatment for sexually transmitted infections. If there is suspected abuse or neglect, child protective services (CPS) and/or local law enforcement should be involved early on.

Assent and Consent

Assent is the agreement of someone not able to give legal consent. Ideally, minors more than 7 years old should receive developmentally appropriate information about their care and be asked for their assent before any tests or procedures are performed. Over the age of 14, the process should be similar to seeking informed consent, even if the legal decision-making rights are not theirs to make.

Informed **consent** is traditionally given by the parent/guardian. It can be provided by a minor if they are emancipated, the care falls under the mature minor doctrine, or for the above condition-specific exceptions.

If someone who is not authorized to provide legal consent accompanies a child, a provider should refrain from providing nonurgent testing and treatment to these children. Unless a minor's right to consent has been legally established, the provider should attempt to notify the legal guardian as soon as possible.

If an EMC is identified, consent is presumed, and all care relating to that emergent condition should be performed without delay. There is no need for two-physician consent for this treatment unless separately required by your institutional policy. If it is not an emergency, care should be delayed until consent can be obtained unless the minor meets one of the other criteria mentioned above.

The parent or guardian has the right to refuse consent for emergent evaluation and treatment, but at the same time is required to act in the best interest of the child. If the medical care in question is necessary and likely to prevent death, disability, or serious harm to the child, law enforcement, and/or CPS involvement will likely be required. Temporary protective custody may be indicated while this care is being provided. Early involvement of the hospital legal and/or ethics team might be helpful.

KEY POINTS

- See everyone even if they are unaccompanied, but only treat emergent conditions without appropriate consent.
- Most requirements vary by state, so make sure you are knowledgeable about how your state defines emancipation, mature minor exception, and condition-specific exceptions.
- A minor is a person. Explain to them what you are doing and why it needs to be done in an age-appropriate manner.

Suggested Readings

Benjamin L, Ishimine P, Joseph M, et al. Evaluation and treatment of minors. *Ann Emerg Med*. 2018;71(2):225-232.

Committee on Bioethics. Informed consent in decision-making in pediatric practice. *Pediatrics*. 2016;138(2): e20161484.

Committee on Pediatric Emergency Medicine and Committee on Bioethics. Consent for emergency medical services for children and adolescents. *Pediatrics*. 2011;128(2):427-433.

Guttmacher Institute. An overview of consent to reproductive health services by young people. https://www.guttmacher.org/state-policy/explore/overview-minors-consent-law. Accessed April 30, 2019.

Retting P. Can a minor refuse assent for emergency care? *Virtual Mentor*. 2012;14(10):763-766.

APPLIED PRACTICE

Evidence-Based Medicine: Have the Tools to Test Wisely

Eddie G. Rodriguez, MD and Fernando Soto, MD, FACEP

"Throughout our medical training, we are taught the 'classic presentation' of diseases and common interventions" but "half of what you learn in medical school is wrong or outdated…unfortunately we don't know which half." Evidence-based medicine (EBM), through the use of basic standardized tools, helps to keep our practice current by applying the best evidence available to clinical care.

Most of the required information to interpret studies may be derived from understanding 2×2 contingency tables. The standardized approach is to arrange the disease on top (x axis) and the test or "gold standard" on the side rows (y axis) with the true positive (TP) in the left upward corner (Table 189.1).

TP is when the patient has the disease and the test is positive. False positive (FP) occurs when the patient does not have the disease but the test is positive. True negative (TN) is when the patient does not have the disease and the test is negative. False negative (FN) occur when the patient has the disease but the test is negative. Prevalence describes how often the disease is present in the study population. It is calculated by taking those with the disease divided by the total of study subjects— (TP + FN)/(TP + FN + TN + FP).

The key terms: sensitivity (sn), specificity (sp), and positive and negative predictive values may be aided with the mnemonic: "Truth above all." Sensitivity and specificity are not impacted by disease prevalence; however, the positive and negative predictive values are. Since much of the time disease prevalence is unknown or variable, many prefer the likelihood ratio.

Sensitivity is the probability that a test will be positive in those with the disease. Tests with a high sensitivity may produce false-positive results but are usually good screening tests. It is calculated by dividing the number of TP by the total of those with the disease—(TP/TP + FN).

Specificity is the probability that a test will be negative in those patients who do NOT have the disease. Tests with high specificity may produce false negatives, but it can be used to confirm or diagnose disease. It is calculated by dividing the TN by all those without the disease—(TN/TN + FP).

Positive predictive value (PPV) is the probability of actually having the disease in all those with a positive test result. It is calculated by dividing the value of those with a positive test and the disease by all those with a positive test (TP/TP + FP).

Negative predictive value (NPV) is the probability that those with a negative study do not have the disease. It is calculated by dividing those disease free with a negative test by all those with a negative test (TN/TN + FN).

Positive likelihood ratio (PLR) is the probability of a patient with the disease having a positive result compared to the probability of a patient without the disease of having a positive result. PLR = sensitivity/1 − specificity.

Negative likelihood ratio (NLR) can be defined as the probability that a patient with the disease has a negative test result compared to the probability of a patient without the disease of having a negative result. NLR = 1 − sensitivity/specificity.

Table 189.1 ■ 2 x 2 Contingency Table			
	Disease		
	+	−	
Test/Exposure +	TP	FP	PPV = TP/TP + FP
−	FN	TN	NPV = TN/TN + FN
	Sn = TP/TP + FN	Sp = TN/TN + FP	

Demonstration of calculations for Sensitivity (Sn), Specificity (Sp), Positive predictive value (PPV), and Negative predictive value (NPV) using 2x2 table with Disease on the X axis and Test/Exposure on the Y axis

Other commonly used EBM tools are absolute risk reduction (ARR), number needed to treat (NNT), and kappa value. The first two terms are extremely useful in describing treatment interventions to patients and colleagues. The last one is used to evaluate the variability in an observation.

ARR, also known as risk difference, is used to describe the magnitude of the effect of an intervention. For example, if a condition is seen in 25% of patients in the control group, but occurs only 5% of the time in those taking a specific drug, then the ARR is 20%.

NNT is the inverse of ARR (1/ARR). It is a way to express how many interventions must take place in order to have the desired outcome. In the above example, the ARR is 20%, so NNT = 1/0.2 = 5. This means that for every 5 treatments provided, 1 event of the desired outcome will be observed.

Kappa value is the interobserver agreement. It measures variations between observations or data points gathered by different people. Kappa may range from 0 to 1 (from no agreement to perfect agreement). A kappa value of 0.25, for example, means weak agreement, whereas a value of 0.75 means very good agreement.

KEY POINTS

- Basic tools of Evidence-based medicine (EBM) will help to keep our practice up to date.
- Sensitivity and Specificity provide us with the probability of a positive or negative test on an individual with or without the disease
- Positive predictive value (PPV) and Negative predictive value (NPV) is the probability of actually having or not having the disease depending on the test result.
- Absolute risk reduction (ARR) and Number needed to treat (NNT) help us share treatment options with patients and colleagues

Suggested Readings

https://bestpractice.bmj.com/info/us/toolkit/ebm-tools/statistics-calculators/
Irwig L, Irwig J, Trevena L, et al. Chapter 18, Relative risk, relative and absolute risk reduction, number needed to treat and confidence intervals. In: *Smart Health Choices: Making Sense of Health Advice*. London: Hammersmith Press; 2008. https://www.ncbi.nlm.nih.gov/books/NBK63647/
McGee S. Simplifying likelihood ratios. *J Gen Intern Med*. 2002;17(8):646-649.

My Baby Turned Blue: Changing the Terminology From ALTE to BRUE

Supriya Sharma, MD, FAAP and Marianne Gausche-Hill, MD, FACEP, FAAP, FAEMS

What should you do when a baby turns blue? Sudden life-threatening events in infants are frightening to the caregiver and challenging for the emergency clinician. These incidents are often difficult to evaluate and manage based on the number of serious underlying conditions that cause such events. In 2016, the American Academy of Pediatrics (AAP) published a clinical practice guideline suggesting a change in terminology from apparent life-threatening event (ALTE) to brief resolved unexplained events (BRUE). This change was meant to distinguish between sudden life-threatening events in infants, which are brief and nonprogressive for which the evaluation and management can be simplified, from the more severe events that may be progressive, and lead to the need for pediatric critical care.

In this chapter, we will explore the change in the management recommendations from ALTE to BRUE.

A BRUE is defined as an event occurring in an infant younger than 1 year when the observer reports a sudden, brief, and now resolved episode of ≥1 of the following:

- Cyanosis or pallor
- Absent, decreased, or irregular breathing
- Marked change in tone (hyper- or hypotonia)
- Altered level of responsiveness

BRUEs are diagnoses of exclusion, after the emergency clinician conducts an appropriate history and physical examination, and there is no other explanation for the event.

It is important for the clinician to differentiate high- and low-risk patients with BRUEs, as this will determine whether the patient requires further workup or management. Low-risk patients are defined by the characteristics below:

- Age >60 days
- Prematurity: gestational age ≥32 weeks and postconceptional age ≥45 weeks
- First BRUE (no previous BRUE ever and not occurring in clusters)
- Duration of event <1 minute
- No cardiopulmonary resuscitation (CPR) required by trained medical provider
- No concerning historical features
- No concerning physical examination findings

Infants who have experienced a BRUE who do not meet the low-risk qualifications are, by definition, high-risk. Unfortunately, a review of the outcomes from the ALTE literature for high-risk patients did not yield definitive recommendations regarding their management. However, it is imperative that the emergency clinician recognize that patients in the high-risk category may have a recurrent event, a serious underlying condition, the potential for an adverse outcome, and may require critical care. For low-risk BRUE patients, the AAP has evidence-based recommendations for providers detailed below (Table 190.1).

Table 190.1 ■ Management Recommendations for Lower-Risk Patients

Providers should:	• Educate caregivers about BRUEs and engage in shared decision-making to guide evaluation, disposition, and follow-up • Offer resources for CPR training to caregiver
Providers may:	• Obtain pertussis testing • Obtain a 12-lead electrocardiogram • Briefly monitor patients with continuous pulse oximetry and serial observations
Providers need not:	• Obtain viral respiratory test, urinalysis, serum blood glucose, bicarbonate, lactic acid, or neuroimaging • Admit the patient *solely* for cardiorespiratory monitoring
Providers should not:	• Obtain white blood count, blood culture, cerebrospinal fluid analysis or culture, serum sodium, potassium, chloride, ammonia, blood gases, urine organic acids, plasma amino acids, or acylcarnitines • Obtain chest radiograph or echocardiogram • Obtain electroencephalogram • Obtain studies for gastroesophageal reflux disease • Obtain lab evaluation for anemia • Initiate home cardiorespiratory monitoring • Prescribe acid suppression therapy or antiepileptic medication

KEY POINTS

■ New clinical guidelines recommend a change in terminology from ALTE to BRUE for low-risk infants.

■ Higher-risk infants (ie, <2 months, CPR was performed by a medical provider, multiple events, comorbid disease including prematurity, abnormal vital signs, or physical examination findings) are sick infants for which evaluation and management is based on possible underlying etiologies and will require hospital admission.

■ Low-risk infants with BRUE may be managed with minimal testing and discharged with close follow-up.

Suggested Readings

McFarlin A. What to do when babies turn blue: beyond the basic brief resolved unexplained event. *Emerg Med Clin North Am.* 2018;36:335-347.

Tate C, Stanley R. Brief resolved unexplained events (formerly apparent life-threatening events) and evaluation of lower-risk infants. *Arch Dis Child Educ Pract Ed.* 2018;103:95-98.

Tieder JS, Bonkowsky JL, Etzel RA, et al.; for the Subcommittee on Apparent life-threatening events, American Academy of Pediatrics. Brief resolved unexplained event (formerly apparent life-threatening events) and evaluation of lower risk infants. *Pediatrics.* 2016;137:e20160591.

The Technological-Dependent Child

Blair Rolnick, MD, FAAP and Christopher S. Amato, MD, FAAP, FACEP

Medical technology is ever changing, leading to increased frequency and challenge for those caring for these children. As with any caregiver, it is vital to truly hear their concerns, as they are the most reliable barometer of the child's status and any recent changes, any planned contingencies, and additional medical equipment. Furthermore, these caregivers are at risk for burn-out, given the complexity of their child's needs, so be sure to assess for strain.

Tracheostomy

Early complications include (1) accidental decannulation, (2) bleeding, (3) subglottic stenosis, (4) wound infection, and (5) pneumomediastinum.

Late complications include (1) infection, (2) granuloma formation, and (3) fistula (rare). The most common emergencies in pediatric patients with tracheostomy are blockage, displacement, and accidental decannulation.

Those in extremis require high-flow oxygen to both the face and tracheostomy after proper positioning. Suction to determine patency and clear secretions. The size of the catheter (double the size of the tracheostomy) used is key: too short may lead to blockage, while too long may cause tracheal trauma. Inability to pass a suction catheter requires an immediate tracheostomy change.

Stoma formation requires ~7 days to mature, at which point the first tube change will occur. Take care to avoid creating a false tract.

Gastrostomy Tube

Displacement requires timely replacement as the tract closes within hours. Gastrostomy tracts typically mature by 3 months. Manipulation prior to this time can create a false tract, subsequently leading to obstruction or peritonitis. If the maturity of a G-tube tract is unknown, consult pediatric surgery or gastroenterology.

Replace tubes in mature tracts as quickly as possible. Apply lubricant to the ostomy and tube. Apply perpendicular pressure at the stoma and gently insert. Replacement should be painless and without resistance. A Foley may be substituted if no replacement is immediately available.

TRICK: place Foley tip in ice-cold water for 10-15 seconds to firm up the tip leading to easier placement.

After replacement, confirm the position. Aspiration of stomach contents and listening for borborygmi after instilling 10-15 mL of air is sufficient to confirm placement. If any uncertainty exists, a confirmatory x-ray using contrast is recommended.

Other less common complications of G-tubes include peritonitis, pneumoperitoneum, gastric outlet obstruction, and local ostomy infections. Incorrect replacement of dislodged G-tubes may lead to peritonitis and septicemia. Gastric outlet obstruction can occur due to migration of the PEG tube distal balloon to the pyloric or from overfilling the balloon.

Ventricle Assist Device

Ventricular assist devices (VADs) are implantable devices that support circulation in patients with heart failure. Compared to the adult population, pediatric VAD patients have increased mortality and morbidity associated with stroke and other thromboembolic events. VADs can be left ventricular assist devices (LVADs), right ventricular assist devices (RVADs), and biventricular.

The LVAD is the device most likely to be encountered. All LVADs consist of a pump, controller, driveline, and batteries attached to the controller or to a power-base unit. When a patient presents to the ED, regardless of reason, the physician should assess the patient while another team member contacts the patients LVAD coordinator.

Evaluation for a patient with LVAD includes assessing perfusion and mean arterial pressure (MAP). There will be no palpable pulse due to the continuous flow from the LVAD. Provide a fluid bolus if there are signs of poor perfusion. Hypertension in LVAD patients requires immediate attention, as increased afterload can lead to thrombosis and stroke. Auscultate the patient's chest and abdomen for the humming sound of the pump.

The primary device parameters are speed, power, battery charge, and pulsatility index (PI). PI is indicative of the patient's volume status, stretch, and contractility. PI is affected by preload and afterload. Decreased preload leads to decreased PI; volume overload leads to increased PI. Pump speed and PI will be inversely related.

- High power, low PI: changing pump speed could indicate pump thrombosis or hypotension— consider fluid.
- High power with high PI: may indicate volume overload.
- Low power, low PI, steady speed: consider hypertensive or outflow/inflow obstruction.
- Low power with high PI: could indicate a suction event (collapse of the left ventricle)

Battery: Contact the VAD coordinator immediately. The pump will automatically reduce speed to conserve battery leading to syncope and light-headedness.

Standard ACLS protocols should be followed in LVAD patients, but extreme caution is needed with chest compressions due to the potential for damage to the cannula. Defibrillation, pacing, and cardioversion can be performed. However, defibrillator or pacer pads would be placed directly over the pump so all issues with the LVAD itself should first be addressed.

KEY POINTS

- Caregivers provide crucial information, and it is essential to hear their concerns and assess for any strain as they are at risk for burn-out given the complexity of their child's medical issues.
- Tracheostomy—when the patient presents in distress, position, and then deliver high-flow oxygen to both the face and tracheostomy.
- LVAD: no pulse is normal, assess for perfusion and MAP. PALS/ACLS protocols apply in LVAD patients, but extreme caution is needed with chest compressions to prevent damage to the cannula.

Suggested Reading

www.mylvad.com provides links to emergency medical service field guides for various LVAD devices.

192

Well-Child Care in the Emergency Department Setting: Looking for "Goldilocks Moments" by Doing Just the Right Amount

Mark S. Mannenbach, MD

The training for most providers caring for children in the emergency department (ED) setting understandably focuses on early recognition and stabilization of high-stakes diagnosis in an effort to reduce both morbidity and mortality. However, most children presenting for care in the ED require little in the way of acute intervention as most children are healthy and at low risk for decompensation. An estimated 800 000 children seek care each day in the ED setting in the United States including 3.4% utilizing the ED as their source for sick care. Increasing numbers of ED visits have led to longer lengths of stay and a potential for decreased patient satisfaction.

Many opportunities exist for ED providers to improve patient satisfaction through an appropriately thorough evaluation of each patient along with clear instructions for follow-up steps including when to return to the ED as well as to the primary care provider. A clear understanding of well-child care concepts will allow the ED provider to deliver appropriate care and potentially meet or even exceed caregiver expectations.

When caring for children who have been injured, clear acknowledgment of appropriate use of protective helmet and car seat restraint use can go a long way to reinforce the injury prevention initiatives covered during well-child visits. Understanding the recommendations for car seat replacement after a motor vehicle collision helps further guide caregivers in these situations. Capturing teachable moments after falls from changing tables or other heights or after accidental ingestions by curious toddlers are other examples of partnering with primary care in injury prevention.

Acute illness or injury creates a unique opportunity for the ED provider to initiate discussions regarding the importance of immunizations in the overall maintenance of a child's health. Parents and caregivers may reconsider previous opposition to immunizations when faced with the reality of potential for poor outcomes or the need for a more extensive evaluation in the ED.

Attention to the growth and developmental milestones of infants and young children will also allow for a more clearly directed evaluation in the ED. The infant who presents with repetitive vomiting episodes and increased head circumference size may be more quickly identified as having a new diagnosis of hydrocephalus or brain tumor in the ED setting. Failure to attain, or even more concerning, loss of milestones raises suspicion for serious underlying pathology such as physical abuse. Guideline development including an expectation for a complete set of vital signs and growth parameters for the young child has the potential to also reassure both the ED provider and the caregiver of the lack of an urgent need for unnecessary diagnostic studies.

Caregivers may leave the ED with the impression that "nothing has been done" even after the ED provider is satisfied that an appropriate evaluation to rule out the important acute care issues has been completed. As an example, in addition to understanding the need to identify potentially high-stakes diagnosis for the newborn with "spitting up," the ED provider can also offer strategies to optimize feeding. A majority of infants will have some vomiting or spitting up in their first few months of life. These symptoms create a great deal of concern especially for new parents. A review of the nutritional requirements for infants and strategies to ensure avoidance of overfeeding along with consideration of intolerance or allergy to infant formula may also be helpful. For breast-fed infants, discussion regarding the mother's diet or medication use may uncover an explanation for symptoms; elimination of cow's milk, eggs, or other foods from the mother's diet may lead to resolution of symptoms in the nursing infant. Reassurance through utilization of the child's growth curve can be very helpful through demonstration of attention to existing data and further connection with the medical home.

The ED provider would do well to not only become an expert in pediatric resuscitation and procedures but also to develop a working knowledge of the common challenges faced by families caring for children. An understanding of the likelihood of significant illness and more common explanations for a child's symptoms through ongoing education utilizing personal experience, review of the literature, and input from primary care providers is critical to appropriate care in the ED setting.

KEY POINTS

- Opportunities exist for providers to apply well-child care concepts to children seeking care in the ED setting.
- Strategies to incorporate well-child care concepts such as an expectation for growth measurements for all children will assist in the delivery of appropriate acute care for children.
- Providers in the acute care setting have a unique viewpoint and have the potential to deliver impactful messaging to family caregivers in regard to injury prevention.
- Immunization recommendations can be shared with family caregivers in the acute care setting to encourage compliance either in real-time or through follow-up visits.
- ED providers are encouraged to obtain and maintain a working knowledge of well-child care concepts with the goal of application to their everyday practice.

Suggested Readings

Barata I, Brown KM, Fitzmaurice L, et al. Best practices for improving flow and care of pediatric patients in the emergency department. *Pediatrics*. 2015;135;e273-e283.

Chu T, Shah A, Walker D, et al. Pattern of symptoms and signs of primary intracranial tumours in children and young adults: a record linkage study. *Arch Dis Child*. 2015;100:1115-1122.

McCollough M, Sharieff GQ. Common complaints in the first thirty days of life. *Emerg Med Clin North Am*. 2002;20:27-48.

Melzer-Lange MD, Zonfrillo MR, Gittelman MA. Injury prevention opportunities in the emergency department. *Pediatr Clin North Am*. 2013;60:1241-1253.

Zachariah P, Posner A, Stockwell MS, et al. Vaccination rates for measles, mumps, rubella, and influenza among children presenting to a pediatric emergency department in New York City. *J Pediatr Infect Dis Soc*. 2014;3: 350-353.

Psych Outbursts, Pediatric Behavioral Management: Exhaust All Nonpharmacologic Measures Before Chemically or Physically Restraining a Child

Adriana Porto, MD and Whitney Minnock, MD

Introduction

An agitated child who presents to the pediatric emergency department (ED) should be evaluated for potential causes of agitation. The agitated state may be a sign of a life-threatening condition that needs to be addressed quickly. There are nonmodifiable and modifiable psychiatric and physical causes of agitation, which can put the patient and staff at risk for injury.

Initial Evaluation

First, make the environment safe for the patient and the team. A calm and friendly approach can keep a patient from feeling threatened. This will encourage the patient better cooperation and communication. Physical examination should evaluate for signs of direct trauma, any clues of medical conditions, any ingestion of toxins or medications, or any other findings that could be driving the agitation. Patients may demonstrate syndromic appearance or behavior consistent with developmental delay that may be dealt with differently than a psychiatric or substance abuse patient. Early signs of agitation include pacing, rocking, or striking at inanimate objects.

Approach to the Agitated Child

A patient suffering from a psychiatric disorder (with or without an associated medical condition or intoxication) warrants a multidisciplinary approach, ideally with a social worker, a psychiatrist (if available), and the ED staff. Clear and constant communication is the key to give the adequate treatment. If the child escalates, he or she should be moved to a safer room, ideally with protected walls and free objects with a potential harm.

Management

It is important to be familiar with the different nonpharmacological techniques and pharmacological options in the ED. Nonpharmacological treatments are first line and focus on creating a calm environment. This includes minimizing external stimuli such as sounds, smells, temperature, and light in the room. Some hospitals provide sound isolation systems and adjust the colors on the walls in behavioral health rooms. When available, child life is an enormous help, particularly for patients with autism and other developmental disorders. The use of weighted blankets can be helpful for children with autism. Soothing techniques such as a soft voice and minimizing the number of people in a room may help decrease the anxiety. Food, drink, video games, computer apps, books, coloring, and activities that keep the patient distracted can all decrease the stress.

When calming interventions fail, be prepared to escalate to chemical and physical restraints. Data on chemical restraint in children are limited and mostly based on case reports or extrapolated from the adult literature. If the child is already taking psychiatric medications, give the usual oral medications unless toxicity is suspected. If the child is not due for a dose, consider ¼ or ½ the total daily amount if taking a benzodiazepine or antipsychotic. Benzodiazepines, antihistamines, and neuroleptics are the most common medications used, with benzodiazepines being the most common. Oral route is preferred, but if the patient is unwilling, consider intramuscular (IM) route before intravenous (IV) if there is no other reason to place an IV. Intranasal (IN) route is also an option and may be preferred depending on the situation or drug (ie, midazolam).

If these medications are not improving the agitation, haloperidol or other antipsychotics can be used. Ziprasidone intramuscularly has shown some benefit in open-label reports of agitated child psychiatric inpatients. Risperidone has also been shown some improvement in aggression. Keep in mind that most of these have only been studied in adolescents. Antipsychotics can cause extrapyramidal symptoms, especially in patients taking other antipsychotic medications or dopamine antagonists medications. If none of those medications work, ketamine in analgesic doses is implemented in various institutions, mostly in patients older than 18 years of age, though there have been some promising case reports involving adolescents.

KEY POINTS

- Rule out medical causes of agitation.
- Early identification of a potentially aggressive patient can prevent the need for restraints.
- Use calming measures first.
- Approach and management should be multidisciplinary.
- Oral or intranasal medications can be as effective as IM or IV.

Suggested Readings

Adimando AA, Poncin YB, Baum CR. Pharmacological management of the agitated pediatric patient. *Pediatr Emerg Care*. 2010;26(11):856–860.

Barzman DH, Brackenbury L, Sonnier L, et al. Brief Rating of Aggression by Children and Adolescents (BRA-CHA): development of a tool for assessing risk of in- patients' aggressive behavior. *J Am Acad Psychiatry Law*. 2011;39(2):170–179.

Connor DF, Melloni RH, Harrison RJ. Overt categorical aggression in referred children and adolescents. *J Am Acad Child Adolesc Psychiatry*. 1998;37:66–73.

Malas N, Brahmbhatt K, McDermott C, et al. Pediatric delirium: evaluation, management and special considerations. *Curr Psychiatry Rep*. 2017;19(9):65.

Navigating the Complexity of Autism Spectrum Disorder in the Pediatric ED—Work With Caregivers to Individualize Care

Sarah Kleist, MD

Autism spectrum disorder (ASD) is a complex neurodevelopmental condition of variable severity that is typically defined by its impairments in verbal communication and social interactions and its restrictive and repetitive behaviors. Over the past several decades, the incidence of this disorder has increased dramatically; as a result, children with ASD are becoming an increasingly larger proportion of patients seen in pediatric emergency departments (EDs) for acute medical and psychiatric conditions. Children with ASD experience specific challenges in the busy clinical environment of the ED. Thus, understanding the core features and behavioral concerns of ASD can help professionals prepare for these encounters and make visits positive and effective for patients, families, and health care providers alike.

A busy hospital ED, with its unpredictability, bright lights, loud noises, crowds, and long wait times, can be overwhelming for anyone. Children with ASD may react very differently than others to these stressors and therefore require a specialized approach to construct a safe and supportive environment. The autism spectrum is widely variable in phenotype, so each person with autism is unique in the way he or she uses and understands language; navigates social situations; reacts to sounds, lights, and touch; and copes with changes to his or her surroundings or routines. And finally, adding to the complexity of an ED visit, ASD often co-exists with disorders such as anxiety, depression, or aggression, which can further complicate diagnostic tests and health care management for these children.

Communication impairments have been reported as a significant barrier to effective evaluation and treatment, as children with ASD often have difficulty developing language skills, expressing themselves, and interpreting what others say to them. By taking the time to obtain a thorough history of the child's communication skills from the parents or caregivers, the provider can best know how to proceed. Providers should avoid open-ended questions and allow more time for processing and response. It is important to remember that children with ASD can often understand than they can speak. Similarly, nonverbal children may understand language even if they are unable to communicate it. Utilizing tablets with ASD-specific applications, sign language (if applicable), gestures, symbolic play, and pictures boards can help staff communicate in a more effective manner.

Children with ASD may be hypersensitive to certain triggers and hyposensitive to others. It is believed that the repetitive behaviors typically present in ASD may actually be adaptive behaviors to help offload sensory differences that the child is experiencing. Many pediatric EDs are starting to adapt by creating autism-friendly experiences. These changes include providing a separate quiet waiting area for families with children with ASD, having sensory boxes that provide objects with a variety of textures to help patients self-soothe and cope with stress, and providing communication tools that help children express fears and concerns.

Children with ASD bring a unique set of challenges to an ED visit. Providers play a primary role in setting the groundwork for a constructive and successful health care evaluation and management plan. Being prepared and proactive can facilitate a good patient-provider relationship. Communicating effectively, decreasing wait times and sensory stimuli, and actively engaging the caretaker can avoid miscommunication, alleviate frustration, and ease anxiety. Reinforcing cooperative behavior through rewards and praise; ignoring behaviors that appear atypical, such as unusual body movements or unexpected vocalizations; and encouraging caregivers to redirect and reassure are all essential in providing quality care.

KEY POINTS

- Children with ASD react differently to stressors in the ED and require a specialized approach to create a safe and supportive environment.
- Children with ASD have difficulty developing and processing language, so communication impairments can present a significant barrier to effective evaluation and treatment.
- Repetitive behaviors present in ASD are thought to be adaptive behaviors that offload sensory differences the child is experiencing. They can be ignored if they are not harmful.
- Effectively communicating, decreasing sensory stimuli, and actively engaging the primary caretaker can help decrease miscommunication and frustration and lead to a positive and effective visit for patients, families, and health care providers alike.

Suggested Readings

Giarelli E, Nocera R, Turchi R, et al. Sensory stimuli as obstacles to emergency care for children with autism spectrum disorder. *Adv Emerg Nurs J*. 2014;36(2):145-163.

Kalb LG, Stuart EA, Freedman B, et al. Psychiatric-related emergency department visits among children with an autism spectrum disorder. *Pediatr Emerg Care*. 2012;28(12):1269-1276.

Nicholas DB, Zwaigenbaum L, Muskat B, et al. Toward practice advancement in emergency care for children with autism spectrum disorder. *Pediatrics*. 2016;137(Suppl 2):S205-S211.

PHARMACY

Avoiding Common Errors in Pediatric Emergency Medicine: Sedation Adjuncts—Do Not Underestimate the Power of Distraction and Analgesia for Pediatric Procedures

Anita A. Thomas, MD

Children are often distressed in a medical setting. In the first year of life, children go to the primary care physician at least seven times, often punctuated by painful procedures such as heel sticks or vaccinations. They are poked and prodded without an ability to understand or rationalize. The process results in a negative experience, often leading to anxiety and fear of medical providers. It is important to distinguish distress from pain, and while it is important to address pain with targeted analgesia, children who can communicate often feel that their psychological distress is more significant than pain. It can be frustrating for all parties when a child is uncooperative during a physical examination or procedure, but remember to utilize available adjuncts in addition to, or even in lieu of, sedation. Pediatric procedural sedation goals include maintaining safety, minimizing pain/psychological trauma, managing anxiety, and controlling behavior/environment for safe procedural completion. These goals align well with sedation adjuncts.

Addressing Pain

Limit painful procedures such as blood draws. Try to bundle labs, particularly for chronically ill kids, who might require several blood draws. Utilize topical anesthetics such as LET (lidocaine, epinephrine, and tetracaine) for lacerations and EMLA (eutectic mixture of local anesthetics), external cooling (eg, vapocoolant spray, cold pack, or ice), or vibration stimulation for peripheral IV placement, abscess drainage, lumbar puncture, and nerve blocks. Nerve blocks can be considered for laceration repairs and hematoma blocks. Buffering lidocaine with bicarbonate can make for a less painful injection. Oral analgesics such as acetaminophen, ibuprofen, or oxycodone are good options. Intranasal fentanyl is rapid acting and can be useful prior to IV access or to help facilitate physical examination when initially assessing a fractured extremity.

Addressing Anxiety

Distraction, distraction, distraction. There are lots of high tech options such as tablets, virtual reality headsets, mobile devices, or video. However, bubbles are an excellent distraction for infants and beyond and can be used as a tool of the physical examination in assessing hand eye coordination, tracking, and gross motor function. Utilizing a family member or staff member to blow bubbles often calms children. Other adjuncts such as stickers or distracting light up toys are useful as well. Singing can calm children as well. It may be helpful to dim the lights in the examination room or examine the child while they are being held by their parents. Importantly, lowering familial anxiety can improve the patient's anxiety as well. Discussing a procedure with the family and patient sets expectations, particularly in older children. Set it up so the child is not surprised by what you are doing. Positioning a pediatric patient for a procedure such that they are looking away from or cannot see the procedure often reduces distress.

If your facility has child life specialists, utilize that resource. They cater to a child's developmental stage and help come up coping/distraction techniques during procedures such as via video entertainment on a tablet. If your facility does not have child life, use your mobile device to pull up a popular video/game that the patient might enjoy. Or use family members' mobile devices to pull up home videos or photos. Pharmacologically, intranasal or oral midazolam are a great choice for anxiolysis (although warn parents about the potential paradoxical reaction) and potential anterograde amnesia for a procedure. Nitrous oxide can also be used to address anxiolysis and has a quick recovery time of 3-5 minutes.

Ultimately...

If all else fails, or if it is an extensive and particularly painful procedure, deep sedation may be the best option. Just remember to always consider sedation adjuncts first to avoid deep sedation when possible.

KEY POINTS

- Do not underestimate the power of distraction and good analgesia/anxiolysis for a procedure before full sedation.
- Utilize child life (if you have it) and family members for comfort and distraction.
- Pull out your mobile device for distraction in a pinch.
- Topical and/or intranasal analgesia/anxiolysis should be considered in a stepwise fashion and may prevent the need for deep sedation.

Suggested Readings

Drendel AL, Ali S. Ten practical ways to make your ED practice less painful and more child-friendly. *Clin Pediatr Emerg Med*. 2017;18(4):242-255.

Johnston CC, Bournaki MC, Gagnon AJ, Pepler CJ, Bourgault P. Self-reported pain intensity and associated distress in children aged 4-18 years on admission, discharge, and one-week follow up to emergency department. *Pediatr Emerg Care*. 2005;21(5):342-346.

Lawton B, Davis T, Goldsten H, Tagg A. Spoonful of sugar: improving the palatability of emergency department visits for children and their families. *Emerg Med Australas*. 2015;27:504-506.

Pillai Riddell RR, Racine NM, Gennis HG, et al. Non-pharmacological management of infant and young child procedural pain. *Cochrane Database Syst Rev*. 2015;(12):CD006275.

Wait, Are Pediatricians Secretly Mathematicians?: Do Not Forget That All Dosing in Children Is Weight-Based

Matthew Shapiro, MD

Children are not miniature adults! Children have various developmentally associated changes in body composition (relevant to medication distribution) and organ function (relevant to medication absorption, metabolism, and excretion) that necessitate specific dosing considerations. While we may have wanted to leave pharmacokinetics in medical school, we need to remember the pharmacokinetic principles of absorption, distribution, metabolism, and excretion to understand the disposition of medications in pediatrics.

Children have wide variations in intragastric pH and the ratio of total body surface area to total body mass (affecting the absorption of oral and percutaneous medications), extracellular and total-body water spaces (affecting medication distribution and plasma drug levels), enzyme expression and activity (affecting metabolism), and renal function (affecting excretion). While the specifics of pediatric pharmacokinetics can be left to our friends in the pharmacy, the underlying premise regarding variation in medication use by pediatric patients is still important.

So What Do We Do With This Information?

Remember to always double check medication dosing and pay close attention to specific recommendations. Medications are always dosed on the *child's weight in kilograms, not pounds*. Obtaining the child's weight should not be a guessing game—if you are unable to obtain an actual weight, use an approved length-based tape to estimate weight such as the Broselow tape. Pediatric medications can be dosed in milligrams per kilogram per dose (eg, mg/kg q8h) or milligrams per kilogram per day divided into a certain number of doses (eg, mg/kg/d divided bid). When looking up dosing, be cognizant of recommendations regarding per dose vs per day to avoid overdosing.

Because children require weight-based dosing and are often growing rapidly, remember that pediatric patients may have grown out of a previously prescribed dose. This is particularly common in children with epilepsy, as it is very easy for a child to gain weight then be underdosed with a medication that was previously perfectly dosed.

Premature and full-term neonates have even more complicated dosing that depends on both gestational age, postnatal age, and corrected age. These considerations are generally *only important if the corrected age of the child is <40 weeks*. Correct age (aka postconceptual age) is simply calculated by adding the gestational age plus postnatal age in weeks. Therefore, an 8-week-old, former 28 weeks gestational age (WGA) infant has a corrected age of 36 WGA. In the neonatal period, dosing differs based upon both gestational age and postnatal age. An ex-35 WGA neonate, now 12 days old, has different IV gentamicin dosing than an ex-35 WGA neonate that is 6 days old.

Medications have variable maximum doses as well. Because we often rely on weight-based dosing, older children and adolescents can reach adult sized, maximum doses. Also, different diagnoses have different doses! Amoxicillin is given as 90 mg/kg/d divided twice daily for acute otitis media, whereas it is given as 50 mg/kg/d once daily or divided twice daily for streptococcal tonsillopharyngitis.

Oral medications have varying concentrations. When calculating doses, pay attention to the various dosage forms in order to avoid giving either a tiny amount of medicine that is impossible for a parent to consistently administer or an unreasonably enormous amount that a child will not take. Generally, it is ok to round liquid medications to a whole number but be mindful of this in nonliquid medications, as the effect can be much more dramatic (eg, rounding a medicine that is 75 mg/mL is very different than rounding one that is 250 mg per tab).

Particular medications can only be given to children of a certain age and/or in certain circumstances. For example, while doxycycline is typically not prescribed to children under 8 years old because of concern for dental staining, it is still the recommended treatment for children under 8 years old diagnosed with Rocky Mountain spotted fever. The American Academy of Pediatrics, U.S. Food and Drug Administration, European Medicines Agency, and the World Health Organization all recommend against using cough suppressants (codeine, dextromethorphan) in children of varying age based on lack of efficacy and concerns for safety, though they can sometimes be prescribed to adolescents.

KEY POINTS

- Children have different medication absorption, distribution, metabolism, and excretion depending on their age.
- Do not guess! Always look up the dosing recommendations.
- If working with infants with a history of prematurity and a corrected age of <40 WGA, pay particular attention to dosing.
- Good options for checking the appropriate doses for age and weight include UpToDate, NeoFax, and the AAP Red Book.

Suggested Readings

Engle WA; American Academy of Pediatrics Committee on Fetus and Newborn. Age terminology during the perinatal period. *Pediatrics*. 2004;114(5):1362-1364.

Kearns GL, et al. Developmental pharmacology—drug disposition, action, and therapy in infants and children. *N Engl J Med*. 2003;349(12):1157-1167.

O'Hara K. Paediatric pharmacokinetics and drug doses. *Aust Prescr*. 2016;39(6):208-210.

May the Dose Be With You... Focus on Communication to Avoid the 10-fold Dosing Error

Elise Milani, MD and Stephen Lim, MD, FAAEM

Medication Errors

Providing medical care to pediatric patients is a complex process involving many people and multiple systems. Because of this multi-tiered process, medication errors are subject to occur. Fortunately, however, this stepwise process establishes a series of "checks" in which many of these errors may be identified and fixed. A medication error can occur anywhere along the process of ordering, transcribing, dispensing, administering, and monitoring a medication. *Adverse medication errors* are medication errors that harm the patient.

The incidence of medication errors among adult and pediatric patients is similar; however, medication errors in pediatric populations are three times more likely to cause harm. Pediatric patients are particularly susceptible to adverse medication errors because of variable sizes, distinct physiology, and communications barriers. Children vary largely in size, and smaller weights can lead to frequent errors in dosing by factors of 10. Dosing is further complicated by medications that come in different concentrations (eg, 1:1000 and 1:10 000 concentration epinephrine). Additionally, pediatric physiology changes during development such that metabolism of any one medication can vary considerably. For example, trimethoprim-sulfamethoxazole can be safely given to a 5-month-old but could be fatal if given to a 1-month-old due to their immature hepatic metabolism. These nuanced differences have significant consequences and require a great deal of consideration. With this in mind, several tools can be implemented to minimize medication errors.

Reducing Medication Errors

Computer systems have proven critical in reducing medication errors. Computerized provider order entry (CPOE) describes a system in which orders are placed and received electronically. This process has drastically reduced errors in transcription as pharmacists and nurses no longer have to read messy doctor handwriting and interpret vague or absent administration instructions. Similarly, computerized clinical decision support (CCDS) is an electronic system that "double checks" orders. It can alert doctors to patient allergies, duplicate medication orders, adverse drug interactions, and evidence-based reminders. Additionally, dosing parameters built into medication orders help minimize dosing errors.

Providing medical care is a multidisciplinary effort. Doctors, nurses, technicians, pharmacists, and other providers should feel obligated and encouraged to raise concerns when medication orders seem inappropriate. A mistake in dosage, route, frequency, and even type of medication can occur, and all medications should be "double checked" before dispensing and administering medication. Clinical pharmacists specialized in their field can provide focused insight on medical management. Clinical pharmacists stationed in emergency departments, intensive care units, and hospital wards help reduce medication errors, particularly dosage errors. Studies have also shown that incorporating clinical pharmacists into medical teams yields more cost-effective medical regiments.

Many errors can be avoided when one confirms that they have heard an order and then repeats back what they have heard. For example, a doctor tells a nurse to "please give patient in room 'A' 3.375 mg of IV Zosyn." The nurse then verifies that he or she heard the message and says, "Ok. I will give patient in room 'A' 3.375 mg of IV Zosyn, correct?" The doctor then confirms this is correct and says, "yes." This technique permits both the nurse and the doctor to verify the message and allows opportunity to catch any discrepancies. If the hospital culture is one of "the doctor's choices should not be questioned," then a nurse will not speak up if an error is recognized. For patient safety and a cohesive work environment, all medical staff must feel comfortable and encouraged to raise concerns.

Continuous education for health care providers is helpful to reduce medication errors. Frequent, updated information should be provided on current medication guidelines, medication adverse effects, hospital rates of medication errors, and ongoing quality improvement measures.

KEY POINTS

- Medication errors in pediatric patients are three times more likely to cause harm when compared to adult patients.
- Children are susceptible to adverse medication errors because of wide variations in their size, physiology, and ability to communicate.
- Tools that help minimize adverse medication errors include computer systems, clinical pharmacists, good workplace communication, double checks, and continuing education.

Suggested Readings

Fortescue EB. Prioritizing strategies for preventing medication errors and adverse drug events in pediatric inpatients. *Pediatrics.* 2003;111(4):722-729.

Lesar TS. Factors relating to errors in medication prescribing. *JAMA.* 1997;277(4):312-317.

Neuspiel DR. Reducing the risk of harm from medication errors in children. *Health Serv Insights.* 2013;6:47-59.

Poole RL. Medication errors: "neonates, infants and children are the most vulnerable!". *J Pediatr Pharmacol Ther.* 2008;13(2):65-67.

Walsh KE. How to avoid pediatric medication errors: a user's guide to the literature. *Arch Dis Child.* 2005;90(7):698-702.

Just a Taste: Be Aware of Bad Tasting Medicines That Kids May Refuse to Take

Rachel Wiltjer, DO and Jennifer E. Guyther, MD

When we were children, most of us thought that medicine tastes bad. Now, as adult clinicians, many of us have seen or heard of a pediatric patient spitting acetaminophen all over the floor (or onto the unlucky person administering it). We can roll our eyes and encourage better administration techniques, but the taste of a medication can present a real problem with adherence to a dosing schedule. Bribery, begging, and brute force, while frequently attempted, rarely work, leaving doctors in a sticky situation.

Flavor is a combination of taste, smell, and chemical irritation. Taste cells appear at 7-8 weeks of gestation and ultimately serve as protection from poisoning. Within hours after birth, indications of the ability to taste can be observed in many infants as they reject bitter and prefer sweet and savory. Liquid medications are prepared with a variety of additives to chemically take advantage of the taste buds. Sodium is considered a bitter blocker, and sugars enhance the sweet receptors. Individual experience and cultures influence flavor preferences. For example, bubble gum and grape flavors predominate in the United States, citrus and red berry flavors are popular in Europe, and licorice wins out in Scandinavia.

A smattering of small studies have compared the tastes of frequently used medications as well as their effects on adherence. Some of the best tasting medications are amoxicillin, cefixime, azithromycin, amoxicillin/clavulanic acid, and cephalexin. Some of the worst are TMP/SMX, penicillin, clindamycin, and metronidazole. Prednisone solution and dexamethasone also have a bad taste.

Unpalatable medications can have a serious effect on adherence. It is already a high order to ask parents to give medications to children who want nothing to do with, often as many as three or four times a day for as long as 2 weeks. Compliance with an antibiotic prescription drops to 44% by day 3 and 18% by day 9. Medications that are prescribed daily or twice a day have compliance rates of 73% and 70%, respectively, compared with 52% for those three times a day and 42% for four times a day. The need to administer a medication that is particularly foul adds to the difficulty of adhering to both the dosing schedule and the total number of doses. To decrease the physical amount of medication that a parent needs to administer, prescribe the highest appropriate concentration and the lowest number of daily doses.

Some pharmacies offer flavor additives for medications, commonly at a small additional cost. Sweeteners such as chocolate, strawberry, or maple syrup can be given at home before and after the medication. Giving a child a cold treat before and after taking the medicine adds sweetness and decreases the functioning of the taste receptors. A lollipop or hard candy can help age-appropriate children cope with unpleasant flavors. Using nonliquid medications such as chewable or dissolvable tablets or sprinkles from opening capsules can sometimes be helpful. Some tablets can be crushed (after checking with the pharmacist) and mixed into an appealing food such as applesauce, peanut butter, or frosting. For slightly older children with particular difficulties and/or who require medications frequently, pill training with mini candies (progressing to larger candies that approximate the size of the pills they need) presents an option to avoid liquid medications entirely.

The first step toward improving adherence with liquid medications is awareness. Consider taste when writing a prescription. Consider tasting some of these medications yourself. If one of the worst offenders is truly the best agent, consider giving a trial dose in the ED before sending the patient home to make sure it can be tolerated. This approach gives the nurses an opportunity to educate parents about techniques that can help with administration of the medication at home. When two drugs are of comparable efficacy, add taste to your medication decision.

KEY POINTS

- Taste has a real impact on medication adherence. After effectiveness, cost, and dosing schedule have been considered, bring taste into the decision to help with compliance.
- Provide parents with strategies to improve medication administration at home, such as giving cold treats before and after the medication, giving a "chaser" of a sweet liquid, or mixing the medication in food the child likes.
- Some of our favorite medications taste horrible, so consider a tolerability test before the patient leaves the ED.

Suggested Readings

Baguley D, Lim E, Bevan A, et al. Prescribing for children—taste and palatability affect adherence to antibiotics: a review. *Arch Dis Child.* 2012;97:293-297.

Bradshaw H, Mitchell M, Edwards C, et al. Medication palatability affects physician prescribing preferences for common pediatric conditions. *Acad Emerg Med.* 2016;23:1243-1247.

Falagas M, Karagiannis AK, Nakouti T, et al. Compliance with once-daily versus twice or thrice-daily administration of antibiotic regimens: a meta-analysis of randomized controlled trials. *PLoS One.* 2015;10(1):e0116207.

Gee SC, Hagemann TM. Palatability of liquid anti-infectives: clinician and student perceptions and practice outcomes. *J Pediatr Pharmacol Ther.* 2007;12(4):216-223.

Przemyslaw K. Patient compliance with antibiotic treatment for respiratory tract infections. *J Antimicrob Chemother.* 2002;46(6):897-903.

Note: Page numbers "followed by an "f denote figures; those followed by a "t" denote tables.